Information Security in Healthcare

Managing Risk

Edited by
Terrell W. Herzig, MSHI, CISSP

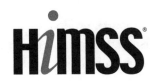

HIMSS Mission

To lead healthcare transformation through effective use of health information technology.

Printed in the U.S.A. 5 4 3 2

Requests for permission to make copies of any part of this work should be sent to:
Permissions Editor
HIMSS
230 E. Ohio, Suite 500
Chicago, IL 60611-3269
mschlossberg@himss.org

ISBN 978-0-9821070-2-7

For more information about HIMSS, please visit www.himss.org.

About the Editor

Terrell W. Herzig, MSHI, CISSP, is Information Security Officer of the UAB Health System, Birmingham, Alabama, the UAB HIPAA Security Officer, and an Adjunct Professor of Health Informatics at the University of Alabama at Birmingham (UAB). Mr. Herzig teaches graduate courses in Information Engineering, Programming, Computer Networks and Information Security in the UAB School of Health Professions. During his tenure at UAB, he has served as Director of Information Technology for the Civitan International Research Center and Director of Informatics for the Pittman General Clinical Research Center. Mr. Herzig has also consulted on numerous informatics projects with external groups, including Southern Nuclear and the US Army Medical Command.

About the Contributors

Mary Anne S. Canant, MBA, CISA, CISSP, is a Senior Information Systems Auditor at the University of Alabama at Birmingham (UAB), for which she provides assurance and advisory services. Her current interests include risk, control and governance of information technologies, and assets supporting UA's Academic Health Center and research enterprise.

Leanne Cordisco, BMET, is the Healthcare IT Program Manager for GE Healthcare. Ms. Cordisco combines 21 years of experience in biomedical engineering with seven years' experience in IT. She works to advance the field of clinical engineering through the development of healthcare IT technical training programs. Ms. Cordisco is a member of the American College of Clinical Engineering, the American Society for Training and Development, and HIMSS. She has authored or presented on more than 20 different healthcare IT-related topics.

Brian Evans, CISSP, CISM, serves as President of Brian Evans Consulting and provides information risk management consultation for clients throughout the United States. He held a similar role as the Principal Risk Strategist for Cardinal Health. Mr. Evans led the Enterprise Computer Incident Response and Forensic Investigations teams for Nationwide Insurance and served as Vice President of Corporate Information Security at Key Bank. As the National Delivery Director and Senior Security Consultant for Computer Task Group, he directed clients on building effective compliance and information risk management programs. Mr. Evans served as Information Security Officer at The Ohio State University Health System and has held positions at the Ohio Department of Health. He also managed Incident Response and Recovery teams in the US Air Force. Mr. Evans earned a master's degree in Public Administration from the University of Cincinnati, Ohio, and a Bachelor of Science degree in Business Management from the University of Maryland, College Park.

Sharon Finney is the Corporate Data Security Officer for Adventist Health System, the largest not-for-profit, Protestant healthcare system in the United States. Adventist Health System currently operates 37 hospitals, 17 skilled nursing facilities, and more than 20 home health, hospice, medical equipment, and infusion entities in 10 states. Ms. Finney is responsible for the data security technology and compliance strategies and data security operations for Adventist Health System. She has more than 20 years of experience in information technology and data security and holds a Bachelor of Science degree in Business Administration.

J. David Kirby, MS, CISSP, CHPS, has served, for more than 30 years, in various roles, developing innovative uses of health information technology with a variety of public, private, state, national, and international organizations. These roles include academic medical center (AMC) information security officer, director of an AMC-based telehealth program, director of an IT innovation center in an AMC, and manager of technology support for an AMC. As current President of Kirby Information Management Consulting LLC (KirbyIMC.com), he provides consulting in innovative health information technology, security, and privacy areas. Customers include healthcare enterprises and information technology vendors of all sizes and types. Mr. Kirby holds Bachelor of Science and Master of Science degrees in Computer Science and certificates in security and privacy, including CISSP, CHPS, and CHS. He is an Adjunct Associate Professor in the Division of Medical Informatics at Duke University Medical Center, Durham, NC.

Mac McMillan is cofounder and CEO of CynergisTek, Inc., a firm specializing in information security, regulatory compliance, and IT audit. Mr. McMillan brings 30 years of security countermeasures experience to his philosophy of managing security programs. He has worked in the healthcare industry since 2000 and frequently contributes to HCCA, AHIA, AHIMA, AHLA, and HIMSS programs. He currently serves as chair for HIMSS' Information Systems Security Work Group. He served as Director of Security for two Department of Defense agencies, receiving both the Silver and Gold Medals for Exceptional Meritorious Service. He holds a Master of Arts degree in National Security and Strategic Studies from the US Naval War College; and a Bachelor of Science degree in Education from Texas A&M University. He was a 1993-1994 Excellence in Government Fellow and is a graduate of the Senior Officials in National Security program from the John F. Kennedy School of Government, Harvard University.

Shelia T. Searson, CIPP, is Program Director in the University of Alabama at Birmingham's (UAB) HIPAA Office. In this role, she has the unique opportunity of working with both the UAB academic units that fall under the HIPAA regulations and the UAB Health System components. Ms. Searson is a member of a UAB team that reports to the UAB Privacy Office and works to ensure compliance with HIPAA privacy and security regulations. Ms. Searson holds a baccalaureate degree in Speech Communications from Shorter College in Rome, Georgia. Her professional affiliations include the International Association of Privacy Professionals, through which she is a Certified Information Privacy Professional, and the American Health Information Management Association.

Tom Walsh, CISSP, is a Certified Information Systems Security Professional (CISSP) and a nationally recognized speaker. As an independent consultant, Tom conducts security training, risk analysis, business impact analysis, business continuity, and disaster recovery planning for clients. Mr. Walsh is also the coauthor of two books, *Medical Records Disaster Planning—A Health Information Manager's Survival Guide* (American Health Information Management Association, 2008) and *Handbook for HIPAA Security Implementation* (American Medical Association, 2003).

Lory Wood is President of Compiled Logic Wares Consulting. As CIO/CSO of Good Health Network (GHN), she deployed a standards-based, secure PKI-enabled Web-based personal health record that is patient owned and controlled and is HIPAA-compliant. GHN is a healthcare certification authority. Ms. Wood is a member of the HITSP Consumer Perspective, Security Privacy and Infrastructure Technical Committee; the Education Communications Outreach Committee; ASTM E31 Healthcare Informatics Committees, including the Continuity of Care Record Technical Workgroup; PDF Healthcare Workgroup; vice chair of HIMSS' PHR Steering Committee; and co-chair of the CCHIT PHR workgroup. She is also Project Manager for the Florida Medicaid Pharmacology Project, which deploys 1,500 PDA/smart phones to physicians serving Medicaid patients. Ms. Wood was lead engineer for DOD T2P2 telemedicine browser-based eConsultation, utilizing secure satellite technology across the Pacific Rim and was awarded the 1999 Technology Excellence in Government Award.

Contents

Preface

Terrell W. Herzig, MSHI, CISSP

It seems like almost every day you read an article regarding the loss of a laptop or a security breach resulting in the loss of patient information. In February of 2009, President Obama signed into law the American Recovery and Reinvestment Act, in effect, creating the first federal breach law. The industry impacted by this law—healthcare. Indeed, ask anyone on the street to list what information about them would be considered the most sensitive if it were publically released, and they would probably answer medical information.

Healthcare presents many unique challenges to information security professionals. First, information must not only be kept confidential, but must be extremely accurate and always available. Second, defining the type and level of access is difficult. Indeed, many people must have access to medical information in order not to impede patient care.

Organizations must use the information they collect to fine-tune operations and cut costs. As the industry embraces new technologies to network and share patient information, it too must secure and guard access to highly sensitive data. Understanding the issues involved can help guide IT expenditures, enable competitive advantages and avoid costly regulatory fines and penalties.

A lot of good information security books are available on the market. Most of these books deal with information security at a low technical level. The intent of this book is to present information security—unique to the healthcare environment—from multiple viewpoints. First, the book is intended to be informative and educational for healthcare managers. From board-level senior managers to front-line management, the book is intended to present healthcare information security practices and concerns in straight-forward language. Second, for practicing information security professionals, the intent is to help them tweak or jump start an appropriate information security management program. Last, but not least, the book should appeal to college education and training programs for healthcare environments.

This book combines the experience and insight of several healthcare IT managers and information security professionals to bring important privacy and security issues to life. Many thanks to each one for providing the readers with tools, checklists, and content to help them build and/or enhance their information security activities. One thing is certain: In this ever-changing information security environment, everyone involved with maintaining privacy and security of healthcare data need continuing support, encouragement, and guidance to remain current and informed. I trust this book will meet some of those needs and provide new and renewed insight into information security as it pertains to healthcare.

Introduction

Shelia T. Searson, CIPP

Why introduce a security book by beginning with a discussion about privacy? A very good question. Privacy should be a critical component of any healthcare institution's strategic vision or operational plan. Most individuals, especially citizens of the United States, assume they have a right to privacy—the right to control the events in their personal lives and the right to keep their personal information secret if they so choose.[1] However, the word *privacy* is not actually included in the Constitution of the United States.[2]

Even so, the right to privacy is viewed as an important component of one's personal freedom, and there is no place that this right is held with stronger conviction than in the relationship between healthcare institutions and patients' personal health information.[3]

Privacy, although not well-defined, is generally understood as the appropriate use of personal information in a range of circumstances. The International Association of Privacy Professionals adds that "what is appropriate will depend on context, law, and the individual's expectations."[4] For our purposes, the terms *privacy* and *information privacy* are synonymous.

Information privacy means that an individual has control of his or her personal information and has reasonable expectations about how this personal information will be used and when it may be disclosed to others.[5] Individuals are sensitive and protective of their personal information, which is generally thought to include address, birth date and age, Social Security number, credit card numbers, salary and debt, and medical conditions. The right to privacy includes the precept that this information will be kept private, confidential and secure.

Depending on a particular situation or environment, an individual may choose to disclose personal information, but this is an individual choice, not an organizational decision. When an individual grants permission for others to use his or her personal information for a specific purpose, that permission includes an expectation that the information, which is private and confidential, will be used only as specified or approved by that individual.

The appropriate use of confidential information is dependent on various privacy laws and regulations that affect such areas as workplace privacy, healthcare, student records and financial information. Each institution must determine those federal laws and sets of regulations with which they are required to comply.

For a healthcare institution, personal information could include patient medical records, employee records, credit or debit card numbers, research data, and passwords or other means of access to its information systems. In the case of an academic health center, add student records to the mix of personal information that must be kept private, confidential and secure.

Healthcare institutions are involved in a careful balance of an individual's privacy rights and the use of the confidential information to perform necessary clinical or business tasks. These tasks have a variety of purposes, ranging from personnel issues related to payroll and benefits to providing direct clinical care, performing laboratory tests, prescribing medications and sharing results with referring physicians. Protecting the privacy of all constituencies within a healthcare institution, including employees, patients, healthcare providers and volunteers, can be a daunting, but reasonable privacy expectation in the current litigious environment. For our purposes, the focus of this book is on personal and health information of patients.

The most encompassing privacy law affecting healthcare institutions is the federal Health Insurance Portability and Accountability Act of 1996, better known as HIPAA. Before HIPAA, the privacy and confidentiality of a patient's health information involved a patchwork of federal and state laws and regulations, professional codes of ethics, standards of practice, and the policies of individual institutions.[6]

Examples of federal regulations affecting healthcare are the Privacy Act and the Federal Policy for the Protection of Human Subjects. The Privacy Act of 1974 was enacted because of concerns related to government misuse of citizen information contained in computerized databases. The act only applies to federal government entities and federal contractors as they use the identifiable personal information of US citizens and legal residents. Therefore, it only regulates healthcare institutions that are federally operated or funded.[7]

The Federal Policy for the Protection of Human Subjects, most usually referred to as the Common Rule, is a set of privacy regulations overseeing federally funded clinical trials and medical research protocols involving human subjects. The Common Rule requires sufficient protection for the privacy of research participants and the confidentiality of the research data. However, the policy relates only to those research projects that are federally funded.[7]

HIPAA provides a broad definition and scope regarding a patient's health information, which HIPAA refers to as protected health information (PHI). PHI includes all oral, written, and electronically maintained information that is created or received by a healthcare provider, a health plan, or a healthcare clearinghouse. PHI includes that information related to an individual's past, present, or future physical or mental health condition or the past, present or future payment for the provision of healthcare.[7]

In essence, PHI is not the actual health or medical record of a patient but rather those data elements that can be used to identify a person when linked with that person's medical information, such as a medical diagnosis or medical condition. PHI data elements, as outlined in HIPAA, include 18 identifiers:

• Names

- All geographic subdivisions smaller than a state, including street address, city, county, precinct, ZIP code and equivalent geocodes
- All elements of dates (except year) directly related to an individual, including date of birth, admission and discharge dates, date of death, and all ages older than 89 years, as well as all elements of dates (including year) indicative of such age
- Telephone numbers
- Fax numbers
- E-mail addresses
- Social Security number
- Medical record numbers
- Health plan beneficiary numbers
- Account numbers
- Certificate/license numbers
- Vehicle identifiers and serial numbers, including license plate numbers
- Device identifiers and serial numbers
- Web universal resource locators (URLs)
- Internet protocol (IP) address numbers
- Biometric identifiers, including fingerprints and voiceprints
- Full-face photographic images and any comparable images
- Any other unique identifying number, characteristic, or code, unless otherwise permitted by the Privacy Rule for re-identification (164.514(c)).[12]

Many of these identifiers are included as necessary measures to ensure patient privacy protections. Name, address, Social Security number, birth date, and account numbers are logical pieces of information to keep private and secure, as these data can easily identify an individual.

However, it may not be immediately evident why certain other data elements are included. Could the serial number or license plate number from an individual's vehicle be used to identify that individual? Why include the serial number from a pacemaker implanted into a cardiovascular patient or from surgical steel used to set a patient's broken ankle? In fact such data elements represent small puzzle pieces that could be investigated and added to other information to identify a patient.

Using or maintaining PHI is not to be confused with using or maintaining a patient's medical record. The data being used or stored must be reviewed in light of these 18 PHI data elements. One of the data elements listed, combined with a medical condition or diagnosis, represents PHI that is protected under HIPAA privacy regulations. For example, information from a database entitled "Former Patients with Lymphoma" (reference to a diagnosis) that includes the patients' names (PHI data element) is considered PHI. Therefore, patient information in clinical and research databases must be used and disclosed in a manner consistent with the HIPAA Privacy Rule.[8]

Healthcare institutions must also comply with state privacy laws and regulations. Of course, these requirements vary greatly from state to state, and HIPAA's privacy protections provide a federal "floor" on which state privacy laws can build.[7] However, the HIPAA Privacy Rule pre-empts state law when the state law is contrary to the Privacy Rule. However, as with most federal regulations, there are exceptions to HIPAA's pre-emption. A common exception is when state law is more stringent than the Privacy Rule in protecting the privacy of PHI.[3] HIPAA represents the floor, or minimum of privacy protections, and allows greater protection provided by the states.

Recent legislation, the American Recovery and Reinvestment Act of 2009 (ARRA), better known as "the Stimulus Bill," signed into federal law on February 17, 2009, significantly enhances and strengthens privacy and security regulations contained in HIPAA.[9] ARRA includes the Health Information Technology for Economic and Clinical Health Act, or the HITECH Act.[10] The HITECH Act promotes the use of health information technology (HIT) and specifically extends the legal provisions of the HIPAA privacy and security regulations. HIPAA-covered entities, Business Associates of covered entities, and some entities previously not considered to be HIPAA-covered entities are affected by these new requirements.[9] The HITECH Act establishes breach notification requirements, further limits the uses and disclosures of PHI, and increases the enforcement of, and the penalties for, noncompliance with HIPAA privacy and security regulations. These requirements represent efforts to keep pace with the new risks to PHI that have emerged since the enactment of HIPAA in 1996. Many HITECH provisions are effective within the first 12 months, while other pieces of the legislation go into effect at later dates.[10] Additional guidance and interpretation regarding the provisions in the law are anticipated, and careful consideration should be given to these emerging regulatory requirements.

So, why is privacy included in any serious consideration of information security? Actually, HIPAA provides regulations to protect both the privacy and security of PHI received and maintained by healthcare institutions. HIPAA's Privacy Rule sets forth regulatory standards for the use and disclosure of PHI, and the Security Regulations, comprised of 18 standards, ensure the confidentiality, integrity, and availability of PHI for business-related purposes.[4]

By definition, *information security* refers to protecting information against loss, unauthorized access, or misuse. It includes assessing the threats and risks to information and assuring confidentiality, integrity, and availability of the data being protected.[1] Therefore, although information privacy and information security are different in concept, they are related in practice. Privacy depends on information security, especially for the confidentiality of the information being protected.[5]

Privacy and security work together in a complementary fashion. For example, strong privacy policies and procedures are worthless if outsiders can break into the institution's information systems and compromise or steal the data. Therefore, privacy and security share a common goal of preventing the unauthorized access, use, and release of confidential information. Sound security practices create audit trails to determine who has accessed confidential, sensitive, or personal information. These audit trails provide the means to encourage adherence to privacy and information security policies and standards and to discourage wrongdoing by enforcing disciplinary actions for misconduct. Both the privacy and security provided to the sensitive data are strengthened.[11]

However, HIPAA privacy and security regulations represent the minimum standards of protection on which management can build policies and practices that are reasonable and appropriate for their institution.[7] The HIPAA privacy and security regulations provide sound minimal guidelines to be followed for the protection of all sensitive or confidential data, not just PHI. An institution's privacy and information security policies and procedures must strike a balance between ensuring privacy for personal and confidential data and permitting important intended business uses of the information.

Once the policies are developed, they must be implemented and enforced. Individual leaders and managers in a healthcare organization must emphasize and reward the importance of privacy and support the interrelationship of privacy and information security. Neither privacy nor information security can exist in a vacuum. Privacy is necessary for today's information-driven, technologically advanced environment. Information security can provide the "privacy" assurance that information technology needs. Administration must strongly support this marriage of privacy and information security, making both important priorities for the institution.

The healthcare workforce needs to know what information is to be kept confidential and the manner in which this is to be accomplished. Knowledge of the institution's policies and operating procedures and understanding business needs and access to the appropriate information are essential at all levels. Formal training about an institution's privacy and information security policies and procedures is an important component of an effective compliance program.

The adage that says "you can have security without privacy, but you cannot have privacy without security"[1] effectively denotes the relationship between information privacy and information security and serves as the rationale for including privacy in any serious consideration of information security. Privacy is the appropriate use of information, and security is the protection of that information while it is being used.[1] The two are explicitly intertwined.[13] The following chapters provide a complete assessment of information security principles and their essential role in protecting privacy and confidentiality of sensitive institutional assets such as PHI.

References

1. International Association of Privacy Professionals. Information Privacy Certification Training Course Book, York, Me: IAPP; 2006.

2. Alderman E, Kennedy C. *The Right to Privacy*. New York, NY: Vintage; 1997; xiii.

3. American Health Information Management Association. *HIPAA in Practice*. Chicago, Ill: AHIMA; 2004; vii.

4. International Association of Privacy Professionals. IAPP Information Privacy Certification Glossary of Common Privacy Terminology. York, Me: IAPP; 2006.

5. Borten K. *The No-Hassle Guide to HIPAA Policies*. Marblehead, Mass: HCPro; 2007.

6. Hughes G. Laws and Regulations Governing the Disclosure of Health Information (AHIMA Practice Brief). Updated November 2002. http://library.ahima.org/xpedio/groups/public/documents/ahima/bok1_016464.hcsp?dDocName=bok1_016464.

7. Boyle L, Mack D. *HIPAA: A Guide to Health Care Privacy and Security Law*. Frederick, Md: Aspen; 2009.

8. Searson S, Hicks J, Cole J, Herzig T, Brooks CM. HIPAA for cancer educators. Accepted for publication by the *Journal of Cancer Education*.

9. American Health Information Management Association. Analysis of Health Care Confidentiality, Privacy, and Security Provisions of The American Recovery and Reinvestment Act of 2009, Public Law 111-5. March 2009.

10. Hirsch R, Fayed R. ARRA 2009 and the HITECH Act: The next phase of HIPAA regulation and enforcement arrives. *The Bureau of National Affairs' Health Law Reporter*, 2009.

11. Swire P, Steinfeld L. Security and Privacy After September 11: The Health Care Example. Copyright held by author/owner. 4. http://www.cfp2002.org/proceedings/proceedings/swire.pdf

12. Department of Health and Human Services. Protecting Personal Health Information in Research: Understanding the HIPAA Privacy Rule.

13. Sealet S. Without security there can be no privacy. November 1, 2001. Available at: http://www.cio.com/article/print30639.

Dedication

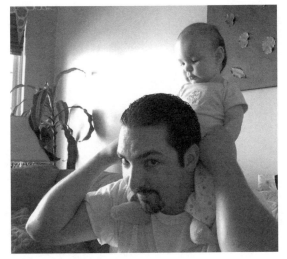

This book is dedicated in loving memory of Matthew Thomas Walsh, a loving and devoted husband and father, caring and loving son and brother, and friend to many. It is also dedicated to his daughter, Scarlet Grace. May she always know that she was the sparkle in her daddy's eyes. www.MatthewWalshStory.com

CHAPTER 1

IT Security Governance

Mac McMillan

Information technology plays a major role in differentiating one health system and its services from the next. In many cases, it becomes a competitive advantage and as such, a part of the organization's persona or image. Consequently, information technology has become a strategic asset, but most boards spend very little time considering it strategically and even less time on the more focused area of data security. This is not adequate in today's reality.

The board's responsibility for ensuring appropriate governance through its oversight flows from the board's fiduciary responsibility to protect the health system's critical assets. That responsibility means ensuring the right structure is established to provide feedback; that the individuals assigned information security responsibilities have the right qualifications; that a culture of continuous risk management is implemented; and that incidents are reviewed and addressed.

In today's economy, the livelihood of the health system is related to how well the enterprise manages with respect to confidentiality, integrity and availability. Confidentiality means controlling access to information as required by law or in accordance with contract or business needs. Confidentiality is an important tenant in healthcare where privacy of patient information is core to the mission of care. Integrity means ensuring that systems and data are reliable, and safe from unauthorized modification or corruption. Having the right information at the right time is undeniably a patient safety concern. Available means making sure the system or data are there when caregivers or support staff need it. Loss of a critical system or information can absolutely impact delivery of services.

Data security incidents can result in real damages to the health system's reputation and business. Negative regulatory findings, litigation and compromised business continuity — which are forms these damages may take — are all board and executive management concerns. Healthcare is fast becoming one of the most regulated industries as it relates to data privacy and security. In addition to the Health Insurance Portability and Accountability Act (HIPAA) and Medicare Security requirements, most healthcare organizations have to deal with a host of other federal and state requirements, such as the Payment Card Industry rules for credit card transactions, FTC rules governing data privacy and state data security beach laws.

In 2008, the Red Flag Rules were amended and broadened to affect many more industries, healthcare being one of them, and in 2009 the American Recovery and Reinvestment Act added to healthcare's challenges by increasing fines for non-compliance, establishing a federal requirement for reporting of breeches, and broadening the scope of HIPAA to include Business Associates. The risk of litigation also is not foreign to healthcare managers. Inadequate controls affecting the privacy and security of patient data can easily lead to a lawsuit. Add to that the risk of not being able to comply under the expanded Federal Rules of Civil Procedure governing discovery of electronically stored information, and the impact and costs to the health system can rise substantially. Last but not least, inadequate controls for data security can lead to a loss of confidence, loss of revenue, can negatively affect bond ratings, interest rates on loans and undermine insurability for business risks. All of these risks, and understanding where the health system stands relative to them, are or should be important concerns for executive management and the board.

Governance Sets the Tone

Security is everyone's responsibility. This is not just a catchy slogan to try to enlist supporters or promote compliance. It is an absolute truth. And the truth is that security, or data protection, is a "top down" phenomena. The tone must be set properly and communicated down through the organization. To do this effectively, not only is there a need for a clear message, but the board and executive management must ensure the right structure is in place to support governance and oversight functions. Security fails more often from lack of managerial support and accountability than all other factors combined.

Data privacy and security start with "top down" policy and end with cultural adoption for proper protection of systems and information. Rules for appropriate access to and use of information facilities must be clearly stated, and to be effective they must be enforced and managers held accountable for failures. Another important way leadership sets the tone is by taking an active role in the selection and placement of those senior staff responsible for carrying out the data security mission for the organization. Just as with other important positions the board or executive leadership should ensure that security personnel are fully qualified and carry the requisite experience and certifications. So too must they be held accountable for performance of the program.

Oversight and Feedback

Many organizations rely on the audit committee to provide oversight for information technology matters. Others use a combination of the audit committee and oversight through compliance. Another approach that provides much better alignment of data protection with business risks is incorporating data privacy and security within a risk management committee. This, however, will require many healthcare organizations to re-think and broaden their view of risk management and potentially the role of the risk manager, who traditionally focused on patient safety and quality concerns.

However, when you take a step back and consider that risks to confidentiality, integrity and availability of information assets can create risks to patient satisfaction and safety, this approach begins to have merit. Whatever the final model chosen, the group should be adequately staffed with membership from the IT, legal, financial, regulatory, audit and business units.

Regardless of the structure adopted, it should accomplish several oversight functions and clearly report to the board and executive leadership. Committees or sub-committees given IT security oversight responsibilities should have as members appropriately qualified technical staff. They should coordinate and recommend information security policy, ensure that measurable criteria are developed for compliance, require consistent employment of useful frameworks within IT and IT security operations such as ISO 27002, ITIL and CIS benchmarks, oversee and receive performance reporting and audit activities, and report to the board and executive management regularly regarding the status of information security.

Boards and their committees also have an important role in determining the qualifications of persons in key roles. Security should be no exception. Information security, like any other specialized focus area, has its own certifications, skills and experience requirements that speak to an individual's ability to perform successfully in a given position. In most health systems, due to the complexity of the enterprise, numbers of systems and users, etc., information security is a full-time endeavor and requires an individual with sound understanding of information security principles and security management experience. Yet in many organizations, information security is still an additional duty.

Lastly, placement of the information security manager in the organization is important. When considering where the information security officer should fit in the organization, the following should be asked: Is the person able to do the job effectively? Is she or he able to be the objective voice that security needs to raise concerns when appropriate? Is he or she provided appropriate resources and time to accomplish the job? An important purpose of governance is to ensure the appropriate environment is created for information security to succeed, with the oversight mechanisms and structure to continually assess its posture, and to ensure that the individuals responsible for security are qualified, resourced and held accountable for performance.

Governance Must Be Visible and Active

The bottom line in information security is that the board and executive management must play an active and visible role if they want the program to be credible and the organization to adhere to its policies. They should establish the requirement for regular program reviews and reporting, clearly articulate roles for audit, legal and compliance in measuring performance, and ask the right questions of those responsible for implementing and overseeing data security. Governance activities should gauge the following:

• Management's involvement in data security.

- Awareness of the organization with respect to current threats and mitigation.
- Implementation of appropriate security controls and their effectiveness.
- Ongoing risk assessment's role as a component of the security program.
- Staff awareness and training efforts and effectiveness.
- Frequency and trends in security incidents, their impacts and remediation.
- Compliance, legal (contractual) and insurance efforts and performance.
- Information security program performance, constraints, budget and resources.
- Overall business risk from data security issues.

Governance and Controls

Ultimately, information security activities should be focused on mitigating risks to the business. Their effectiveness in supporting governance objectives must be measurable. Establishing control objectives can be very useful for identifying metrics for performance. Control objectives are simple statements that express expectations or outcomes of appropriate behavior associated with a particular requirement or goal. Control objectives should allow clear differentiation of appropriate outcome or behavior. To be relevant, control objectives should draw a clear connection between a program requirement and a risk to the business. The following are examples:

- No patient information will be lost or compromised due to laptop loss.
- No person shall gain unauthorized access following termination.
- No system will be adversely impacted by malware as a result of no antivirus protection applied.
- No system outage shall occur as a result of an unauthorized change.

There is no limit to the number of control objectives that can be articulated to express those behaviors or expectations desired to support measurement of the effectiveness of the program. For each control objective, there may be one or more controls that are associated with it. Each of these should be measurable to determine if their effectiveness and the objective has been met. For instance, an analysis of the first control objective above might be assessed by reviewing related controls and relevant information, as depicted in Figures 1-1, 1-2, 1-3, and 1-4.

Security controls applicable reviewed:

- Laptop authentication.
- Laptop/data encryption.
- Physical control of the laptop.
- User awareness.

Risk increased or mitigated:

- Compliance.
- Legal.
- Reputation.
- Patient safety.
- Quality.

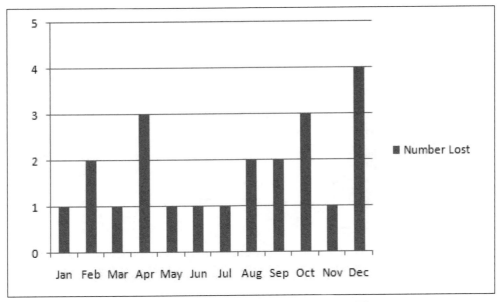

Figure 1-1: Sample of Metric–Number of Laptops Lost Over Time.

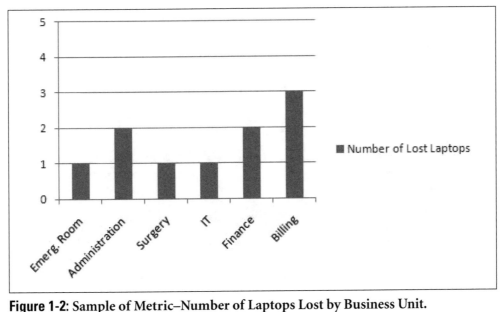

Figure 1-2: Sample of Metric–Number of Laptops Lost by Business Unit.

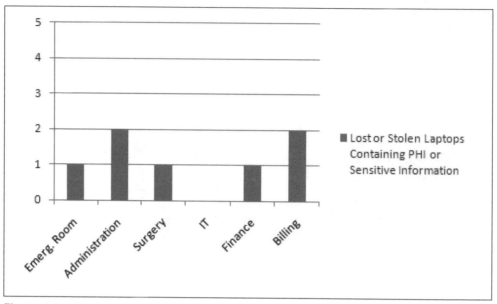

Figure 1-3: Sample of Metric–Number of Laptops Lost with ePHI or Other Sensitive Information by Business Unit.

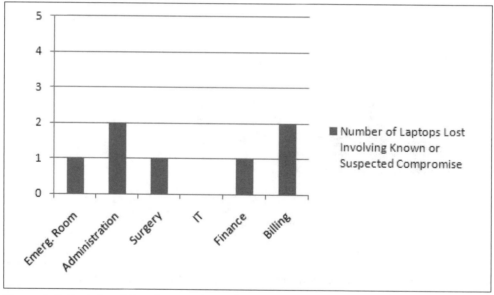

Figure 1-4: Sample of Metric–Number of Laptops Lost Involving Known or Suspected Compromise.

This is by no means all-inclusive. There may be other controls, information or metrics analyzed, but the idea here is to assess risk from an enterprise perspective; to tie actual events, their impacts, the absence/presence and effectiveness of security controls, and accountability back to business risk based on real metrics so governance can be effected. The data presented and answers to the above questions permits the development of a unified picture of the potential business risk of a lost laptop, where and what mitigation may be required, and where accountability lies.

SUMMARY

Governance of information security should seek to direct, inform, assess and measure the performance of people, systems and controls to achieve risk mitigation objectives. Security starts at the top, but effective security occurs when it becomes a part of the culture of the organization and guides behaviors. Sustainable security occurs when rules are clearly communicated, controls are visible and monitored and accountability is enforced. The role of governance is to set the tone, provision leadership and resources, articulate the rules, create appropriate oversight, empower appropriate audit and reviews, and ensure accountability.

Discussion Questions

1. Discuss the importance of IT governance and the role it plays on security.
2. Discuss the recent regulatory requirements for privacy and security in healthcare.
3. How can a breach of privacy impact a healthcare organization?
4. Who is responsible for information security, and why?
5. Who in the healthcare organization is ultimately responsible for information security?

CHAPTER 2

Risk Management and Strategic Planning

Tom Walsh, CISSP

BUSINESS RISKS—YOU DON'T KNOW WHAT YOU DON'T KNOW!

Every business operates with some level of risk. To eliminate all risks would require the elimination of all threats, and that is impossible. Therefore, information security professionals must balance the needs of the business with the need for securing business assets as a part of risk management. Paying too much attention to either security or business needs at the cost of ignoring the other creates an imbalance that ultimately leads to problems.

This chapter focuses on the means to manage risks to an acceptable level and the creation of a strategic plan aligned with the organization's business plans for fulfilling the mission of the organization.

Appropriate management of risks begins with and requires an assessment of information assets and the potential threats, existing controls, and remaining vulnerabilities. An analysis is then conducted to determine the probability of the potential threat circumventing existing controls to exploit the vulnerabilities and to determine the potential impact if the threat is realized.

Although risk analysis is a systematic process, it is far from being a precise science. Assessing risks requires "what if" thinking; it is an attempt to predict the future—a future information security professionals do not want to come to fruition. In some cases, this requires that logically-thinking information security professionals must make their best guess when determining the likelihood or probability of an event occurring, as well as the potential impact.

Several methodologies as well as commercially available risk-analysis tools exist that organizations can use for conducting a risk analysis. Most of these methodologies and tools generally follow the same basic principles for risk analysis.

The National Institute of Standards and Technology (NIST) is a federal agency that develops standards and guidelines. In particular, the Computer Security Division (CSD) is responsible for the creation of the Special Publications (SP) in the 800 series, publications that provide guidance on information security. Within the preamble of the HIPAA Security Rule, there is a reference to the NIST SP 800-30, "Risk Management Guide for Information Technology Systems." Because of that reference, this chapter will use the NIST SP 800-30 as the basis for explaining risk analysis. Figure 2-1 outlines the NIST risk methodology.

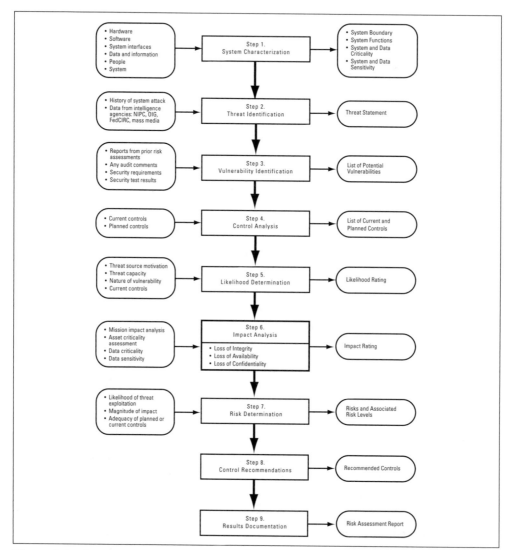

Figure 2-1: The NIST SP 800-30 Risk Assessment Methodology Flowchart.

THE NINE-STEP RISK PROCESS OUTLINED BY NIST

Step 1—System characterization. In order to assess risks, the first step is to identify the information assets that need to be protected. System characterization is the process of identifying the information assets that require protecting either because of their criticality to the business and/or because of the sensitivity of the information that is processed and stored on the system. Eventually all information systems (clinical as well as business operational systems) should be assessed and analyzed. A common practice is to start with the systems that have the highest potential for organizational risk.

System characterization groups, like hardware devices, make it easier to identify the threats, controls, and vulnerabilities, and to assess overall risks. Following are examples of how some hardware devices could be characterized:

- Servers and mainframes.
- Networking components (routers, switches, firewalls).
- Computer workstations (stationary computers used in office and work areas).
- Mobile computing devices (laptops, tablets, hand-held computing devices, smart phones, etc.).

While the threats to these devices may be the same, the probability or impact could be somewhat different. For example, the theft of a mobile computing device is more likely than the theft of a server or an AS/400. Another example would be the failure of a hardware device. The failure of a single computer workstation probably will not have as great of an impact as the failure of a key network component for which there is no failover or backup device. In this example, the workstation failure presumably only impacts one person, whereas the network failure could potentially impact everyone with network access. System characterization allows grouping of similar information assets to make it easier to determine a risk profile.

Step 2—Threat identification. Once "systems" have been grouped or characterized, the next step is to identify threats. For simplicity, threats could be grouped into three general categories: acts of nature, acts of man, and environmental threats. Figure 2-2 lists examples of the possible threats under the three general threat categories.

Possible Threats

Acts of Nature
- Weather – Hurricane, tornado, high wind, ice or snow storm
- Earthquake
- Firestorm

Acts of Man
- Malicious code (Virus or worm)
- Careless, errors, or unintentional acts
- Unauthorized access, software license violations, computer misuse or any other intentional act that violates expected workforce behavior
- Hardware or software tampering
- Denial of service attacks
- Unintentional programming errors, software failures, or bugs
- Hacking
- Theft
- Social engineering
- Fraud

Environmental
- Hardware or mechanical failure
- Power failure, fluctuation, or electrical disturbance
- Communication loss – Cut LAN cable or telecommunications line
- HVAC failure (Data Center) – Overheating or humidity
- Water pipe break

Figure 2-2: General Categories of Threats, with Examples.

Acts of nature imply some type of disaster beyond our control, whereas acts of man are normally intentional or accidental actions committed by people that perhaps could be controlled. Environmental acts are also events that could be prevented or at least, a response could be planned to minimize their impact.

Going overboard with threat identification is a common mistake. The term, "reasonably anticipated" as it pertains to threats or hazards is used three times within the HIPAA Security Rule (twice in the Preamble and once in the actual rule). Therefore, when determining which threats to include or exclude during the risk analysis process, the true test should be, "Is this a reasonably anticipated threat or hazard?" The answer is usually based on things such as geographic location and past experiences, or is based on the type of information asset involved, as explained in the example in the previous section.

Step 3—Vulnerability identification. Vulnerability identification determines whether flaws or inherent weaknesses exist in a system. Vulnerabilities can be associated with hardware or software design as well as weaknesses in operational practices. They are usually expressed as the lack of a safeguard or control. Many information security professionals find that it is easier to first assess existing security controls and then determine the vulnerabilities that remain.

Step 4—Control analysis. Control analysis identifies existing security safeguards and controls to determine whether they are adequate in either preventing or detecting a threat. When a threat cannot be prevented, such as an earthquake or a tornado, then the control analysis determines whether systems can be adequately recovered and restored to their original functionality. Assurance testing or validation may also be used to determine whether existing controls are adequate.

Step 5—Likelihood determination. Once the threats, controls, and vulnerabilities have been determined, the next step is to determine the likelihood of a potential threat exploiting the vulnerabilities. Likelihood can be rated by expressing it as either high, medium, or low. The definitions of these ratings are described in NIST SP 800-30 and are listed in Figure 2-3.

Likelihood Level	Likelihood Definition
High	The threat-source is highly motivated and sufficiently capable, and controls to prevent the vulnerability from being exercised are ineffective.
Medium	The threat-source is motivated and capable, but controls are in place that may impede successful exercise of the vulnerability.
Low	The threat-source lacks motivation or capability, or controls are in place to prevent, or at least significantly impede, the vulnerability from being exercised.

Figure 2-3: Likelihood Levels and Definitions.

Step 6—Impact analysis. The next step in the process is to determine the potential impact that could result from threats successfully exploiting vulnerabilities. Figure 2-4 lists categories of impacts, along with examples.

Possible Impacts

Confidentiality

- Disclosure of PHI
- Disclosure of Social Security numbers (patients or employees)
- Unauthorized access to sensitive or proprietary information

Integrity

- Data alteration
- Data synchronization errors

Availability

- Business interruption
- Replacement of lost information

Opportunity or Financial

- Loss of business
- Equipment repair or replacement
- Fines for noncompliance

Reputation

- Loss of patient confidence
- Decreased employee morale

Litigation

- Criminal charges
- Civil suit

Figure 2-4: General Categories of Impacts, with Examples.

Because it is challenging to quantify impacts (for example, how can an organization assign a dollar value to the impact of a tarnished reputation as the result of a breach?), it is sometimes easier to express impacts with ratings of high, medium, or low. The definitions of the ratings are derived from NIST and are described in Figure 2-5. Rating of impacts should take *resiliency*—how quickly the organization could recover from an incident once a threat is realized into consideration. The criticality and sensitivity of the information stored and processed on an information asset would also be a factor in determining overall impact.

Magnitude of Impact	Impact Definition
High	Exercise of the vulnerability (1) may result in the high costly loss of major tangible assets or resources; (2) may significantly violate
Medium	Exercise of the vulnerability (1) may result in the costly loss of tangible assets or resources; (2) may violate
Low	Exercise of the vulnerability (1) may result in the loss of some tangible assets or resources or (2) may noticeably affect an organization's mission

Figure 2-5: Impact Levels and Definitions.

Step 7—Risk determination. The purpose of this step is to assign a risk score that is determined by likelihood and impact. The scoring of risks provides a prioritization and focus for the limited resources allocated for information security. One of the ways risks can be scored is through the OCTAVE[SM] Approach, as described in Figure 2-6.

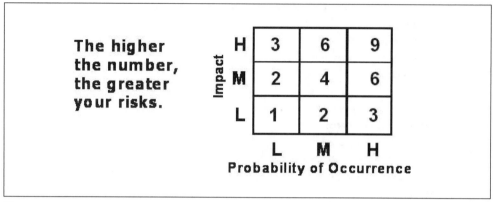

Figure 2-6: The OCTAVE[SM] Approach for Determining Risk Score. (The OCTAVE[SM] Approach. Used by permission.)

Step 8—Control recommendations. Control recommendations are made by examining the vulnerabilities. Where a vulnerability is written as the lack of a control or a weak safeguard, the control recommendation is essentially the opposite. For example, Figure 2-7 lists examples of how a stated vulnerability can be translated to a control recommendation.

Vulnerability	Control Recommendation
Audit logs are not regularly reviewed and are primarily used for problem solving.	Create procedures to randomly audit users; formalize log review responsibilities and procedures.
User's account is not disabled after a predetermined number of unsuccessful logon attempts.	Consider locking out a user's account after five consecutive unsuccessful logon attempts.
Disaster recovery plan has not been created; a formal business impact analysis has not been conducted.	Conduct a formal business impact analysis (BIA); create a disaster recovery plan that outlines a systematic approach to recovery based upon the needs of the business as documented in a BIA.

Figure 2-7: Samples of Control Recommendations.

Step 9—Results documentation. Once risks have been scored, the executives and/ or those directors or managers, also known as *data owners,* directly responsible for the business operation supported by the information asset must be made aware of the *residual risks*—the risks that remain in light of the existing controls and safeguards. The residual risks, the key findings (vulnerabilities), and the control recommendations for reducing risks are documented in the final risk analysis report. To keep the report from becoming too detailed, the executive summary should only focus on the vulnerabilities and control recommendations for which the overall risk score exceeds the organization's level of acceptable risk, also known as *risk appetite*. For most organizations, risk scores of 1 or 2 are acceptable, which means there is no added value in investing additional resources to reduce the risks. Risk scores of 3 or 4 are marginal and usually need some level of remediation to manage the risks appropriately, depending on the system's criticality of the sensitivity of the data. Risk scores of 6 or 9 represent unacceptable risks that exceed the organization's risk tolerance, and they must be remediated immediately. Figure 2-8 is an example of how risks are rated using a green, yellow and red dashboard approach.

Rating (Score)	Probability (Likelihood)	Severity (Impact)
Red (9 or 6)	H H M	H M H
Yellow (4 or 3)	H M L	L M H
Green (2 or 1)	M L L	L M L

Figure 2-8: Risk Dashboard.

The larger risk scores indicate the areas in which additional security safeguards and controls may be beneficial to reduce risks to an acceptable level. Some controls, considered to be "low hanging fruit"—something that does not require significant resources (budget, staff, time, etc.), might be recommended—even when the risk scores are below the organizational threshold of risk tolerance—because they make good business sense.

Once the executives and/or data owners are aware of the scoring of residual risks, they need to make one of the three following decisions:

• **Remediate**—Apply controls to reduce risks to an acceptable level.

• **Transfer**—The risk could be transferred by purchasing insurance or, in some cases by outsourcing, such as subscribing to Software-as-a-Service (SaaS) and having an application and the data remotely hosted.

• **Accept**—Because the cost to remediate may be too expensive, or if the system will be replaced soon, or if it would not be feasible to implement any additional controls then the risks should be accepted by executives or the data owner.

Whatever the decision, it needs to be documented in the risk analysis report. The written risk analysis becomes the evidence that an organization took a systematic and business approach in applying security controls.

Tips for Success

With the basics of risk analysis covered, it is time to go deeper with a couple of topics.

Divide and conquer—Risk analysis can be a daunting task, especially when you do not know where to begin. That is why system characterization is the first step. Dividing up the risk analysis into smaller manageable components saves time and makes the process far easier. For example, an overall assessment of a system, which includes assessment of the physical and environmental controls in place, is conducted in layers. Figure 2-9 outlines some of the general layers of security that would be assessed when conducting a risk analysis for a major application or system. Since organizations have multiple applications and systems, theoretically, these assessment steps would be repeated over and over again.

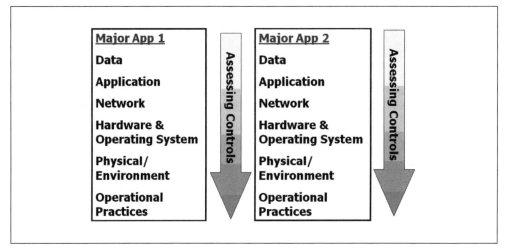

Figure 2-9: Assessing Major Applications.

If the system is hosted in a data center (also called a computer room or server room), then the system would more than likely share all of the same physical and environmental threats, controls, and vulnerabilities as all of the other systems in the room. Therefore, it is easier to do one risk analysis of the data center rather than repeating that portion of the assessment each time a risk analysis is conducted on a major application or system. Likewise, most systems share the same internal network. A single assessment of the network would eliminate the need for repeating a network assessment as part of each system's risk analysis.

Listed next are some of the common areas of assessment for which it would make more sense to break up the risk analysis into smaller parts. Figure 2-10 illustrates how to use shared risk profiles for some of the security layers to streamline the risk analysis process for each major application or system. By using this approach, the risk analysis for a major application would be focused on the security controls implemented within the application and the controls used to protect the data.

Guessing game—Determining what are reasonably anticipated threats as well as their likelihood and impact are, for the most part, educated guesses. That is because there is no accurate source for determining likelihood and impact. Sure, there are computer crime surveys and news stories about organizations that have suffered breaches, but one must question the accuracy of that information. For every computer crime or breach presented in the news, how many are not? In fact, most executives want to keep these types of events from making the news. As mentioned earlier, some impacts are not tangible such as reputation and therefore, cannot be easily measured.

Major App 1	Assessing	Major App 2	Assessing	A hierarchical approach to assessing controls and risks
Data		Data		
Application		Application		
Network		Network		Risk Profile
Hardware & Operating System		Hardware & Operating System		Risk Profile
Physical/ Environment		Physical/ Environment		Risk Profile
Operational Practices		Operational Practices		Risk Profile

Figure 2-10: Using Shared Risk Profiles. (**Tom Walsh Consulting, LLC. Used by permission.**)

Additionally, each organization will have a different probability, or likelihood of a breach occurring, based on several factors, including the types of controls, type of business, and geographical location. Certain government agencies in Washington, DC, for example, may be targeted for political reasons more so than a rural community-based hospital.

History may help us predict future events. For example, it's clear that if the data center is located in the basement of a hospital, and the basement has flooded in the past, unless something drastic has been done to prevent it, there is a good chance it might flood again. Incident reporting, which is required under HIPAA's Security Rule (§164.308(a)(6)(i) and (ii)), is also useful when determining the probability and potential impacts of events. The downside? IT people are notorious for lacking documentation. Therefore, many incidents go unreported or if they are reported, lack enough detail to be helpful.

One last thing regarding the educated guess: people who are good at predicting the future could probably make their fortune doing other things besides information security, such as betting on horses or other sporting events.

Get it in writing—The risk analysis report should offer recommendations for reducing risks to executives and data owners. However, it is still their decision as to how the risks will be handled. The risk report is there to help them make an informed business decision. By getting executives and data owners to sign off on the risk analysis means the process is complete and the information security officer has done his or her job in communicating risks. As vital as this last step is, getting sign off, it is often forgotten. Remember, "If it's important, get it in writing."

Other challenges—Technical people tend to be binary thinkers and detail-oriented to the degree that often they suffer from the "paralysis of analysis." To help overcome this challenge, it is important to remind them that the risk analysis is a "snapshot in time." Threats change, systems and applications are constantly being updated, and new vulnerabilities are discovered daily. That is why a risk analysis needs to be updated periodically. The good news is that once a risk analysis has been conducted, updating the risk profiles and reports is far easier than the very first time the risk analysis is conducted.

Assessing controls is normally done through the use of some type of checklist or by a survey of questions. Finding the right balance is important. Ask too many questions and no one will have the time to complete the checklist or survey. Ask too few questions and you may not feel sure you were thorough in your assessment.

I HAVE A FIREWALL SO I AM SECURE…RIGHT?

Well… not quite. Perimeter security: firewalls, intrusion prevention or detection systems, router configurations, segmented networks (DMZ, extranets, etc.) secure gateways, e-mail filters, etc., all work to prevent or detect the unauthorized outsider from hacking in or attacks that could disrupt business operations. Most organizations have done an adequate job of preventing outsider attacks. Otherwise, they would have a difficult time staying in business.

In today's computing environment, it is challenging to define the perimeter or boundaries of the network. Information sharing and electronic transactions with Business Associates and other covered entities make the perimeter more of a fuzzy line rather than the sure boundary of a fence. Holes are punched in the firewall as business needs require ports to be opened and various protocols allowed to pass through the firewall. Therefore, internal systems cannot solely rely on perimeter security.

In what is known as "Tootsie Pop" security, organizations often focus the majority of their information security budget on hardening the perimeter of their network (hard outer shell), while leaving the information assets on the "inside" of the perimeter somewhat vulnerable (soft and gooey filling). However, as pointed out in a previous section of this chapter, there is a tremendous importance in knowing what information assets need protecting and identifying the reasonably anticipated threats. Based upon that, most security professionals would agree that today, the greater threat is the insider threat—emanating from employees and other authorized users—rather than threat from the outsider. Instead of structuring security based on a Tootsie Pop, the focus should be on hardening the more vulnerable information assets on the inside. The results of the risk analysis would indicate points at which additional internal controls are needed.

The Information Technology Infrastructure Library (ITIL) identifies the three areas that need to be considered to improve services and align with business requirements: people, processes, and technology.

People—Security experts agree that the greatest threat to information security is the carbon-based interface units—people. Therefore, when assessing and later managing risks, the potential risk from people must be one of the highest priorities. Is it coincidence that in Figure 2-2 there are more examples under the general category of "Acts of Man"? I think not! People do crazy things—intentionally and accidentally. Policies, procedures, and technology sometimes are no match for the dogged determination of a misguided person.

With that said, any security safeguard or control must first consider the human element.

Processes—Clinicians' primary focus is patient care. Anything that stands in their way of meeting the objective of quality care, including security, is bypassed. This is especially true when doing things securely places more obstacles in their way than doing things insecurely. People take the path of least resistance. If a security process takes 10 steps and two days to do things right or two steps and 10 minutes to do things the wrong way with the same outcome, for them at least, why wouldn't a busy healthcare worker take the easy way? The overused expression to describe the ease of use, accessibility of information is, *transparent*. A CIO once described that the word transparent really means to users, "they never saw it coming." Using Thesaurus.com as reference, the word *understandable* comes up as suitable substitute for transparent. It makes sense. When people understand why security processes and controls exist, they are more willing to follow the process (policy or procedure) rather than trying a work-around. A good information security officer will spend a great deal of time promoting understanding of the security process by being prepared with a risk-based or compliance-based answer to the question "why?" "Because I said so" does not work with kids; why would we expect that it would work with adults?

When developing security processes, information security professionals often look to best practices. Best practices imply there is a best way or process to achieving a desired outcome that is far better than other processes. These practices are determined by the majority of professionals within a field or area.

A practice is something that is customarily used or which is repeated, such as a process. For example, managing users' access to information systems is a process. A best practice incorporates a process so that, for example, IT or the system administrator is automatically and immediately notified by the HR/payroll system when an employee's account should be changed or inactivated because he or she leaves the organization, transfers (changes jobs internally), is on medical leave, or is placed on disciplinary suspension.

Two considerations worth noting:

- Although best practices may provide guidance, keep in mind that there is no penalty for choosing not to implement best practices.

- The second word in the expression is *practice* and not *technology,* although the latest and the greatest technology is what IT people often think when they hear the expression *best practices.*

Terms or phrases such as *generally accepted* or *common practices* mean that this is what most other organizations are doing. In healthcare, few organizations can afford to be the leaders or trendsetters of best practices in information security. But organizations do, however, want to keep pace with their peers by following what is commonly practiced among the majority of healthcare organizations that are similar in size and mission. Returning to our previous example about access control, the common practice in healthcare today is for the IT or the system administrator to receive e-mail notices from the HR/payroll system every other week to coincide with pay periods. The notices generally do not include those on medical leave or those placed on disciplinary suspension, such as three days' leave without pay. Keep in mind, the employee that is placed on such disciplinary leave is a potentially disgruntled employee.

Technology—When all else fails, technology can sometimes be deployed to enforce security policies. Using technology for this purpose, however, brings about a whole new set of management problems, making it both a blessing and a curse. With the introduction of each new technological device, a group of people exist who are determined to find a way to circumvent it. Technology should be viewed as a part of the whole solution rather than the only solution. Figure 2-11 lists some of the things to consider when selecting technical controls.

For information security controls, the three areas that need to be considered are people, processes, and technology—in that order.

- Current technology and network environment
- Future infrastructure plans
- Impact and organizational culture
- Budget
- Balance between security controls and the ease of use by users
- Balance between cost of the security control versus the value of the information systems and data being protected
- The specific threats and vulnerabilities that the control will address in consideration of the overall risk score

---

Figure 2-11: Things to Consider When Selecting Technical Controls.

IT'S 2:00 A.M.—DO YOU KNOW WHERE YOUR INFORMATION IS?

Once a risk analysis has been conducted on the major applications and the general support systems, such as the network, it is time to assess other areas that may contain potential risks to confidential information. These other areas include departmental applications or systems, mobile computing devices, portable media, backup media, and Business Associates.

Islands of data—Departments create their own documents, spreadsheets, or even databases that contain confidential information such as protected health information (PHI), Social Security numbers, credit card data, or cardholder information, and other sensitive or proprietary information such as financial or personnel information. Each department independently creates and manages their confidential information, often with little understanding of the risks or security process used to govern IT. This arrangement can be thought of as having created "islands of confidential data" with little or no protection of the shoreline.

Because of its simplicity, a user can create his or her own Access database without IT involvement. Often, the database starts out as a small project or as a job aid. Later, it grows and user dependency increases. Before long, the simple database becomes a critical application for the department. If the database contains confidential information, then it begs the question: What security controls have been implemented to protect the data stored within the database? Access controls? Audit trails? Encryption? Chances are that few, if any, of these controls have been implemented, meaning that the database may violate regulatory requirements.

Confidential information may sometimes be extracted from larger, organization-wide applications or systems and then placed into Excel spreadsheets, making it easier for users to work with the data. Again, what security controls are in place in this arrangement, and does management understand the residual risks? How is data integrity preserved? This is especially important if the data from the spreadsheet are used to make key business decisions.

Mobile computing devices and portable media—Mobile computing devices and portable media pose a significant security risk because they may contain confidential information and, being mobile and portable, they are at greater risk for loss, theft, or unauthorized access. If media or a mobile device is lost or stolen, the information stored on the device potentially becomes available to anyone who comes into possession of the device. This represents a serious risk.

Mobile computing devices refers to devices such as laptops, tablets, hand-held computing devices, and other types of smart phones, such as a BlackBerry. *Portable media* includes plug-in memory devices (USB-flash drives, thumb drives, jump drives, etc.), CD-ROMs, DVDs, optical disks, external hard drives, removable disk storage system (Zip drive), backup tapes, and floppy disks. As the memory capability on these devices has increased over the years, so have the risks. The challenge is to secure and centrally manage mobile devices and portable media, as well as maintain accountability to comply with §164.310(d)(2)(iii) of HIPAA's Security Rule.

In July 2008, Providence Health & Services had to pay a $100,000 "resolution" fine to the Department of Health & Human Services (HHS) as a result of five incidents that occurred between September 2005 and March 2006. The incidents involved laptops, backup tapes, and optical disks that contained the PHI of 386,000 patients that were lost or stolen. The data stored on these devices were unencrypted (Source: Health Data Management, www.healthdatamanagement.com). In addition to fines, organizations may have to pay for identity theft insurance for individuals whose privacy was breached. The cost of this insurance, along with the time spent to investigate and respond to an incident, can significantly impact the bottom line for any organization. For example, in September 2007, the state of Ohio estimated that the total cost to respond to the data theft of a computer backup tape stolen from a state employee's car was expected to exceed $3 million dollars.

Business Associate Agreements (BAA)—The complexity of healthcare requires patient information to be shared with other organizations as part of treatment, payment, and healthcare operations (TPO) and also to government agencies when required by law. Sharing patient information is similar to sharing a secret with a friend to whom you say, "Don't tell a soul." The friend may agree to your request, but there is no way you can actually prevent him or her from sharing the secret and, in most cases, no way of detecting whether he or she shared your secret. That is why a BAA alone is not enough.

The HIPAA Security Rule Preamble[1] outlines five things a Business Associate must do when sharing patient information:

1. Implement safeguards that reasonably and appropriately protect the confidentiality, integrity, and availability of the electronically protected health information that it creates, receives, maintains, or transmits on behalf of the covered entity;
2. Ensure that any agent, including a subcontractor, to whom it provides this information agrees to implement reasonable and appropriate safeguards;
3. Report to the covered entity any security incident of which it becomes aware;
4. Make its policies, procedures, and documentation required by this subpart relating to such safeguards, available to the Secretary for purposes of determining the covered entity's compliance with this subpart; and
5. Authorize termination of the contract by the covered entity if the covered entity determines that the Business Associate has violated a material term of the contract.

In addition to these five stated requirements, the following is stated within the Preamble to the HIPAA Security Rule, "Business Associates must be made aware of security policies and procedures, whether through contract language or other means." In this regard, two questions information security professionals must ask are:

- How will the requirements for Business Associates be verified, keeping in mind that requirement #5 states that the covered entity has to terminate the contract with the Business Associate if they discover a material breach or violation of the contract?

- How will the requirements be implemented? For example, #3 requires the Business Associate to report an incident but offers no details on how this would be accomplished. Who does the incident get reported to? When does the incident have to be reported? Within 24 hours? 72 hours? How does the incident get reported? By telephone? Certified mail? These are just a few examples of what a BAA does not typically address but needs to address in order to manage risks appropriately.

Because of the American Recovery and Reinvestment Act of 2009, Business Associates must now comply with the HIPAA Security Rule and are subject to the same civil and criminal penalties for violations. As a result, most organizations will need to update the wording in their BAAs.

DO YOU HAVE A STRATEGIC PLAN FOR SECURITY?

Once the risk analysis is completed, a plan needs to be created to track remediation tasks. For the plan to gain organization-wide support, it should be aligned with strategic business initiatives as well as regulatory requirements.

Wherever possible, an information security professional should link each planned security control to a business initiative. This requires a careful review of both the organization's strategic plan as well as the IT strategic plan. For example, a single sign-on based upon strong authentication could be linked to the organization's strategic objective to "improve physician satisfaction" and an IT objective to increase "physician use of computer systems." Physicians who practice at multiple hospitals or healthcare facilities may have several user IDs and passwords. The single sign-on could reduce the number of user IDs and passwords within an organization to one, thus, making it easier for them to use the various computer systems.

Besides business objectives, security controls should also be linked to regulatory requirements. And the list of regulatory requirements keeps growing. Figure 2-12 highlights some of the key federal legislation and industry requirements of which information security professionals should be aware.

Regulation	Known As	Requirements
The Health Insurance Portability and Accountability Act of 1996	HIPAA	(Security Rule) To provide standards for administrative, physical and technical safeguards for the protection of electronic patient health information (ePHI).
Payment Card Industry Data Security Standard*	PCI DSS	A set of comprehensive requirements for improving security developed by the five major credit card companies.
FTC's Identity Theft Red Flag Rules (part of part of the Fair and Accurate Credit Transactions (FACT) Act of 2003	Red Flags Rule	Creditors with covered accounts must have identity theft prevention programs in place to identify, detect, and respond to patterns, practices, or specific activities that could indicate identity theft.
Sarbanes-Oxley Act	SOX	Requires: • Internal control monitoring • Records management • Whistleblower protection • Companies to meet a higher standard of ethics and best practices for controls
Federal Information Security Management Act of 2002	FISMA	A set of requirements, including annual audits, to improve information security within the federal government and other parties such as government contractors.

Figure 2-12: Key Regulatory Requirements.

Four of these are worth further detailed explanation as to how they may apply to healthcare organizations.

- **PCI DSS**—Any business that accepts credit cards (merchants) must comply with the rules set forth by the PCI Security Standards Council, a limited liability organization formed by the five major credit card companies. Failure to comply could result in fines, liability for damages, and loss of merchant status (no longer able to accept credit card payments).

- **Red Flag Rules**—Under FTC rules, many healthcare providers will be considered creditors with "covered accounts" because they sometimes permit deferred payment for services, or payments to be made in multiple installments, which is considered to be an extension of credit.

- **FISMA**—Healthcare organizations that conduct research under a federal government grant may also be required to prove that the computer systems used meet the requirements of Federal Information Security Management Act (FISMA) of 2002.

- **SOX**—There are rumors of similar legislation being passed for non-profit organizations. There has been other legislation that applies to all corporations, including non-profits. Financial auditors typically use the Sarbanes-Oxley Act (SOX) requirements for internal controls as basis for their annual audits of healthcare organizations.

HIPAA requirements for risk analysis and risk management—When the original proposed HIPAA Security Rule was released in August 1998, the authors decided to list the implementation specifications within each of the three categories of safeguards (administrative, physical, and technical) in alphabetical order. But for the final HIPAA Security Rule, released in February 2003, the updated implementation specifications were listed more so in the order of priority for establishing an information security program. Therefore, it is important to note that the first two implementation specifications in the administrative category are:

- **§164.308(a)(1)(ii)(A) Risk analysis** *(Required)*. Conduct an accurate and thorough assessment of the potential risks and vulnerabilities to the confidentiality, integrity, and availability of electronically protected health information held by the covered entity.

- **§164.308(a)(1)(ii)(B) Risk management** *(Required)*. Implement security measures sufficient to reduce risks and vulnerabilities to a reasonable and appropriate level to comply with §164.306(a).

But risk analysis is not a one-time event. Security controls must be validated and risks must be evaluated. HIPAA's Security Rule also requires:

- **§164.308(a)(8) Evaluation** *(Required)*. Perform a periodic technical and non-technical evaluation, based initially upon the standards and implemented under this rule and subsequently, in response to environmental or operational changes affecting the security of electronic protected health information, that establishes the extent to which an entity's security policies and procedures meet the requirements of this subpart.

Besides HIPAA, risk analysis is either required or referenced in the other regulatory requirements listed in Figure 2-12.

To wrap up this section, here are the steps for creating a strategic plan for security.

1. Completing a risk analysis for major applications and general support systems.
2. Having executive management and data owners determine what controls will be implemented to reduce risks to an acceptable level, and sign off on the risk analysis reports.
3. Compiling the remediation tasks into a plan for information security.
4. Aligning information security controls with business strategic plans and IT business objectives.
5. Aligning information security controls with the appropriate regulatory requirements.
6. Creating a prioritized plan of action.
7. Publishing and sharing the plan with others.

SUMMARY

Information security professionals must identify the reasonably anticipated threats and prioritize the risks to help business executives make an informed business decision. Once decisions are made by the executives, the information security officer creates a plan so that the limited resources dedicated to security can be used efficiently and effectively.

Information security is less about the elimination of risk and more about the appropriate management of risk.

Discussion Questions[2]:

Selected questions from the CMS white papers on the HIPAA Security Rule, "Sample questions for covered entities to consider":

1. What are the human, natural, and environmental threats to information systems that contain ePHI?
2. What security measures are already in place to protect ePHI (i.e., safeguards)?
3. Is executive leadership and/or management involved in risk management and mitigation decisions?
4. Are security processes being communicated throughout the organization?
5. How often should an evaluation be done? For example, are additional evaluations performed if security incidents are identified, changes are made in the organization, or new technology is implemented?
6. Is an internal or external evaluation, or a combination of both, most appropriate for the covered entity?
7. Are periodic evaluation reports and the supporting material considered in the analysis, recommendations, and subsequent changes fully documented?
8. Have existing Business Associate contracts created and implemented for compliance with the Privacy Rule, which involve ePHI, been reviewed to determine if Security Rule requirements are addressed?
9. To minimize additional work efforts, can existing Business Associate contracts, which involve ePHI, be modified to include Security Rule requirements?

References

1. The Health Insurance Portability and Accountability Act of 1996 (HIPAA) Security Rule §164.314, 2. (1996).

2. Source: Department of Health & Human Services. Security standards: administrative safeguards. HIPAA Security Series 2. May 2005.

CHAPTER 3

Data Management and Portability

Terrell W. Herzig, MSHI, CISSP

THREATS TO INTERNAL DATA MANAGEMENT

Healthcare generates an enormous amount of data daily. To adequately represent the health of an individual, it is necessary to have these data available and accessible whenever the patient presents for treatment or care. This often requires healthcare organizations to invest in expensive data storage solutions and rapid retrieval systems. This requirement, however, lends itself to exposing the organization to a greater risk of a breach. The volume of information, coupled with the number of healthcare individuals needing access to the information, adds increased risk of data leakage or a breach of patient information.

Storage, energy and facility costs are consuming an increasing amount of the healthcare IT budget. Healthcare organizations must examine the need to maintain such large information vaults and evaluate current information management strategies. The purchase of storage-related products and services should be driven by carefully developed information life cycle management strategies.

This chapter explores issues related to data management practices within healthcare organizations. It examines the legal requirements for healthcare information retention and the appropriate methods for its destruction at the end of the life cycle. This chapter also takes a brief look at emerging trends in information governance and the impact they can have on healthcare organizations.

With the increased amount of data available and the ease with which information can be transported, healthcare organizations find themselves open to increased liability. It is imperative that these organizations understand their internal data management activities and the new threats they face if they do not establish formal information governance policies and procedures.

Privacy Laws and Their Impact on the Use of Personal Information

People are often surprised to learn that privacy is not traditionally stated within the United States Constitution as a right. Instead, privacy rights have largely been developed within the 20th century, possibly as a result of the rapid development of technology capable of collecting, storing, and distributing vast amounts of personal data. The development of technology often outpaces the ability of society to police and govern its use. Indeed, most privacy rights in the United States have come by way of a mixture of state law, federal statutes, and Constitutional law.

Many individuals may incorrectly think that the establishment of HIPAA in 1996 was the first federal legislative act to establish an individual's privacy. Actually, numerous federal laws have been established for this purpose and also for the sharing of sensitive information. The following are some of the more notable laws and regulations:

- 1974: The US Federal Privacy Act: Applies to federal agencies as it provides for the protection of information about private information that is held in federal databases.

- 1980: Organization for the Economic Cooperation and Development Guidelines (OECD): Provides for limitations on data collection, specifications for the purpose of collecting data, limitations on data use, information security safeguards, and participation by the individual on whom the data are being collected.

- 1984: US Medical Computer Crime Act: Addresses attempts to illegally access or alter computerized medical records, either by phone or computer network.

- 1984: First US Federal Computer Crime Law: Covers classified defense or foreign relations information, records of financial institutions or credit reporting agencies, and government computers. This law made it a misdemeanor to knowingly access a US government computer without or beyond authorization.

- 1986: US Computer Fraud and Abuse Act: Clarifies the 1984 law and added use of a federal computer with intent to fraud; altering, damaging, or destroying information in a federal-interest computer; or preventing the use of the computer or information that causes a loss of $1,000 or more or could impair medical care; and trafficking in computer passwords if it affects interstate or foreign commerce or permits unauthorized access to government computers.

- 1994: US Computer Abuse Amendments Act: Modifies the previous fraud and abuse laws by changing certain definitions and terminologies to update the law's applicability. This included changing the phrase "federal interest computer" to "a computer used in interstate commerce," added coverage for viruses and worms, included intentional damage done with "reckless disregard of substantial and unjustifiable risk," and provides provisions for civil actions to recover damages.

- 1996: US National Information Infrastructure Protection Act: Amends the Computer Fraud and Abuse Act. The amended act is patterned after the OECD Guidelines and addresses the confidentiality, integrity, and availability of ISs.

- 1999: Gramm-Leach-Bliley Act: Originally passed in 1999 and then amended in 2003, the act provides protection of non-public information, including healthcare information.

- 2000: US Congress Electronic Signatures in Global and National Commerce Act (ESIGN): Facilitates the use of electronic records and signatures in interstate and foreign commerce by ensuring the validity of electronic contracts. This legislation was intent on protecting and preserving consumers' rights under consumer protection laws.

- 2001: USA Provide Appropriate Tools Required to Intercept and Obstruct Terrorism (PATRIOT) Act: Establishes and permits the subpoena of electronic records, monitoring of Internet communications, and the search and seizure of information on live systems (including switches, routers, and servers), backups, and archives. Communications can be intercepted under a delayed search warrant.

- 2002: E-Government Act: Establishes a comprehensive framework for security controls over information resources impacting federal operations and assets. It also provides coverage for the coordination of information security efforts throughout the civilian and law enforcement communities.

Until the development of HIPAA regulations, protection and safeguards related to patient information were primarily determined by state laws, which were often written based on controlling liability. Most states have laws that address privacy issues for sensitive health information. With no national model from which to draw, state laws are often inconsistent. On occasion a state law may conflict with a federal law when an entity expands operations across state or national geographic boundaries.

HIPAA may pre-empt conflicting state laws but usually within a certain set of circumstances. A state law is not preempted if it is "more stringent" than the federal rules, meaning that the state law offers more privacy protection to an individual. State laws are not pre-empted if they relate to the reporting of a disease, injury, child abuse, birth, death, or the conduct of a public health investigation, licensure of facilities, or an individual.

As identity theft, medical fraud, and other incidents continue to increase, both state and federal governments continue to develop and enhance privacy legislation. In January 2008, California enacted AB1298, which expands California's breach law to include unencrypted medical histories, information on mental or physical conditions, medical treatments and diagnoses, unencrypted insurance data, and other related information. This means that almost any medical-related information disclosed in a breach would require the notification of the patients involved.

In October 2008, the Healthcare Information and Management Systems Society (HIMSS) commissioned a study by Kroll Fraud Solutions to survey the security of patient data.[1] During this study, several issues related to the data collected and stored by healthcare facilities were identified. The following are their findings:

- Patient data collected and stored in hospitals and healthcare facilities are the most valuable and content-rich for fraudulent use and profitability. In addition to name, Social Security number, and date of birth (the golden combination), records in these facilities contain mailing address, insurance policy information, medical history, and, in some cases, credit card and financial information to expedite billing and payment. The data contained in one record represent more than that of any other source, including banks, schools, or human resources departments.

- Hospitals are aggregators of birth and death records, valuable resources for identity theft crimes. These records are often used for identity theft in which an identity is fabricated from multiple sources. The thefts are harder to detect and restore, and the victims include those persons who are not likely to have any prevention measures in place, such as minors and the deceased, which would extend the life of the identity theft cycle.

- Patient data breaches cause difficulties beyond financial damage and are the most difficult to resolve. Patients whose data are used for medical fraud (i.e., the perpetrators use stolen information to receive treatment) suffer from insurance eligibility/application issues, as well as misdiagnosis due to misinformation on their health records.

The study also discloses that in the period between 2006-2007, more than 1.5 million names were exposed during data breaches that occurred in hospitals alone. This figure did not include the other categories of healthcare facilities and services, such as home health providers, physician offices, and pharmaceutical companies.

THE PERFECT STORM

In December 2006, the United States Federal Rules of Civil Procedure were amended to address the difficulties in producing electronically stored information during discovery in litigation. Although the rules apply to issues in the US federal court system, they have served as templates for nearly every state and local jurisdiction. Local jurisdictions can adopt the changes to the Federal Rules of Civil Procedure.

Today nearly every court case involves some form of legal discovery of electronically created documents or digitally stored information. "E-discovery" is the term referring to the legal discovery of electronic-based documents. E-discovery requires that a party to a legal proceeding produce, in a timely manner, any electronic documents the court may deem relevant to that case. As with healthcare, the integrity and relevancy of data are critical.

The vast amounts of information preserved by healthcare organizations are required, in part, due to laws that govern how long the organization must retain certain documents. The American Health Information Management Association (AHIMA) has compiled many relevant retention schedules into a practice brief entitled "Retention of Health Information."[2] This practice brief is available at the AHIMA Web site.

When reviewing the types of data available within the healthcare environment, including diagnostic images, disease index, fetal heart monitor strips, patient health and medical records, and the length of time they are to be retained (some permanently); the risk involved in appropriately managing this information is immediately evident. In an academic medical center engaged in research, the volume of information and risk exposure increase dramatically. Healthcare is also one of the most litigious industries. When combining the vast data storehouse of an academic medical center with the healthcare industry tendency toward lawsuits, the environment becomes ripe for invoking e-discovery processes.

E-Discovery

E-discovery can be costly and resource-intensive, but the ramifications for failing to adequately prepare for e-discovery can be disastrous. Organizations that fail to preserve electronically stored documents can face sanctions and fines. As e-discovery costs become more widely known, executives will take appropriate steps to ensure that they are ready to fulfill discovery requests for digital information.

Preparing for e-discovery means planning, training the appropriate IT personnel, establishing the appropriate technologies, and developing liaisons with legal staff. The following points can help your organization deal with discovery requests:

- **Create a liaison between IT and legal staff.** My organization began its efforts to prepare for the e-discovery changes almost immediately after the modifications were announced. A series of joint meetings with legal and risk management staff were held. During these exchanges, one IT person was assigned to work with the legal and risk management team. This individual is the designated resource person on whom the legal team would depend for information regarding IT topology and system architecture; identifying records and retention practices, hardware and software architectures; and the accessibility to data. If necessary, this individual can speak to the facility's practices of backups, archiving, and transporting data.

- **Identify experts.** Most IT staff do not have the background or special training required to collect and preserve evidence for court proceedings. Whereas a substantially large organization may have the resources to train such individuals, many smaller companies may have to employ outside resources to assist in this function.

- **Establish appropriate tools and technology.** While assessing your technical staff for the competences to collect and preserve possible electronic evidence, and assess the availability of technology and tools to fulfill a request. E-discovery professionals use specialized software to enable the fast and accurate collection of data. Once collected, specialized tools are employed to filter the information to the relevant specifics. Specialists, who provide external services, often maintain a robust collection of software and hardware to facilitate retrievals from systems that are obsolete. This provides discovery options with the minimal risk to damaging operational systems and storage devices. These specialists can also provide a variety of court-approved output techniques.

- **Prepare for depositions.** Many organizations are preparing IT individuals to act as FRCP 30(b)(6) witnesses. These witnesses may be asked to provide depositions regarding the organization's technology infrastructure and its data retention practices.

- **Create and maintain a record retention policy.** As evidenced in this chapter, medical establishments have many retention requirements. Therefore, healthcare organizations must adopt policies and procedures that adequately manage the life cycle of the information in their safeguard. Policies must be comprehensive and provide for adequate destruction and disposal of obsolete information. The policies should be developed in cooperation with representatives from the legal, risk management, and health information management (HIM) departments. IT should never be left to determine the retention policies for the organization. Once litigation starts, IT is potentially the group that will hold and preserve the documents. The IT and legal departments must communicate as the litigation proceeds to establish that responsibilities are being completed correctly.

- **Watch the e-mail.** Try to reduce the volume of digital data that may be subject to discovery. Counsel employees to use systems such as e-mail for business purposes only. Many people will include in e-mail things that they would never say in public. Establish and enforce appropriate e-mail use policies.

What Do I Do When I Receive a Litigation Hold?

A litigation hold is the suspension of an organization's document retention/destruction policies for documents that may be relevant to a lawsuit. The lawsuit may have been filed or a lawsuit is "reasonably anticipated." A litigation hold ensures that relevant data are not destroyed and key employees are notified of document preservation requirements. Litigation holds have the potential to disrupt routine maintenance and information management practices, such as recycling tape backups.

The requirement to preserve information arises when a party is alerted that certain information is likely to be sought in discovery. This could occur upon receipt of a complaint, a demand letter, or a letter expressly requesting the preservation of certain documents.

Successful litigation holds will require a managed process by both legal and IT staff. The first step is the identification and preservation of potential responsive documentation. Within the IT department, the CIO, application managers, security and compliance staff, e-mail managers, database managers, and data center managers must understand the processes and technologies involved in identifying and preserving evidence.

Approaches to Litigation Hold

Ways to perform litigation holds are many and varied. One approach to collecting and preserving electronic evidence is a custodian-based collection approach. In this approach, the people who work with the records and data on a daily basis are most frequently the best qualified to know where and how to find the data. This approach is still valid today for small organizations with small record collections and little litigation action. A modern day derivative of this approach is to have IT operations suspend routine file deletions throughout its various systems. Suspension of file deletions should always be part of any litigation hold process.

A more esoteric method in custodian-based approaches to litigation hold is to have forensic images made of the hard drives for systems subject to collection, as illustrated in Figure 3-1. This approach can be costly and requires specific skills to establish the appropriate chain-of-custody practices.

A forensic copy of a hard drive is the process of obtaining a bit-for-bit copy of the original drive at the time of imaging. This technique usually requires generating special hash codes to show the data were not modified after copying. The data management issues related to these tasks can compound the issues of collection.

Another form of litigation hold is the preservation of evidence in place. This approach involves working with IT to decide which documents are needed and are considered important. In such methods, Boolean searches are conducted against large collections of data to identify and locate relevant documents. Search criteria are usually decided in prediscovery meetings with both legal parties. Using this approach depends on the availability of enterprise search tools and associated mechanisms.

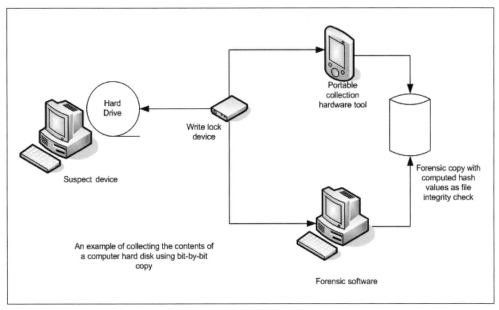

Figure 3-1: An Example of Forensic Imaging.

Once the required files have been identified, they must be preserved. The files should be locked down so they cannot be altered or deleted. Files may be locked and made read-only or removed from the search indexes or systems so they cannot be located. The benefit of this action is not having to reproduce the files in other storage locations. However, holding files in place can interfere with IT operations and, in some cases, software applications. Remember litigation suits can last for weeks, months, or even years.

A second method of files preservation involves the creation of "forensically sound" copies of files in a separate data store location. By making forensically sound copies, the files' metadata are preserved when they are copied to the alternate location.

A third form of litigation hold involves the use of record management systems and archives that have the native ability to support litigation holds, as illustrated in Figure 3-2. The use of systems to place and maintain litigation is straightforward. Records can be searched, and the resulting collection set can be electronically placed on hold. The caveat to this process is that only records that have been archived in this method can be held this way. Organizations using this method may find that such record management systems only support certain file types, such as office documents and e-mail. For information systems to operate successfully in healthcare, the vendors of the systems will need to supply adequate connectivity in their systems to support the diverse information needs of patient care.

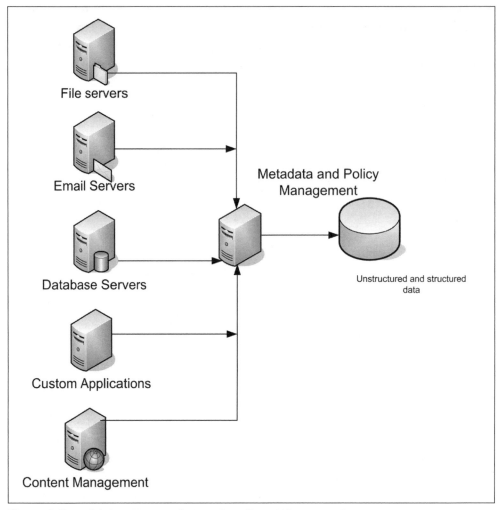

Figure 3-2: Archiving Data and Metadata for e-Discovery Purposes.

DATA RETENTION

Many healthcare providers maintain patient records online, or what is commonly referred to as *tier-1 storage*, much longer than is necessary. For example, the records of patients who have had elective surgery and have not experienced any abnormalities and have no near-term follow-up may be in tier-1 storage indefinitely. As a result, information storage grows continuously and not only impacts annual IT budgets but can jeopardize disaster recovery and backup strategies. Many providers back up patient records using processes that make complete copies of information stores each week (or more frequently) and store these copies on expensive tier-1 storage.

Current healthcare trends, business models, and quality and performance improvement processes all demand statistical analysis of healthcare data. Easy access to large amounts of healthcare information is required to support these analysis practices. Providers must streamline access to information to support these functions. While storage needs are growing, the how, when, and where the data are stored is changing. A hierarchy of storage mediums may be needed to cost-effectively match the information's relevancy and accessibility to the appropriate storage technology.

Software systems built on policy-based rule sets can automate the movement of information to different storage tiers at a specific point in time, based on predetermined thresholds. Storage management solutions can co-locate medical information in redundant physical locations to enable rapid, efficient disaster recovery solutions.

Healthcare organizations continue to face both state and federal legal requirements to maintain various forms of patient and financial data. For example, HIPAA requires covered entities to "establish and implement procedures to create and maintain retrievable exact copies of electronic protected health information."[3] While organizations may define maximum retention periods for data, certain minimum retention times are defined by various state and federal laws. The following list is an example of minimum retention requirements:

- Patient financial data—Seven to 10 years.

- Federal payor audit records—Five to seven years.

- Private payor audit records—Six to seven years.

- Medicaid data—Five years.

- OIG (Office of Inspector General) audit data—10 to 15 years.

- Clinical data (nursing, pharmacy, laboratory)—Seven to 10 years.

- Radiology data—10 years.

- Surgery data—Seven to 10 years.

- Mental health information—Seven years.

- Neonatal (fetal heart monitoring)—Age of majority, plus statute of limitations.

- Register of births, deaths, surgical procedures and adoptions—Permanently.

Document retention policies and enterprise content management systems are no longer niche systems. Healthcare organizations should review the state of controls and risk factors related to information governance practices. A thorough review will include all "shadow IT" systems. Examine mission-critical information stored in unsecured spreadsheets and desktop database files. Document controls on access, record retention, database security, and external data transfers and data integrity. With the signing of the American Recovery and Reinvestment Act in February 2009, the nation's first federal breach notification law became reality. Under section 13402 of Title XIII of that act, covered entities must notify patients of a breach if their information is accessed by an unauthorized party and the information was not rendered unusable, unreadable, or indecipherable. The HHS secretary was mandated to issue guidance specifying the technologies and methodologies to be used to comply with the new law and avoid patient notification in the event of a breach. As a result, HHS issued a guidance on April 17, 2009.[4] This guidance indicates two acceptable means of rendering ePHI as unreadable or indecipherable: encryption and destruction. The guidance specifically points to documentation from NIST[5] to be used when implementing encryption and destruction of PHI (both electronic and print forms). The call for encryption applies to data at rest as well as data in transit. This requirement makes data management and data retention policies and procedures even more critical.

Data Leakage

Many organizations focus on keeping external sources away from their internal data. Some fail to consider the activities of their most trusted asset, the employee. As employees become more mobile and consumer devices continue to creep into enterprise operations, data leakage, the movement of information resources outside organizational boundaries in methods not approved by management, has become prevalent. (See Figure 3-3.) I like this definition of data leakage, incidentally, much better than the standard trade press definition of "the unauthorized use of information outside of an organization." Vendors that want to sell data loss prevention products will attempt to convince management that their issues with data leakage are occurring because of weak controls or the lack of their particular "tool of the month."

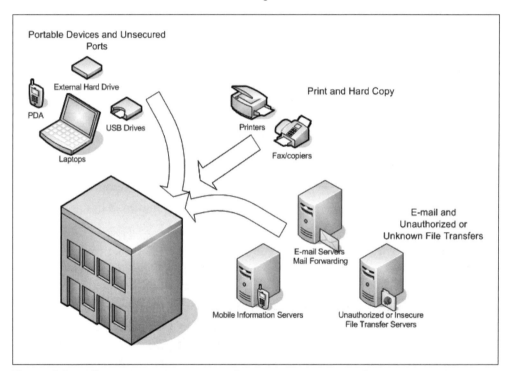

Figure 3-3: Different Ways Sensitive Information Can Leave the Organization.

Few employees understand the threats mobility brings to the security of information resources nor do they have adequate knowledge to securely operate the devices. The number of employees taking work home is increasing. As a result, information such as e-mails, paper records, and other data moves around outside organizational walls. Medical transcriptionists practically all work from home. Physicians and other clinical staff take calls from home or other off-site locations. Home health providers carry laptop computers filled with patient information. How many articles have been written about personal computers being sold at auctions and garage sales that contain sensitive information? The primary population to leak data is that group who has been given explicit access to it. Therefore, the group with the greatest risk of being involved with a data leak is our own people.

Data format can also affect information accessibility. Standard and easy to use formats, rather than specialized software, are much more likely to be used by someone outside an organization to access information. Clinical and hospital staff are more likely to download, recreate, and remove information to personal devices (such as cell phones and personal digital assistants [PDAs]) if the data could be useful to them by being on that device. While the use of the information by the workforce member may be perfectly legitimate, the freedom to load the data on a personal device represents a loss of organizational control over the information if the device is lost or stolen. Most individuals do not understand the real issue in the loss of information on a device: that is, if the information is not under organizational control, the organization cannot account for its use. There is no means to ascertain the level of access to the information, only the likelihood that the information will be accessed.

Automation improves accessibility by making it easier to collate and retrieve relevant data. If the organization has search tools, repositories, data warehouses, or ad-hoc reporting mechanisms, then the likelihood of sensitive data walking out of the door increases dramatically.

The easier it is to copy data, the greater the likelihood of it occurring, and the harder it becomes to control. In healthcare, this becomes a double-edged sword. Patient lives can depend on the rapid access to data. Granting access to data and balancing the appropriate amount of access control is a delicate balance.

With the increased availability of high-speed communication channels like the Internet, huge outflows of information can occur from a variety of sources. Specially crafted malware can install system backdoors and make the computer available from anywhere on the Internet. E-mail administrators continue to raise attachment sizes to facilitate the rapid movement of patient data to a particular physician. Finally, the proliferation of portable storage devices, such as hard drives and thumb drives, make it possible to literally walk out of the door with gigabytes (or even terabytes) of data. The mobility of data is particularly challenging in healthcare.

When a data storage medium (such as tape, hard drive, thumb drive, CD, DVD) is lost, the chances of the information actually falling into hostile hands is probably quite low. However, the conservative conclusion is that when the data are out of the organization's control, a data leak beyond the organization has occurred. Following the same philosophy, a growing number of regulatory bodies are placing the burden on corporations to treat lost data as having been stolen, which forces the corporations to notify individuals whose data might have been lost. Three forms of control are becoming increasingly important to control data:

- Reduce data accessibility.

- Control the ability to copy data.

- Improve the detection of data flow.

Controls that can reduce accessibility, especially in the case of a data loss or theft, are encryption tools. Any portable device that may transport sensitive information should be encrypted. If the device does not support an encryption option, do not use it. This simple rule applies to laptops, PDAs, smart phones, portable hard drives, thumb drives, and CD/DVDs.

The amount of sensitive information that is copied or reproduced should be identified through policy and user education. Unfortunately, some users will continue to ignore policy or not appropriately understand the nature of sensitive information. As a result, technical controls that restrict USB ports and Internet protocols are becoming increasingly necessary.

When preventive controls fail, the damage may be reduced through the use of controls such as content monitoring. Content monitoring works by instantly classifying data as it flows through a connection point and dynamically applies controls that may take the form of an advisory message or a block in transmission.

THE UNHOLY TRINITY: E-MAIL, GOOGLE, AND MYSPACE

Does your organization currently operate a Web content management solution? If not, try this experiment. Monitor the content passing through your firewall for a period of time. The results will be more revealing if you examine all ports and not just Web-based traffic on port 80. You may be shocked to discover the amount and type of sensitive information leaving the organization. You will probably discover large amounts of billing data, credit card numbers, credit reports and bank account numbers transversing the perimeter on its way across the Internet—unencrypted.

Next, examine the traffic that is being passed on traditional unencrypted protocols such as telnet and FTP (File Transfer Protocol). You will probably detect users moving sensitive data using these unsecure protocols. Even though your organization may have a secure gateway for file transfers, you must take action to promote its use. Users can't use the proper tools if they are not aware they exist. Have you blocked the unsecure outbound protocols so users can't easily use unsecure protocols such as FTP? This is an example of how overlapping security controls can pay off. Security awareness and training along with VLAN management can effectively reinforce the issue of secure information transfer.

Recently, when I examined the logs from our Web content management system, I discovered an increasing use of Google applications. Using the data reconstruction feature of the software, I was able to rebuild the spreadsheet uploaded to Google documents. Upon opening the document, I immediately recognized it to be a research database. Fortunately, it contained only a randomly assigned study number and several copies of non-descriptive laboratory values.

Each of these cases represents data leakage. Each had good intent, and when the situations were discussed with end users, they were not aware of the risk at which they had placed themselves and the organization. In the Google case, the researcher was unaware that he could not store PHI on Google applications. He was adamant it was password protected and shared only with the individuals authorized in the study.

The issue with storing PHI on Google applications or any other Internet file-sharing site is that of loss of control. To reiterate a basic chapter tenet and describe a data leak: information stored outside the organization's control is assumed to be compromised. Although I doubt Google employees would rummage through this researcher's files, no formal business relationship existed with Google, so they were not bound within a trusted legal relationship.

When these findings were shared with senior management, policies and plans were established, with the assistance of risk management, to enable content management. Since the implementation of the content management solution, few requests for exceptions are presented, and most of these exceptions arise from misclassified content.

Social Computing

One of the ugliest incidents I have ever witnessed involved personal MySpace pages. I will not divulge the details except to report that the incident involved inappropriate pictures that were subsequently posted on MySpace.

MySpace and Facebook are but two examples of a new generation of software called *social software*. Social software services provide communication channels for collaboration, marketing, recruitment, and customer services. These services can also serve as portals for information exchange and privacy invasion and can put organizations at risk for discrimination, harassment, and crimes against persons.

Using social software services for business activities involves the uploading of corporate information into the social environment. It could be uploaded intentionally as part of a marketing campaign or as a malicious or erroneous activity. As user profiles within social software sites can be accessed and managed through corporate and non-corporate networks, this limits the effectiveness of content controls.

The corporate use of social software sites requires that staff maintain profiles within the social software environment. Communications are then initiated, received, and managed in the social software services. Staff profiles are the conduits through which corporate information can flow. Access to information on profile pages is controlled by utilities in the social software and is configured by the owner of the profile. I recently read about one incident in which the ER nursing staff made derogatory remarks and complaints about the hospital physician and administrative staff on a social software site. This resulted in a number of legal actions and litigations.

The result of these information exchange activities is that significant amounts of information about the inner workings of an organization are publicly exposed. Once information is made public on the Internet, it cannot be recalled and made confidential again.

Media Handling and Data Transfer

When discussing data mobility, management, and leakage, it is important to discuss the availability of mass storage devices and the need to move large files. Healthcare is ripe with the need to move large datasets among both internal and external locations. Diagnostic images, billing materials, quality control documents, registries, and data exchanges with business partners are required daily.

With the explosive availability of inexpensive computer hardware, what used to be expensive storage devices are now included with every PC as it is shipped. CD- and DVD-ROM drives are now as much a part of the standard PC configuration as an internal hard drive and monitor. Most modern PC operating systems incorporate burning software directly into the operating system. A user, in most cases, only has to drag the files where they should be copied on the CD/DVD drive icon, and a few seconds later the files are on the media and ready for shipment.

Recently, while walking into my office from the parking deck, I found a CD with a label attached indicating it contained diagnostic information for an individual who was obviously a referral from an out-of-state facility. The label contained the patient's name, date of birth, age, medical record number assigned by the referring facility, and Social Security number. I suspected the patient had dropped the CD as he or she was moving through the parking deck.

When I arrived at my office, I dropped the CD into my CD drive and was immediately bombarded with multiple CT images, history and physicals, and pathology reports. The referring physician had also scanned vital components of the patient's medical record into PDF format. All material was selectable via menus, designed to execute on autorun. No passwords or encryption was utilized. Anyone finding this CD would have been able to access this individual's medical information. After a little more than two hours, I had successfully tracked down the patient and was able to return the materials. Clearly, while convenient, such transfers are fraught with risk. In this case, the data were relevant to a single patient, but DVDs are capable of holding gigabytes of data.

Transfers using CDs are reviewed as routine by clinical staff, and our help desk routinely receives calls to support autorun CD programs that do not execute properly. These tools are often ActiveX controls and do not behave well on a managed desktop due to tightened security controls.

All healthcare organizations must define acceptable protocols for transfering information within the appropriate policies and procedures. Each organization must understand its information life cycles and the associated workflows to reduce the risk of data leakage through inadvertent media handling. Organizations may find that managed file-transfer products will satisfy most of their needs.

Managed file transfer systems can replace both the one-off transfer situations and the requirements for routine file transfers between business entities. Most solutions offer Web interfaces configured similarly to a typical Web portal deployment. Users can authenticate to the portal and be notified of data transfers awaiting movement. Files can be sent and received securely. Audit trails are retained to indicate transfer dates and who transferred which files. The portal solution enforces security policy requirements for encrypted file transfers and non-repudiation.

User accounts are easily managed and can be integrated into corporate directory structures. The more sophisticated managed file transfer systems allow multiple roles within the administrative structure, allowing the distribution of responsibility and account controls. Shadow copies of the transferred data can be compressed and retained for records. The more secure solutions will use Web-based, front-end appliances that inhabit the perimeter de-militarized zone (DMZ) and maintain private firewall connections to the data store inside the secure network. By passing the data being transferred through such firewall mechanisms, the data can be analyzed for possible malicious content and undergo additional security checks. The internal data store is encrypted while at rest and secure from the general user population. This makes managing file transfers from untrusted outside entities safer.

By being able to quickly handle the need to send individual files, the solutions can greatly reduce the dependency of burning CD or DVD disks and mailing them to Business Associates. With these safer solutions in place, end-point security tools can be allowed to control write operations to workstation CD/DVD drives, which will reduce the chance of inadvertent CD/DVD burns. Practices that combine this technique with astute control of access to data will minimize the risk of large, unauthorized data transfers.

DATA DESTRUCTION AND MEDIA SANITIZATION

This chapter has discussed data and data management practices and the importance of managing the life cycle of information. Like other IT life cycles, information management has an end to its life cycle. Information that is no longer utilized must be disposed of in ways that will permanently remove the data and leave the organization with a lower level of risk exposure. Many organizations dispose of equipment no longer needed by sale, auction, or landfill.

Healthcare operations are particularly vulnerable as they have multiple devices that store sensitive information. New biomedical devices and bedside monitoring equipment can cache data locally prior to sending it upstream to the electronic record.

The continued creep of consumer devices into the IT corporate infrastructure can increase risk of data leaks when users operate portable devices and do not follow appropriate information destruction procedures. Corporate IT shops routinely have to deal with sanitizing sensitive media inside rental or leased equipment and on products that break and need to be returned to the manufacturer.

In addition to devices that are explicitly meant for storage, a growing variety of devices contain persistent storage media. Storage devices that are taken out of operation and are no longer under the direct control of the data custodian can potentially allow the data it contains to leak to inappropriate parties within or outside of the organization. Healthcare organizations need to be particularly sensitive to devices that may carry residual data. These devices include IT appliances, server hard drives, printers, copiers, fax machines, PCs, laptops, PDAs, smart phones, compact flash cards, solid state memory devices, USB drives, CD/DVDs, zip drives, backup tapes, and even the near-obsolete floppy drive.

Many organizations will sell, auction, or donate old equipment. The best practice is to ensure that no discarded or re-used equipment contains any readable or recoverable data.

Overwriting

Overwriting is the process of replacing data on a storage device so that the data cannot be recovered, but the device can still be reused. File deleting and reformatting do not remove the data. Forensic recovery tools can quickly retrieve deleted files and formatted drives. To make the data completely unrecoverable requires fully overwriting the data. To properly overwrite the data means that every area of the media carrying data must be overwritten. Due to the quality of the magnetic surface and the sophistication of recovery techniques, this process will require multiple overwrites to make sure the data are unrecoverable. The number of overwrites needed is still a hotly debated topic, but the current best practice is to base the number of rewrites on the sensitivity of the information it contains. For example, the US Department of Defense (DoD) standard 5220.22-M requires overwriting each block of data with a pattern, then its complement, and finally another bit pattern. The 5220 standard requires a minimum of three overwrites, but other standards often call for seven or more rewrites.

Virtually all Advance Technology Attached (ATA) hard drives in operation today contain a technology called "secure erase" (**Note**: Not Small Computer Systems Interface-SCSI drives). With the exception of certain PC bios configurations, secure erase can be initiated from a software utility used on a bootable CD. Secure erase can be more thorough and performs faster than block overwrites. Consult NIST Special Publication 800-88[8] "Guidelines for Media Sanitization" for additional information.[5]

For overwriting to be successful, the drive must be in working order. Inoperable drives will need to be physically destroyed. Physical destruction is also the only appropriate method to sanitize magnetic tapes and write-only media, such as CD and DVDs.

Most data recovery laboratories are equipped to recover information from nonfunctional hard drives, even if a hard drive has suffered water or fire damage. A case in point: in May 2008, it was announced that a data recovery engineer had successfully recovered data from the burned and melted hard drive aboard wreckage from the ill-fated space shuttle Columbia.[6] (See Figure 3-4.)

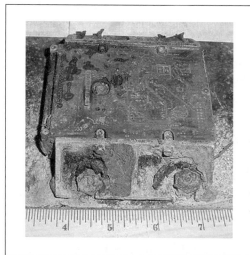 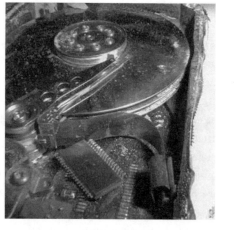

Figure 3-4: Photos from NASA Showing the Recovered Hard Drive Wreckage from Columbia. (Images reprinted with permission from Kroll Ontrack Inc.)

Two forms of physical destruction are capable of sanitizing hard drive storage:

- **Degaussing**. The hard disk surface is subjected to strong magnetic fields. This requires special equipment and frequent testing to ensure that the degaussing is effective. Media such as CD/DVDs are not affected by degaussing.

- **Total disk destruction**. This method involves disintegrating, incinerating, pulverizing, shredding, or melting the device. CDs and DVDs can be destroyed in-house by using a cross-cutting shredder. Larger devices, such as hard drives, may require a contract with an outside service that is capable of destroying drives in bulk quantities and providing a certificate of destruction for accountability.

Data Destruction Best Practices[5]

- Ensure all media that will be reused in house are sanitized before being reused.

- Ensure that all media not being reused are securely stored in locked facilities.

- Verify that sanitizing methods were successful. By the quality control process, we recently discovered issues related to the degaussing of hard drives.

- If you are degaussing in-house, make sure the equipment is calibrated and functioning correctly. Ensure that all personnel who will operate the degausser are appropriately trained.

- If outsourcing data sanitization, request a detailed and documented process-flow indicating how the device will be handled and tracked from pickup through final disposition. If at all possible, tour the facility. Periodically audit to confirm the documented processes. Retain certification documents indicating the destruction of the device.

SUMMARY

Healthcare organizations are struggling with the challenges of data management. Explosive data growth is consuming expensive storage resources and system administrator's time. Data silos throughout the organization are compounding the problem by consuming expensive data storage devices, competing for burdened resources and hampering IT from delivering added value to healthcare business.

Healthcare organizations must develop management systems that will facilitate the automatic transfer of data between storage tiers, while compressing and de-duplicating the data. Such solutions must accommodate a wide variety of data, such as DICOM images and scanned patient documents. Clinicians and administrators must be able to access the stored data at any time. The appropriate selection of such systems can reduce the total cost of IT ownership and enhance the use of backup systems.

Organizations that are growing through acquisitions or through the formation of Health Information Networks (HIN) will face issues of interfacing different systems. During mergers and acquisitions, it is not uncommon to have different systems performing the same function. To facilitate the exchange of data within the environment or convert to one system can prove costly. Previous information management focus was on one entity. This is no longer the case. Changing healthcare and transforming information require the reorientation of organizational responsibilities and policies regarding information management.

Discussion Questions
1. Discuss the progression of privacy laws and their impact on patient privacy.
2. How are conflicts between state laws and the HIPAA regulations handled?
3. Discuss the ramifications of "e-discovery" on health organizations.
4. Explain litigation hold and possible methods for performing a hold.
5. Discuss ways to avoid data leakage.
6. What are the things that need to be considered during data transfers?
7. List the various ways to destroy data and explain the positives and negatives of each method.

References

1. 2008 HIMSS Analytics Report: Security of Patient Data. Commissioned by Kroll Fraud Solutions. April 2008.

2. American Health Information Management Association. Practice brief: retention of health information (updated). Available at: http://library.ahima.org/xpedio/groups/public/documents/ahima/bok1_012545. hcsp?dDocName=bok1_012545.

3. *Federal Register.* February 20, 2003;68(34):8377.

4. *Federal Register.* April 27, 2009;74(79):19008.

5. NIST Special Publication 800-888, 800–111, Guide to Storage Encryption Technologies for End User Devices. Federal Information Processing Standards (FIPS) 140–2. NIST Special Publication 800–888, Guidelines for Media Sanitization.

6. Minkel JR. Hard drive recovered from *Columbia* shuttle solves physics problem: an experiment that flew on the *Columbia* shuttle achieves closure. *Scientific American* [online]. Accessed July 13, 2009. Available at: www.sciam.com/article.cfm?id=hard-drive-recovered-from-columbia.

Chapter 4

Audit Logging

Terrell W. Herzig, MSHI, CISSP

LOG DATA STORAGE

Ask five people to define audit logging and you will get five different answers. Because an audit trail is a record of system activities, each IT person will define audit logs in terms of the systems they deal with on a daily basis. Health information professionals will define an audit log as a record of activity in the patient chart. A network person will explain that it is a log of all network activity. An information security officer will describe an audit log as a log of a user's activity within a system.

All of these definitions are correct, yet each deals with different data. Besides differences in data, no standard format for audit data exists; therefore, each system will have its own method for storing records and content. Information security staff must not only contend with the different forms of audit data available to them on a daily basis but must be able to correlate events among the different logs and be able to do so in near real-time operations.

Computer systems can generate enormous amounts of log data. Electronic health records (EHR), network activity, user accounts, workstation systems, remote access logs, and server logs are but a few of the many different logs needed to reconstruct a picture of what a user may be doing, what information was accessed and from what point was the information accessed, and what was done with the information.

Log data require careful storage and management if the data are going to be relevant for detecting activity or responding to an incident. Log management functions have become a substantial business requirement due to a number of factors:

- Regulatory compliance often mandates the retaining of log data but lacks guidance on what needs to be captured, thus creating a need to collect, store, and index large amounts of log data. Recent regulatory compliance efforts are focused on the management of identity fraud.

- ARRA adds additional requirements for accounting of disclosures. The new requirements specifically include disclosures for treatment, payment, and healthcare operations.

- Researching incidents and security breaches requires useful, detailed historic log data.

- Information must be retained for evidence or record purposes.

LOG COLLECTION AND MONITORING

To create audit trails, systems must be configured to capture and record events across various system activities. Collecting data generated by a system, application, network, or user is essential for reviewing and analyzing the security state of a system. System events are activities generated by the particular hardware or operating environment. User events are generated by user interactions or activities, such as logging into an application or the network.

Audit trails can be used to examine the sequence of events that occurred on a system or within an application or across a network. These data are useful to identify attacks, intrusions, or misuse of computer resources. A properly configured logging system should provide the following:

- Alerts to the administrator or security personnel regarding suspicious activities.

- Details on the extent of an intruder's activity.

- Information necessary for legal proceedings and evidence of regulatory activity.

Today's modern computer systems can generate tremendous amounts of log data. Sometimes, determining the events to monitor and record can be one of the most difficult parts of establishing a logging program. Most systems contain the ability for a system administrator to enable or disable logging, determine the events to log, and offload those events to a central system. It is critical for log events to be moved to a central log collection location. Individuals with intent on compromising a system will attempt to cover their tracks by removing evidence from the system's log files.

Consider the typical Windows XP desktop system. By default, the system does not log events. The system administrator must enable logging and then determine the appropriate events to collect. This requires detailed experience on the part of the administrator to understand what events are relevant and meaningful vs. items of little value. Once logging is activated within Windows, three logs are created by default: application, system, and security logs. Depending on the version of Windows and the installed applications, additional logs may be installed on the system. A recent examination of these three logs listed on my workstation yielded 6,200 logged events over a 30-day period.

Audit trails can hold individuals accountable for their actions. As indicated in Figures 4-1 and 4-2, an operating system can allow objects to be configured for audit, such as configurations of successful or failed logon attempts. This audit trail can help resolve incidents involving individuals inside the organization. Audit data can indicate who logged into a system and accessed certain files, the time of the access, and the type of access.

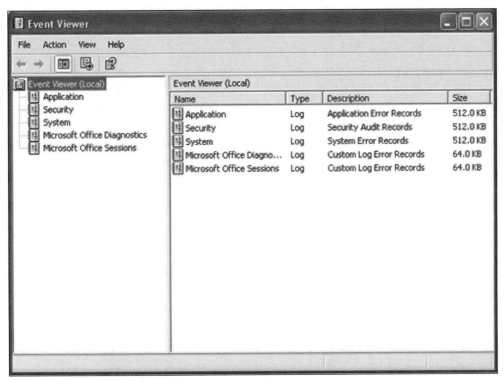

Figure 4-1: Windows Event Viewer Showing Log Files Available on the Current Workstation.

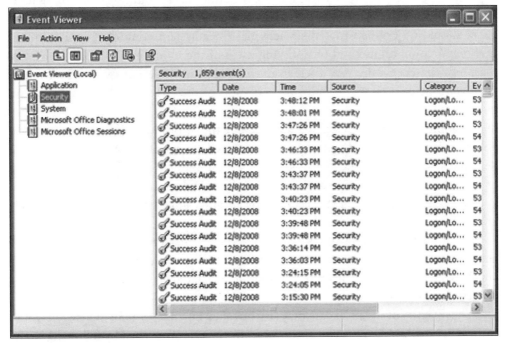

Figure 4-2: Windows Security Event Log.

Configuration of audit capabilities is critical. Audit trails generate tremendous amounts of data. Left unmanaged, event data can overwhelm a system and, in some cases, cause it to shutdown. Data left on the device being monitored are subject to tampering and deletion. Depending on how the audit system is configured, the number of users on the system, and the number of systems, audit data could grow into tens of thousands of events to be captured and recorded.

With such volumes of data, the audit logs may exceed administrative time and the skill to review and investigate events. Organizations will quickly discover the need for intelligent management and analysis software to correlate and alert operators to events that need investigation. These systems are capable of "learning" and correlating common events to establish baselines. When activities or events occur outside the baseline, operators and security staff can be alerted to potential problems. Procedures must be established in advance and personnel must be trained to understand what details within the logs are pertinent.

Because audit data can identify an intrusion attempt or misuse of a resource, it is common for an unauthorized user to either disable the auditing or clear and delete the logs. To prevent this abuse, control mechanisms should be in place to allow only authorized system administrators to read, print, and delete audit log files. Log storage locations should be protected and should not be available to anyone except authorized investigators. Log file locations should be encrypted and protected against overwrite or deletion. To prevent log files from being altered or overwritten, they are often stored on write-once media, such as CD, DVD, or other optical media.

LEGAL IMPLICATIONS OF AUDIT LOGGING

Equally important as properly configuring the auditing capabilities is informing users that a system is being monitored. Regardless of the particular work environment, users should be notified that their activities on a system could be monitored and audited. A common method of notifying users of the monitoring process is to place warning banners on the user's screen during login. In the event of an investigation, the data generated by the monitoring and audit of the system could be used in legal proceedings.

In some organizations, logging may include the recording of keystroke activity by the user. Keystroke monitoring can be performed on specific activities or keystroke sequences. Regardless of the type of logging or the amount of auditing to be conducted, organizations should always make sure that they (1) document audit and logging in organizational security policy; (2) communicate and train the workforce; and (3) apply the policy to all workforce members.

Additional legal implications can stem from the need to use audit trails during incident investigations. In the event audit information is to be used in court proceedings, it will be necessary to demonstrate that the audit material was properly handled with a sufficient chain of custody.

The integrity of the audit data may also be called into question. In this case, it will be critical to establish the integrity of the logs, which is accomplished by following sound procedures and using integrity monitoring tools to prove the logs were not tampered with in any way. This may mean the logs have to be handled to strict forensic standards. IT staff with the responsibility of managing audit logs should receive training on the appropriate methodologies for the forensic handling of audit data.

Another area of growing legal concern is the preservation of audit data and the implications it can have with e-discovery. As with other types of critical information, audit log data should be documented in the organization's data retention policies. Policies should be clear on which logs are subject to which retention time periods.

Because log data varies from application to application and system to system and because of the potential impact of e-discovery, many organizations are examining the use of formal archiving systems. Archiving systems take data from different applications and maintain the data in databases that are easy to search in the event of a litigation hold. The organization's retention policy will monitor the data and appropriately destroy data upon expiration. In the event of a litigation hold, the data can be flagged in the archiving system, and the retention policy is suspended for the information in question until it has been released from hold.

In healthcare, many larger organizations have built data repositories to house audit data. By feeding the audit data to a relational database system (perhaps SQL Server or Oracle), data can be cross-linked, in many cases, to provide a more informative picture of events during incident investigations. Such "audit marts" can then easily feed archiving systems for long-term storage requirements, and the retention policies can be enforced as part of the archiving system.

BUILDING AND MAINTAINING A LOGGING INFRASTRUCTURE

Given the amount of data involved with logging activities, organizations must carefully plan to implement a workable log strategy. Once the organization has determined the logging requirements and the events to monitor and create policy, attention must be dedicated to the proper design and fit of the logging infrastructure.

The log management infrastructure should include centralized servers and repositories to accommodate both the current and future needs of the organization. (See Figure 4-3). Major factors to consider include the volume of log data to be stored and processed, network bandwidth, online and offline storage, integration with archiving systems, the security requirements of the log data and how they are to be protected, and the time and resources needed to analyze the logs. Staff resources to accomplish these tasks must be considered as well.

In healthcare, the types of events to log and analyze tend to be more complex than standard IT department operations, partially due to the audit requirements from the IT perspective and the requirements to audit a wealth of data from the patient support infrastructure. The major operational processes typically include configuring log sources, performing analysis and event correlation, initiating response and investigation of identified events, and the long-term management of storage. Additional IT administrative responsibilities include monitoring of the logging status of log sources, the rotation of logs on the devices, management of upgrades and patches to the logging system, the synchronization of time clocks, and the maintenance of policy.

A frequently missed nuance of a logging infrastructure is the issue of common time tracking and synchronization. Healthcare organizations may be ahead in some aspects of this critical infrastructure need. Many healthcare operations already require time clocks and computer clocks to be synchronized to one central time source (usually an atomic clock-based system). It is absolutely critical that IT maintain the synchronization of all IT systems, including workstations and medical devices, within its logging infrastructure. Failure to do so can result in difficulties reconciling events or correlating the events in response to an incident or during real-time monitoring.

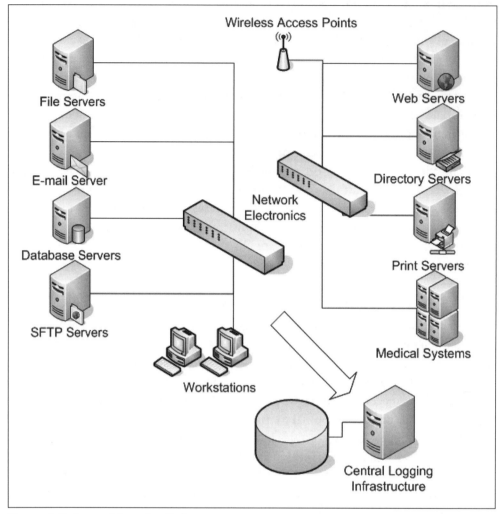

Figure 4-3: Central Logging Infrastructure.

Types of Logs and Log Data

Most organizations use many different network-based and host-based applications. In healthcare, an institution will maintain hundreds if not thousands of workstations, servers, network devices, and applications. Each may generate security logs or application logs. For example, as previously discussed, a Windows workstation can generate security events, application events, and system events. Add to this the logs generated from applications and the amount of traffic generated can be substantial. The following are examples of logging traffic:

- **Workstation logs**. Events include security events such as successful logins, login failures, attempts to elevate privilege, etc. System events, such as hard-drive space issues and additional information, may be collected.

- **VPN and remote access**. VPN systems log successful logins, failed logins, dates and times users connect, the security state of their system, and information about each session.

- **Application logs, such as antispyware and antimalware**. Logs and alerts are created to report infections and remediation actions. Some packages will log administrative detail regarding the download and installation of updates and new virus signature files.

- **Web proxies and content monitoring**. Reports the URLs and use of the Internet. Details include the end points involved in the connection, the URLs visited and the classification of the site, who visited, and the traffic transferred.

- **Authentication servers**. Directory servers and single-sign-on systems log authentication attempts, usernames, date and time, and success or failure.

- **Network devices**. Network devices are capable of logging packets as they pass the various devices.

- **Intrusion detection systems**. These systems typically record details on suspicious behavior, attack detection, file integrity checks, and other forms of information related to attempts to gain access and violate network policy.

- **Vulnerability management**. These systems typically produce details regarding installed software and the vulnerabilities of systems. Informational items include missing patches and software reports of out-of-version installations, as well as information regarding a host's configuration.

- **Clinical information systems (CIS)**. Details regarding who has accessed patient records, date and time stamps, and what was altered, viewed, or deleted. These systems can generate sufficient numbers of events to warrant their own central collection and analysis systems.

- **Firewalls**. Activity regarding the movement of traffic from within the organization and attempts to gain access from outside the organization. Examples include traffic denials, protocol, and port activity.

- **Network Access Control (NAC) servers**. NAC systems examine a host's security posture and record log details related to the findings and remediation of deficiencies.

- **E-mail systems**. Generate logs detailing e-mail statistics and usage patterns.

As discussed, many factors contribute to complicating log management. One complicating factor is dealing with the many types of logs and log sources. As this chapter has discussed, any application can generate multiple events and, in many cases, multiple logs.

Each log source records certain pieces of information. Standard formats for the output of logs and consistency in log messages do not exist, so it can be difficult to link logs and events from different sources. Log files may also represent common values differently. For example, date formats could be formatted as MMDDYYYY in one log and MM-DD-YY in another.

Log sources can use different output formats. Typical formats include ASCII comma delimited files, tab separated text files, Access databases, Syslog, Simple Network

Management Protocol (SNMP), Extensible Markup Language, and proprietary binary files. Some logs are created for local storage. Others, like the SNMP messages, are formatted to be transmitted to another system for processing.

When an application or system generates a log or event, it uses the system's time clock to timestamp the event. If a clock is inaccurate, the timestamps will be inaccurate. Analyzing the logs becomes more difficult, particularly when multiple hosts and/or applications are involved.

To facilitate the use of logs and subsequent analysis, an organization will often need to implement some automated method of converting logs with differing content into something with a standard format and consistent data field representation. Most organizations have access to some form of a high-end relation database management system. Its use is a practical answer as the collection point for log data.

Log Analysis

Log analysis is often left to the individual system administrator or application owner which results in the task being given a low priority due to the other duties of administrators, such as handling operational issues. Administrators usually do not receive training to adequately and effectively understand the log detail, nor do they have the appropriate tools to sift, script, or analyze log data. Many administrators consider log analysis to be boring and unproductive and treat logs in a reactive manner. To maintain the value and integrity of logs, sound strategies are needed for analyzing logs.

A log management infrastructure consists of several key functions. Log data must be acquired from different hosts or systems. The first issue facing IT operations staff is the limitation of the logging systems themselves. Some clients will provide functionality for the central collection of logging data based on scheduling, while others may only offer to feed data on a continuous basis. Better products will provide the capability for administrators to throttle bandwidth or set reporting schedules to not burden network operations.

Whether on the host, application, or central log server, the log files have to be parsed and aggregated. Some clients send audit events downstream and require processing on server-based collection systems. Other applications and systems may have the intrinsic tools to aggregate events before sending them to a central collection device.

The processes of parsing, event filtering, and aggregation will need to be planned for each system that will generate log data. As noted earlier, accomplishing these processes may require significant IT resources. There is no standard to log formats and output files, so IT operations will often spend time parsing many different file formats in order to view and process the logs. During parsing, it may be necessary to filter or suppress some log entries from analysis, reporting, or long-term storage because they contain useless data.

It is critical to have software that effectively correlates events within log data. Event correlation is the process of finding relationships among multiple logs or log entries. The most common form of event correlation is rule-based correlation, which matches multiple log entries from single or multiple sources based on values such as event types, IP addresses, or timestamps. Additional methods of event correlation may include statistical analysis or the use of visualization tools. Once the analysis software has identified relationships among the data and correlated events, it must be able to generate alerts based on the new information. This, in turn, may generate audit data from the analysis system.

SUMMARY

Healthcare organizations generate a tremendous amount of audit data daily. Combine this audit data with the data produced from IT operations and the volume can be overwhelming. The management of these data is critical and requires a substantial management infrastructure. Log management helps to ensure that security records are stored with sufficient detail and for the appropriate time period. With an increase in regulatory requirements for log management, healthcare must be proactive in its log analysis routines. Without routine analysis, it is difficult, if not impossible, to identify security incidents, policy violations, fraudulent activities, and operational issues.

The fundamental problem with log management is striking a balance between management resources with the supply of log data. This difficulty is compounded with a large number of log sources and the daily volume of information contained in multiple formats and record descriptors.

Readers interested in learning more about audit logs and the establishment of an adequate audit infrastructure should consult the NIST guide SP800-92, *Guide to Computer Security Log Management*.[1]

Discussion Questions

1. Explain the information an audit log should provide.
2. What security measures should be taken to prevent the unauthorized access or use of audit logs?
3. Discuss the legal implications of audit logging.
4. Explain what must be considered when developing and maintaining a logging infrastructure.

Reference

1. Kent K, Souppaya M. *Guide to computer security log management: recommendations of the National Institute of Standards and Technology*. National Institute of Standards and Technology. SP800-92. Available at: http://csrc.nist.gov/publications/nistpubs/800-92/SP800-92.pdf.

CHAPTER 5

Identity and Access Management

Terrell W. Herzig, MSHI, CISSP

PROVIDING SECURITY SERVICES

Identity and access controls are the collection of control mechanisms that specify what users can do on a system, the resources they can access, and the operations they can perform. They serve as safeguards, ensuring that only users with both a specific "need to know" and the appropriate authority can access a system. These controls help determine the programs the user may execute and the types of information they can read, edit, add, or delete.

The identity and access management process is not new to security management programs. However, managing users' rights across a healthcare organization has become increasingly complex. Users' access rights are typically based on their roles in the enterprise and/or the groups to which they belong. Clinicians usually have multiple roles and frequently rotate among organizations. In today's healthcare environment, the notion of a "single role for any one individual" is absurd. It is important to think in terms of process-oriented roles. Management by process-oriented roles allows for users' rights to be based on the processes users perform. However, today, most healthcare facilities still take a silo application-based approach to access management. Therefore, the identity process is often specific to the application or environment in which it is required.

As healthcare entities continue to expand their business over the Internet, the number and types of users with which they must contend will increase as well. Consequently, more users will need access to IT resources; platform environments will remain complex and heterogeneous; and Web services will drive access to applications and data. Thus, the healthcare enterprise must adapt its perceptions of identity and access management to account for change.

To rapidly adjust to such change, healthcare IT must consider incorporating a range of technologies, including user provisioning, privilege management, password management, single sign-on, and external account management products. IT will need to implement these technologies in combination across all platforms and applications.

This chapter will focus on identity and access management within the healthcare environment. It will discuss how your security environment should offer security services such as authentication, authorization, role management, and identity provisioning.

IDENTIFICATION AND AUTHENTICATION

Healthcare IT systems contain enormous amounts of sensitive information. As a result, this information must be protected, of the highest integrity, and available when needed. To adequately protect this information, we must be able to control who is allowed to add, edit, or delete the information within each system. One of the first steps to securing a system is to provide the ability to verify the identity of its users. In fact, a system without the ability to identify and verify users would have no informational integrity. Granting access to a system resource is the process of identifying and authenticating each user and system process with a need to consume the particular resource.

Many of you will recognize the most common identification and authentication process used in healthcare today: a user ID and password. In the user context, the first step is to *identify* the user to the system. The second step involves *authenticating* the first step. Authentication is the process of verifying the identity of the user. Passwords are the method most often used for authenticating users. When used as the sole means of authentication, however, this approach proves inadequate in preventing unauthorized access to a computer resource. Also, it is important you not confuse authentication with authorization. *Authorization* is the process of establishing what a user can do once the user has been identified and authenticated to the system.

Identification is the cornerstone of an information security program. All system entities must have a unique identifier that differentiates them from other entities. This is the key component to the access control process. User identification provides accountability when combined with audit trails. This enables activities to be traced to an individual, and, as a result, individuals can be held responsible for their actions.

Authentication is the process of associating an individual with his unique identifier; that is, the manner in which the individual establishes the validity of his claimed identity. There are three basic authentication methods (commonly referred to as "factors") by which an individual may authenticate his identity:

- Something an individual *knows* (e.g., a password, personal ID number, or PIN.)
- Something an individual *possesses* (e.g., a token or a card.)
- Something an individual *is* (e.g., a fingerprint or biometric.)

An important concept of authentication is one-factor or two-factor (sometimes referred to as multifactor) authentication. One-factor authentication requires the use of one authentication method, such as something you know, like a password. Two-factor authentication would be a combination of two methods, such as something you know, the password, and something you have, such as an access card. Another example of two-factor authentication is the combination of a PIN and a biometric fingerprint scan. When an authentication system uses two or more factors, it is said to provide "strong" authentication. As we will soon see, strong authentication techniques should be used for access to sensitive information types, especially for ePHI.

PASSWORDS—SOMETHING THE USER KNOWS

The most common type of user-known authentication is a password. The password is a protected word or string that authenticates the user to a system. The theory is that a user has a secret password that only he or she knows. When the individual enters the password into a system, the entered password is compared to a password on file. If they match, the user must be authentic because the user is the only one who knows the secret password. The problem in this theory is maintaining the secrecy of the password! Users often write down the password, taping it to their monitors or placing it underneath the keyboards. Healthcare workers often share their passwords or make them so simple that they are easily guessed. Therefore, a discussion of increasing security based on passwords must begin with a dialog on selecting an appropriate password. The password must be easy to remember, but difficult to guess.

Password Selection—Why All the Fuss?

So why do security professionals always stress the importance of selecting passwords? First, most operating systems (OS), applications, hardware, and database management systems are shipped with default passwords, or worse, no passwords at all. The products are required to be shipped in this state initially for IT staff to gain system access in order to configure and install the product. The vendors depend on the IT personnel or the end user to change or set the password from its default setting. Like IT staff, outside attackers have access to these default passwords and, if given access to the device, can break into the systems.

Users tend to select common words or something that is simple for them to remember. This makes it easy to either guess the password or launch some form of an attack against the system in an effort to guess the password. This is often easier than it sounds as most individuals will select a password based on something with which they are familiar and will remember easily, such as the name of a spouse, child, or pet. A street address, birth date, anniversary date, phone number, or Social Security number are often choices an individual will hurriedly select when creating a password. As this information is associated to the individual, little research about the user is needed to guess his or her password.

Several tactics exist to attack passwords. One of the more common is a brute force attack involving the use of a dictionary or exhaustive attempts at character combinations. To reduce the effectiveness of such attacks, a user can misspell words, include numbers, or add punctuation. Another password security consideration is the length of the password. The longer the password, the longer it will take to generate exhaustive searches to decode it.

Another common password attack utilizes the password hash and a rainbow table. This technique works by obtaining a copy of the password hash. So, what is a *hash*? Operating systems and applications store user passwords in a format that makes them unreadable to humans. This sounds complex, but is not difficult to accomplish. Programmers use cryptographic techniques called *hashing* to produce an encrypted output. The technique works in a single direction and is based on a mathematical function. (See Figure 5-1.) To create a hash code, pass a piece of plain text to a subroutine that in return gives a code that is unique for that piece of text and will always be unique for that exact text expression. Since the hash is nonreversible, the hash value cannot be "decoded" to determine the original text. This provides a method to encrypt user passwords. The password can then be stored on disk or in a database without much concern that a system administrator or other user can examine the encrypted text and derive the user's password. The theory is that the user will be prompted for the password, which is passed through the hash function, and the result is compared against the password database for a match. The password text and its associated encrypted hash are never stored together in the password database. At first glance, this sounds secure.

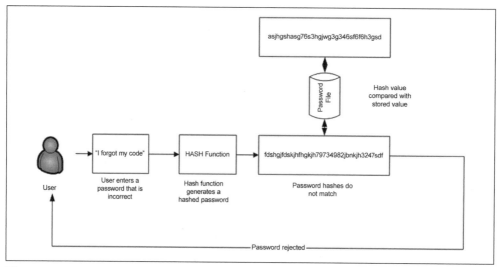

Figure 5-1: How a Hash Function Is Used to Store and Validate Passwords.

You do not have to be in IT long to understand that computing power gets cheaper and more plentiful each year. Advances in computer power often mean more sophisticated software and gains in productivity. To the hacking community, the increased productivity equates to an increased potential for cracking passwords. Several years ago, an enterprising group of individuals came together to develop a technique to crack passwords based on the hash output. Hash algorithms are quite varied, but all are built around standards that monitor and test their ability to generate unique hash values for a given text. Software vendors use these same hash algorithms. The idea behind the hash attack is to use many computers to generate possible password values, such as that of exhaustive guessing. These "randomly generated" passwords are then fed to the hash programs, storing the resulting encrypted text into a large database system. This time, the random text and the result codes are stored in the same database. Now, to determine a user password, one needs only to get the stored hash value from the OS or application and do a reverse lookup in the database. Therefore, the key to cracking a password using this technique is as follows:

• Have access to a large database of prehashed possible passwords with their resulting hash value (called a *rainbow table*).

- Gain access to the hashed password on the user's system or application.

- Compare the user's hashed password against the prehashed database and look for a match.

The text string associated with the hash value will be the user's password. Although the process may sound simple, it is not. Operating systems and applications usually maintain file locks on the password files, preventing even administrative users from copying them. This, however, assumes you are attempting to gain access to the hash files with the system in operation. It is possible to "boot" a system with an OS other than the one installed on the device. Since the system is being booted under a different OS, the password hash file of the native OS is no longer locked. Attempting this process may seem unlikely and too complex a task to warrant concern in daily operations. However, give a motivated individual one hour of time searching the Internet, and he can download a tool that can carry out the attack.

I recently executed this attack as a test on a sample of 10 workstations. I was able to derive the user password on every workstation in an average time of five minutes and eight seconds. The fastest speed to crack a single password was two minutes and 40 seconds. The password was nine characters long, included upper and lowercase letters, a number, and a punctuation symbol. There was a common characteristic of the passwords which were cracked: each was a string of one or more words found in a dictionary with either letters or punctuation marks added to the end of the string. So, with this type of technology readily available and free on the Internet, what should we be doing to counter the threat?

ENTER THE PASSPHRASE

A passphrase is a sequence of letters and numbers used as an alternative to a password. Think of it as an anagram of the first letters in a sentence. For example, choose a simple phrase that is easily remembered, "I live at 223 White Hat Road." From this statement, create the password "IL@223whrd." Note this password contains all the usual strong password requirements, such as upper and lowercase letters, numbers, and special characters. It is also 10 characters long, making a bit tougher to crack. The use of a passphrase instead of a word reduces the likelihood of the resulting password being found in a dictionary. As the passphrase appears to be a meaningless combination of characters, breaking it would require a "brute force" method to generate all permutations of the letters in the phrase.

However, as most systems in existence today are reliant on passwords, shouldn't we make every effort to increase the integrity of how we create and maintain passwords? Here are some recommendations that you should implement regarding password management:

- Educate your users about the strengths and weaknesses of passwords. Remember, a good information security program is a layered program. Never forget: often the weakest link in a system is the human link. You can only reduce this risk through proper training, awareness, and education.

- Advise users to create passwords that are not dictionary words or proper names.

- Guide users to choose passwords that are a mixture of alphabetic, numeric, and special characters.

- Direct users to create longer passwords, which tend to be more secure. The shorter the password, the easier it will be to brute force attack.

- Consider using passphrases.

- Last, but not least, restrict the lifetime of a password.

This final recommendation does not come without controversy. The last thing clinicians want to do is maintain multiple passwords with multiple expirations. Honestly, I hate changing passwords, too. But, considering the weaknesses of passwords, keeping and reusing a single password invites problems.

Consider that an attacker with the motivation to steal a password in order to gain access to a system will not readily disclose the fact he has done so. Once an attacker has assumed a user's identity, he is free to exercise the access privileges of that user. Preserving a secure environment in this case now shifts to controls in areas such as auditing, logging, event correlation, and intrusion detection systems. This is why security must be implemented as a layered approach to information security.

Current "best practices" promote the changing of passwords every 90 days, depending on the sensitivity and type of application or system. I have found this does not work well in large healthcare environments with numerous ISs. Depending on the IT environment, strive to find a balance between the use of strong password characteristics, discussed earlier, and longer times without forced change. Consider the use of password filters that force longer passwords and a mix of numbers and special characters in exchange for a longer time period between required changes.

Automated attacks against password systems are not the only forms of attacks raising concerns. Other methods for gaining access to a user's password are becoming more effective and easier to implement. These methods include:

- **Key-logging malware**—viruses and other forms of spyware that may arrive in e-mails through spam or by visitation of an infected Web site. Users are tricked into installing software that collects usernames and passwords as they attempt to login. In some cases, they may receive an innocent looking e-mail redirecting them to an infected Web site, where the malware is downloaded without the user's knowledge. The infected computer then opens a connection to an Internet site or Web chat room and begins transferring the stolen credentials.

- **Phishing schemes**—social engineering attacks that rely on fake Web sites and forms to trick users into supplying their user ID and passwords. The phishing scheme usually attempts to convince the user he or she needs to update some vital account information and provides a link to click on to update information. Unknowingly, the user is actually redirected to a fake Web site where they are entering their credentials into a hacker's database.

Password-gathering malware is a well-documented threat, and its use is increasing at an alarming rate. The healthcare enterprise depends heavily on timely access to its healthcare delivery systems. Every desktop must have active spyware and antivirus controls. However, although such software tools can reduce the risk of key-logging malware, they provide little defense against the social engineering techniques, for which defense depends on a security-aware organizational culture. Therefore, readers should take note regarding security awareness programs, as depicted in Table 5-1. This is the mechanism to educate and continually inform all members of the workforce. Security training is not a one-time event. It must be continual.

Table 5-1: Password Vulnerabilities.

Weak password	Poor password choice. Use of dictionary words. Password too short.
Phishing attack	Tricks users into supplying their credentials in response to a fake message or Web site.
Sharing of password	Users share their passwords with coworkers.
Shoulder surfing	Another user is actively watching users type their passwords and remembering them for later use.
Social engineering	Manipulates users to reveal their password.
Keylogging	This is usually installed by malware. The software captures the users' keystrokes and uploads the captured data to a malware site.
Brute force attacks	Attempts at trying all possible password combinations, or the attempt to crack a system by guessing the password.
Password cracking tools	Use of special tools to launch automated brute force attacks, or the use of tools such as rainbow cracking.
Password re-use	User continues to use the same tool and circumvents re-use restrictions by appending a sequential number to the end of the password.

The astute security professional reading this text may have noticed an omission in the bulleted password management list. This item is the recommendation to establish account lockouts after a limited number of unsuccessful login attempts. However, I have personally witnessed denial of service attacks focused on deliberately locking user accounts by attempting to login with a list of invalid passwords. This could be disastrous in a patient care setting. The attacker would only need knowledge of the organization's standard account-naming convention or a listing of the employee directory.

One objective of the organization's identity and access management (IAM) program should be to ensure that users have access to the minimum resources necessary to perform their jobs—a practice known as the "principle of least privilege." Utilizing the principle of least privilege limits the scope of a breach and can reduce the incidence of internal tampering and data theft. Ensuring that users only have access to the minimum amount of information necessary to do their jobs is an ongoing process that requires care and can be facilitated by using roles as a basis for access control.

Another IAM objective is the capability to rapidly, and at any time, remove or disable all accounts for a user through a centrally triggered process. No user should continue to have access to a system when his or her duties no longer require the access or, if, for some reason, suspension is required. Another effective method of eliminating unneeded access is to automatically lock or disable accounts that go unused for specified periods of time. Be mindful, however, to consider these strategies in relation to practice habits and on-call situations. So critical are these basic IAM functions, they are featured predominately in the HIPAA Security regulations.

Organizations may try to address authentication weaknesses by increasing password length and complexity. As already illustrated, stronger passwords are hard to remember, and therefore, users will write them down, adding to risk. Further, increasing the length and complexity will only remediate a few of the many attacks against passwords. Healthcare organizations must recognize that additional controls are needed to mitigate the risks against passwords and evaluate the use of stronger authentication options.

Two-Factor Authentication

An option to counter the inherent vulnerabilities of passwords is to use another method of authentication or require two authentication methods (two-factor authentication). The two-factor authentication method is often described as utilizing something the user knows with something the user has on his person to gain access to a system.

Technical solutions include one-time passwords or solutions involving memory or smart cards. These options reduce the vulnerabilities associated with traditional password use. Smart cards require the user to apply both a PIN code (something they know) and the card (something they have) to gain access to a system. Therefore, even if the card is lost or stolen, other users could not gain access unless they knew the PIN (assuming the user does not write his or her PIN code on the back of the card!)

One-Time Passwords

A one-time password (OTP) is not like a traditional password that is used multiple times. The OTP is used once and changed after each use. One of the attractive security features of this solution is that, if the transmission of the password is intercepted, it cannot be re-used. Because the OTP is only valid for one access, a captured OTP would be denied. Most OTPs are managed through the issuance of an authentication mechanism called a *token*, which is a small piece of hardware with a built-in clock and a factory-coded random key.

Two key types of OTPs are commonly found in the healthcare environment. One type uses a secret key to encrypt an internal value that yields a password that works only once. This type of OTP is often referred to as synchronous OTP. Another type uses a challenge-response technique, in which the tokens encrypt the challenge to yield a single-use password, sometimes referred to as *asynchronous OTP*.

Synchronous Tokens

There are two general methods for generating a synchronous one-time password. The first is a counter-based token that combines a secret key with a synchronized counter to generate the password. The second method uses a synchronized clock to generate the password. New passwords combine the secret key with an arbitrary value, such as a counter or a clock. The server and the token remaining synchronized regarding the passwords generated is what makes this process synchronous. If the token and server lose synchronization, the user will not be able to authenticate to the system. Clock-based tokens usually will search a few minutes on either side of the time to find a match and can resynchronize with every use.

To use a counter-based token, an administrator must first set a secret key and an internal counter into the token and copy this information to the authentication server. The owner of the token pushes a button on the token to activate the OTP service. The token then increments the internal counter, combines it with the secret key, and computes a hash result.

The clock-based token uses internal clocks instead of counters. An internal clock value is combined with the token's secret key to generate a time-based password. The token device displays the generated result for use when logging into the system. The server performs a similar process by combining its own clock value with a copy of the token's secret key. In case of time delay between the token and the server, the server can be programmed to accept any password derived from the clock value within a specified time window.

Asynchronous Tokens

This type of token generates a password, based on a challenge from the authenticating server, that is combined with the secret key on the token. The user, in response to the challenge, applies the result of this combination as his or her reply. To begin the sequence, a challenge number is sent to the user's workstation. The user enters this challenge number into the token device. The challenge number is combined with the token's secret internal key to generate a result that is displayed on the token's display. The user enters the generated token result. The server, which also has the token's secret key, performs a similar computation. The server's result is then compared with the result that the user entered.

An advantage of the asynchronous method is that the servers and tokens do not need to maintain synchronization. By generating a random challenge each time, the server ensures that previously valid passwords will not be valid for future sessions.

Tokens may also come in the form of software used on workstations and PDAs, such as the Palm organizer. This software is often referred to as a *soft token*. Using a soft token, the server site generates the initial base secret key and sends it to the user as a data file. Once the user has properly installed the data file, the soft token will work the same as the physical token.

Smart Cards

A smart card is credit card-sized, but unlike a credit card, contains an embedded chip that can accept, store, and send information. It can hold more data than the magnetic strip on the back of an ordinary credit or debit card. Most smart cards today are hybrid cards and contain both a semiconductor chip and a magnetic strip. The semiconductor chip can be a memory chip or contain a complete microprocessor with an internal memory.

Smart cards most often come in two forms, contact and contactless. The embedded chip either communicates directly via a physical contact or remotely via some type of electromagnetic interface. Contact-based smart cards must be inserted into a reader. Data, encryption, and information are transmitted via the contacts in the reader. A key security feature of the smart card is that the data are stored in an encrypted format.

A contactless card makes use of an electromagnetic signal and a built-in antenna on each card to create the link between the card and a reader. Power for the card's electronics are derived from the microwave signals used to communicate with the card. As the power is very low, the card must be within a certain proximity of the card reader for the card to work. Cards of this type are most often used in transportation sectors for fare cards.

A third category of smart card is the hybrid or combo card. These hybrid cards contain both a contact and contactless interface.

Cards with memory chips are simply storage devices that cannot process information. They usually provide between four and 300 megabytes of data. The chip in a memory card consists only of storage and a small amount of hardware to prevent access to the stored data. The authentication aspect of the memory card is to store and manage passwords.

Smart cards containing microprocessors can do much more. Essentially, they are small computers on a card. The microprocessor can store information and manipulate the data in memory. The value of the smart card is its ability to store personal data with a high degree of security and portability. The smart card can isolate functions such as digital signatures, key management, and authentication. Because such functions can be delegated to card operations, the smart card can be an integral part of an enterprise-wide authentication system.

Like all technology, smart cards come with inherent weaknesses and vulnerabilities. Because the smart card is essentially a computer, similar types of attacks can be used against the card. The attacks may be invasive or noninvasive. In an invasive attack, the attacker will attempt to analyze the card to gain information about the card and chip. An invasive attack will likely render the card inoperable in hopes of gaining enough insight to conduct a noninvasive attack. Another vulnerable aspect of the card is the interface to the reader. The smart card must have the capability to resist unauthorized instructions via the software interface.

Authentication Based on Physical Attributes—Something the User Is

The most common form of authentication based on physical attributes is through biometric devices. Each individual has physical attributes about their person that uniquely identifies him or her from the remainder of the population. The physical distinctions that you use daily to recognize a friend can be used to verify that friend's identity to electronic systems. Biometric identification uses a physical attribute, such as a palm print, a fingerprint, or an iris pattern; or a behavioral trait, such as voice inflection or signature, to uniquely identify the user. Physical traits are more stable over time, but tend to be more expensive to use than behavioral traits, which are subject to change and require frequent updates to the enrollment data. Three important elements of biometric devices are accuracy, processing speed, and user acceptance.

Accuracy is considered the most important characteristic of biometric devices. The IS must be able to separate authentic users from imposters. Processing speed is related to the processing capability of the system. In other words, how fast is a user's authentication accepted or rejected by the system? This is usually measured from the time a user presents the physical characteristic to the time the data are matched and a reject/accept decision is signaled.

Because users must be comfortable and willing to use the system, the biometric device needs to be acceptable to the users. This generally means that the system should be safe and convenient to use and provide fast enrollment without the need to update often. Finally, users must be assured that their data will not be stored and used without proper permissions and safeguards.

Single Sign-On Technologies

Users typically need access to many different computer systems and applications to accomplish their work. The login password architecture could result in many different login IDs and several passwords. It could also mean that the user has to cope with various concepts of password length and strength requirements if careful identity management practices are not in place. The key term is identity management.

As organizations grow, so usually does the application count. In healthcare, this is the operational norm. Consider the amount of information generated on a daily basis for patient care and billing: lab systems, radiology systems, telemetry devices, bedside devices, diagnostic equipment, to name a few. This wide range of access could easily require users to maintain multiple sets of login IDs and passwords. Most savvy users will quickly revert to using the same password, where possible, in all the differing systems. This need for multiple user IDs and passwords could cause the user to practice poor password protections and revert to practices described previously, including writing passwords down.

In a single sign-on (SSO) solution, the user logs in one time and is then authenticated to all remaining disparate systems automatically. (See Figure 5-2.) SSO minimizes the number of times a user logs in, and in some cases, the number of authentication characteristics. An alternative to SSO is single login in which the user has a single user ID and password on every system in the organization. Users must still authenticate to each application, but simply use the same password and login ID.

As an access control mechanism, SSO addresses the identification and authentication needs across multiple platforms. The need for SSO is motivated by the following factors:

• Multiple entry points, including Internet access.

• Management of large numbers of workstations with the need to control how they are to be used.

• Multiple applications being used daily by a significant cross-section of the organization.

• The need for simple and efficient management of access control.

If these factors apply to your healthcare delivery organization, you should consider implementing SSO technology. Clinicians need fast access to data to care for patients. As a result, login and password management becomes frustrating and helps to perpetuate security as a barrier, rather than an enabler, to business operations. This being said, please note that information technology cannot solve every problem. One of my favorite expressions is "paving a cow path." IT sometimes focuses too heavily on automating processes instead of studying the process itself. Single sign-on brings both advantages and disadvantages to authentication and access management. An organization should carefully study the use cases prior to deciding to implement an SSO solution.

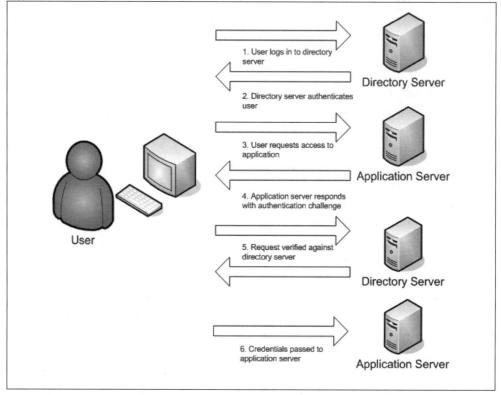

Figure 5-2: Basic Single Sign-On.

The advantages of an SSO are as follows:

- A more efficient user login experience is provided. Users only need to authenticate once.

- Because fewer passwords must be remembered, stronger passwords are created.

- The need for multiple passwords and password change synchronization can be avoided.

- The effectiveness and timeliness of disabling and deactivating user accounts are improved. SSO systems can allow a single administrator to add, delete, or modify accounts across the enterprise from a central point.

Disadvantages of SSO are as follows:

- If a user's ID and password are compromised, an intruder will have access to all of the resources for which the employee authenticates.

- Security policy becomes critical. It must be followed precisely to ensure access is granted and limited to appropriate users.

- Implementation can be difficult. SSO products are improving, but problems still exist with integrating legacy applications, mainframe interfaces, and application incompatibilities.

In most SSO systems, the user provides a user ID and password to a primary system that authenticates the user against a master system. When a user requests access against a target system, the SSO system retrieves the user's password for the requested application and begins a session with the new system using that password. In some systems, the user would only see a list of applications for which he or she has been authorized to use.

In healthcare, the barriers to implementing an SSO solution can be daunting. Legacy applications may exist that do not have the technological support to facilitate SSO. In some healthcare organizations, the IT department may not maintain sufficient IT experience or carry sufficient influence to convince supporting business units to adapt or purchase new systems that fit current identity and authentication management architectures. Finally, integrating stronger authentication with legacy mainframe applications can be difficult.

Healthcare organizations must carefully analyze the set of known and anticipated initiatives and balance them against the competing complexity patterns to determine whether the results will provide an acceptable solution. It may be more cost-effective to first employ your analysis and determine alternative or intermediate methods to reduce password management headaches. For example, consider use of the following:

- Self-service password reset and synchronizations.

- Evaluation of password policies, combining and consolidating when appropriate.

- Lightweight Directory Access Protocols (LDAP) or Active Directory implementations.

SSO solutions serve as "proxies" between the end-client devices and target systems. These target systems still maintain independent credential stores and present specific unique sign-on prompts to users. SSO products must detect the unique prompts and respond appropriately. Difficult-to-integrate applications will add time to implementations and may require custom development. As healthcare delivery organizations continue to gravitate to Web products and Web technology systems, SSO products can experience difficulties recognizing graphical user content. In certain instances, SSO authentication can fail due to system upgrades. The SSO product may be relying on a text prompt that will fail if the application text is changed and not reflected to the SSO system.

Before purchasing an SSO solution, organizations should carefully evaluate potential products before making a final purchasing decision. At a minimum, organizations should complete the following checklist:

- Determine how the SSO product will provide core functions. Does it contain tools that can provide graphical "wizards" to help recognize GUI interfaces and prompts?

- Conduct proof-of-concept testing. Try different scenarios in "your" target environment. Test Windows, Macs, Web applications, and Java-scripted systems, along with terminal-based mainframe applications.

- Study and evaluate the SSO backend. How are the identity attributes and credentials stored/processed? Are the credentials encrypted? What are the administrative tools and options? How are the security policies created and managed? Is the repository based on directories, databases, or file systems? If it utilizes directories, are they based on Microsoft Active Directory or LDAP? If it is a database, what type of relational database management systems (RDBMS) product is used?

- Clarify whether the SSO solution supports fault-tolerance strategies. Do these strategies coincide with your current operational plans?

- Determine whether the SSO solution is two-tiered or N-tiered. In a *two-tier system*, the SSO clients interact directly with the directory structure. In an *N-tier approach*, SSO products use both physical and logical middleware to interact with clients. They will also broker interactions with the RDBMS. Some two-tier approaches may require directory schema extensions to add administrative and credential caches. This could result in performance issues within larger organizations.

- Confirm the SSO solution provides for strong authentication. Can the SSO integrate biometrics, token, or smart card technologies?

- Decide whether third-party integration toolkits or application-programming interfaces (API) are required to make the product functional. Does the product require software drivers? Are they provided or purchased separately?

- Find out whether the SSO solution can handle multiple authentication events. Some applications may have the requirement for the user to complete two or more authentications to reach the application.

- List the key events that are logged by the SSO system. What are the auditing capabilities? What is the granularity of the reports? Are additional reporting tools available? Can custom reports be created?

- Determine the logout policies allowed. Can the SSO logout target applications after a period of inactivity? Can the SSO enforce single login policies for specific applications?

- Confirm whether certain target applications can be accessed offline. In other words, can an application locally authenticate without attaching to a server?

- Clarify what user provisioning tools come with the SSO.

Most SSO systems can obfuscate the target application password and negotiate a password change with the target application. A user provisioning system can aid the setup and maintenance of users, as well as the password obfuscation tasks.

Web Access Management Solutions

Web access-management (WAM) solutions provide SSO to Web-based applications and other resources via custom integration. WAM solutions do not require the deployment of client software. Typically, WAM solutions are most often deployed for large user groups and can be used internally or within a mixed environment. WAM solutions can and are often supplemented with federation security models or capabilities. This allows the use of standards-based SSO among different trust and identity management domains.

FEDERATED SECURITY—THE NEXT BIG STEP IN IDENTITY AND ACCESS MANAGEMENT

So what are Federated Identity and Access Management? Healthcare organizations today face the challenge of managing an ever increasing number of internal and external user identities. With the formation of regional health information organizations (RHIO) and health information exchanges (HIE), the need to communicate outside traditional healthcare borders is increasing. I routinely receive requests from radiologists who have acquired contracts with outside health providers, and referring physicians who want to follow their patients and vendors, needing to support their products for access to our systems. This does not take into account the contractors and suppliers who revolve through the facility on a daily basis. Indeed, the walls of the traditional healthcare delivery organization are in the process of evaporating. Filling the vacuum will require the philosophy of building identity and access management solutions that are easier to manage and can accommodate the need for "access from anywhere."

Federation identity fits into the overall identity management scheme by attempting to limit the management burden caused by requests from external identities. The fewer times an identity must be managed, the more efficient the entire system becomes.

Federation, in somewhat technical terms, is a perimeter mechanism that sits on the network edge and shares identity information with other federation mechanisms. For this to operate, each participating organization must have an established "trust" relationship. The federation technology creates or gathers the trust assertions that must be made when an internal user wants to access an external resource, or vice versa. Therefore, federation can be viewed as an extension of identity management beyond the traditional borders of the healthcare organization.

Federated identity management offers a standards-based approach by allowing an organization to provide information about a managed identity to another organization (an identity consumer, service, or resource provider). Each organization in the "community of trust" keeps track of the identities of those individuals central to it—its employees and workforce members. Once individuals have been authenticated by their own organizations, they can access other organizations' resources without re-authentication.

Obstacles to Implementing Federated Identity

Implementing a federated identity management project within an organization will only be undertaken if the cross-domain access to resources proves of significant value to the organizations participating in the project. While federated identity projects are in the works, most are large federation initiatives, such as the US government's e-Authentication Initiative. Such projects are complex undertakings, involve multiple organizations, and are usually slow to deploy.

Many organizations may find they have already provided access to internal resources using traditional methods (for example, creating user IDs on behalf of external users and establishing remote access methods). Because of this effort and the cost to implement federated identity, it may be less expensive to continue with the current status quo.

Another potential barrier to implementation is that the creation of a federated security model still presents many of the control and liability issues that were common in daily management efforts. Each participant must trust the other participants to perform their identity management functions and to protect issued identity credentials. The establishment of interorganization agreements to establish the necessary trust can be a difficult challenge. Healthcare organizations must consider the legal, process, and technology consequences of creating federated identity models. A thorough risk assessment should be conducted to identify the potential damage that could result from a misused trust relationship. Listed next are questions that the risk assessment must answer:

- How will each participating healthcare delivery organization or partner confirm the identities of individual internal users before issuing them credentials that can be used both internally and across the federation?

- How strong must the online authentication and technologies be within each participating organization? Will all organizations select and use the same strong password techniques? Will stronger forms of authentication be required?

- Which organizations will be liable (and to what extent) if a member's identity credential is used to commit fraud or improperly access the resources of a partner organization?

Federated Identity and Distributed Public-Key Infrastructure

For an authentication system to be viable with a large number of users, the management system has to be distributed, with many organizations handling identity and credential management for local users. Establishing direct trust between large numbers of organizations is an uphill battle. Therefore, with a large number of organizations, it is practical to have a central entity with which each organization establishes trust. This seemingly insurmountable task could be accomplished by utilizing a distributed public-key infrastructure (PKI).

What is a PKI? Without getting too technical, PKI is based on a technique called asymmetric cryptography. Asymmetric cryptography works by using public and private keys. As an individual who wants to exchange information with someone in a secure manner, I may wish to encrypt the message. In the past, I would use an encryption program and send the message to its intended recipient. I would then send the password or "key" to the individual in a different message so they could decrypt it. In this technique, both parties would use the same key to encrypt and decrypt the message. If the key is intercepted or compromised, the message can be easily decrypted.

Asymmetric encryption uses a key pair. A key pair comprises a "public" key and a "private" key. The key pair would be established when I first install my encryption software, and it is unique to my identity. My private key is stored somewhere securely, perhaps on a smart card or encrypted on my hard drive. I can use my private key to create digital signatures and decrypt documents. My public key is published to the Internet and shared widely. My public key can be used to verify a document I have digitally signed. My public key can be used by anyone to encrypt a document that only my private key will decrypt.

This basic cryptography and verification provided by public and private keys does not necessarily require a public key infrastructure. To understand the need for PKI, one needs to consider the trust assumptions behind the digital signature verification. Suppose I receive a document sent to me by someone named "John Doe." The document was purported to be signed by John using John's public key. I can verify that the public key John provided was used to sign the document. The important question is "How can I be certain that a particular public key actually belongs to John?" How can you establish trust that a given public key is owned by a particular person or entity? This is the problem PKI sets out to solve and is fundamental to using digital signatures on a large scale.

The basic building block of a PKI infrastructure is the digital certificate. An entity creating a certificate is called a certification authority (CA). The core components of a certificate include:

- The name of an entity or person. This may include several names, as well as e-mail addresses and LDAP directory names.
- The public key (e.g., John Doe's public key).
- A digital certificate created by the CA (using the CA's private key). This signature is bound to the components of the certificate (remember the hashing process).

By creating such a certificate, the CA is stating that it has verified that public key in the certificate does indeed belong to John Doe. Certificates and CAs enable a chain of trust to be created. The beginning point is that the CA is trusted. This trust leads to trust of certificates issued by the CA because the digital signature on the certificate can be verified using the CA's public key.

PKI is needed to support large-scale deployments. For example, PKI is instrumental in the following examples:

- Verification that a document or message was created by the person claimed.
- Validation that message or document has not been tampered with.
- Confirmation that the contents of a message or document can only be read by the intended recipient.
- Nonrepudiation services. The creation of a document or message cannot be subsequently denied.

The requirements for large-scale PKI come from situations in which services such as those listed must be implemented or supported across multiple organizations.

This discussion so far has considered authentication, or the validation of identity. In most situations, authorization is needed by an entity or service provider performing the authentication to establish the rights of the authenticated user. Federated identity and distributed PKI provide three common authorization scenarios:

- **Implicit authorization**. The fact that the user has authenticated is taken at face value. This is only appropriate in low-risk applications that take on the model "use is allowed, provided I know who you are."
- **Local authorization**. An example is an application that permits a restricted number of users with role-based access. This local information could form a list of local or remote users who are authorized to access the application.

- **Authorized via certificate**. Digital certificates allow additional information to be included and used for authorization. Groups could agree on arbitrary attributes to be included in the certificate to be used for authorization purposes.

   Both federated identity and distributed PKI models can be used for smart-card authentication. Both require an infrastructure to operate. With federated identity, a common infrastructure can be used for password and smart card-based authentication.

   Distributed PKI can be used for applications other than Web services. Applications can make direct use of PKI-based authentication, such as secure login. Other applications might include physical entry systems. Because the authentication is done locally, it is straightforward for the local organization to apply its own security policies to the authentication. PKI can also support verification by digital signature. Because the PKI model can support applications beyond Web services, it would be preferable for many types of deployments.

Homeland Security Presidential Directive 12/HSPD-12

On August 27, 2004, President George W. Bush issued a Presidential Homeland Security Presidential Directive/HSPD-12,[1] "Policy for a Common Identification Standard for Federal Employees and Contractors." This Presidential Directive mandated a common security access policy and technical infrastructure across the entire federal government. To implement this policy, the federal government directed the General Services Administration (GSA) to develop a federal government trust model and a secure infrastructure to exchange sensitive information. GSA and NIST have worked together to develop a general-purpose PKI infrastructure, which is codified in Federal Standard 201. This standard requires a common access card be developed using a federally organized PKI, which will allow common access procedures across all government levels.

   GSA and HIMSS proposed the e-Authentication pilots to validate the technical concepts of using this model in healthcare. The project chose to use Access Certificates for Electronic Services (ACES) credentials to demonstrate the capabilities of using PKI within multiple healthcare settings. The ACES Program provides digital certificates and PKI services to enable electronic government applications requiring access control, digital signature, and/or electronic authentication. The program also supports the sharing of health information in cross-organization and RHIO and HIE data exchange. The pilot focused on the following security measures:

- Strong authentication to securely and privately transmit data among RHIOs.

- Trusted federal PKI credential service provider to provide digital certificates for authorized end-users in each RHIO.

- Local registration authorities trained and certified for each RHIO.

- Standard certificates used for single-factor authentication and digital signature.

- Tokens in the form of smart cards, used for security and multifactor authentication, generate digital signatures and secure data storage and transport.

- Federal PKI architecture employing multiple certificate-validation protocols.

The project met its objectives of having the RHIOs and HIEs leverage the common authentication infrastructure provided by the GSA's e-Authentication Service Component.

- Multiple RHIOs can agree and implement a common framework for the policies, procedures, and standards for federated identity authentication across multiple use cases.

- The federal e-Authentication infrastructure is relevant and applicable to use-cases for RHIOs in diverse operational environments.

- PKI, as a standard for strong authentication, can be deployed uniformly across multiple RHIOs.

- The federal PKI and its trusted Federal Credential Service Providers can be leveraged for use in multiple use-cases across multiple RHIOs.

- For RHIOs, local registration authorities and local enrollment are viable for large-scale deployments to provide for strong authentication using federal e-Authentication components.

- Hardware tokens (i.e., smart cards, flash drives) are viable for RHIO deployment of level-4 authentication assurance.

- The service was usable, tested, and implemented regardless of the RHIO or HIE use-case realization.

- The GSA's risk-assessment process for identification of the sensitivity level for information exchanged was learned and understood by the participants.

SUMMARY

An effective and appropriate identity management solution is an initiative that can have substantial impact in today's healthcare market. Healthcare institutions need to be concerned about identity management for a number of reasons, including the following:

- As hospitals and healthcare centers turn to wireless networks and roaming desktops to improve employee productivity, the potential for unauthorized access grows. Now you do not need a hard-wired connection access to sensitive information.

- HIPAA regulations require network administrators to effectively safeguard access to patient information.

- Information access management is complicated by the fragmented nature of healthcare provisions. Some records may be held centrally in a hospital, others in an off-site unit, and still more in outlying pharmacies or clinics. How do you ensure they are all managed securely?

- A busy hospital is packed with employees, contractors, patients, friends and relatives, and other visitors, any of whom may have a reason to access the network. Administrators need to make sure this access is restricted.

Clinicians can save significant amounts of time normally spent in front of a computing device doing entry or review and can harvest this newly available time to devote more attention to patient care. Non-clinical users can also leverage identity management to solve many of the costly password and account-related issues that would normally require a call to the Help Desk to resolve.

A decline of overall Help Desk traffic will enable staff to be more responsive to the remainder of the calls and tickets it receives. Furthermore, IT can take advantage of identity management (IDM) to streamline and automate the user provisioning and decommissioning processes, adding extra levels of security and end-user satisfaction, while at the same time, freeing up application specialists from having to manually run through the account creation process.

And finally, IT can also leverage the enhanced security and auditing capabilities to ensure compliance with stringent healthcare information protection regulations. IDM is complex; it is complicated; it is difficult to implement correctly and effectively. However, it can also produce a marked positive impact on patient care.

Discussion Questions

1. Describe the differences between "identification" and "authentication."
2. What is "strong" authentication?
3. Discuss methods to strengthen password security.
4. Discuss the various types of password attacks and how to protect against them.
5. Describe token systems and their benefits.
6. Discuss the attributes of "single sign-on" technologies.
7. Define federated identity.
8. Describe when the use of PKI and a PKI infrastructure might be necessary.

Reference

1. Healthcare Information and Management Systems Society. HIMSS/GSA: national e-authentication white paper. June 2007. Accessed October 13, 2008. Available at: www.himss.org/content/files/GSAwhitepaper.pdf.

CHAPTER 6

Sharing Patient Information

J. David Kirby, MS, CISSP, CHPS

HEALTH INFORMATION SHARING: ENVIRONMENTAL FACTORS THAT INFLUENCE SECURITY RISK MANAGEMENT

Sharing information sounds like a good thing. Most people who work in healthcare gladly share information with patients and colleagues on a regular basis. Providers are comfortable with how patient privacy is managed, and they also know how to manage their own business interests in sharing these data. But consumers and providers of healthcare services may not be as comfortable with the notion of sharing patient information electronically. Health information exchanges (HIE), regional health information organizations (RHIO), and personal health record (PHR) systems are the key new tools that are challenging providers and patients to rethink how health information is shared.

For most people, the prospect of using HIEs, RHIOs, and PHRs raises both great hopes and concerns. The hopes are focused on providing access to protected health information (PHI) to empower patients, improve care, and lower costs. The concerns are focused on three risks: What if the PHI is not handled confidentially? Will the data provided have the level of integrity that I need (i.e., will they be sufficiently complete, current, and correct)? What if the data are not available when I need them?

These three concerns in managing PHI are the traditional central topics of interest in information security risk management. Security professionals call these topics confidentiality, integrity, and availability (CIA). Information security and privacy practitioners in healthcare organizations (henceforth called practitioners) typically work in these three areas, though they may not use these exact terms. Viewing these new concerns, related to sharing PHI electronically, through the CIA prism puts practitioners on familiar turf. Still, new challenges arise in applying the CIA of security to HIEs, RHIOs, and PHRs.

In this chapter, we cover information security risk management concepts and issues associated with the use of health information for HIEs, RHIOs, and PHRs. This chapter includes guidance for practitioners; however, a tried and true formula for success in this area has not yet emerged. This means that practitioners building or connecting to these new health information-sharing vehicles will have to think through the issues to effectively manage risk.

The names and acronyms for health information exchanges change from time to time. Today, health information exchanges, regional health information organizations and personal health records are the typical names given to health information-sharing enterprises. We will stick with these names and add a way of referring to them collectively, calling these enterprises health information networks (HIN).

HINs have to manage all of the information security risks that are present in operating a traditional health information system (e.g., a Hospital Information System [HIS]). But, an HIN is not just a larger version of an HIS. HINs must also contend with factors that are new to the information security practitioner. These new factors present some challenges and opportunities in managing information security risk. Let's review these new key factors for HINs.

Risk Distribution

The typical practitioner for a single healthcare enterprise (e.g., a hospital) makes risk management choices by considering the costs and benefits of various choices available to him or her. For example, will the extra protection offered by a more expensive intrusion detection system be worth the extra cost to the hospital? By contrast, an HIN must consider how the information security risks are to be *distributed* among a large number of parties. The HIN must have a suitable *risk-sharing* model for the HIN to succeed. Without this, the needed parties (e.g., hospitals, medical practices, patients) will not participate in the HIN.

Let's look at an example of the risk distribution issue. How will the HIN distribute the risk of the inappropriate disclosure of PHI among the various parties? These parties are PHI providers, PHI recipients, and PHI subjects (patients). There is an established tradition for sharing PHI on paper. But, we can't simply apply the risk-management model used in the paper process to an HIN because an HIN presents new problems (but also opportunities) to consider. For example, the paper PHI-sharing model includes processes carried out by humans that, if used routinely in an HIN, would produce work and delay in PHI-sharing that would threaten the success of the HIN.

Managing the risk of inappropriate PHI disclosure in an HIN will have to be done in a way that will satisfy *each* of the parties involved. As each party considers whether and how it will participate in the HIN, it will try to balance its benefits and its risks. For example, many patients want the ability to control the flow of their PHI in the HIN—without a large burden put on them. Even consumers who don't want to control PHI flow directly do want to be protected but at what risk/benefit tradeoff level? PHI providers must discover benefits that make the costs of sharing PHI reasonable to bear. For example, a physician might provide patient demographics gathered at his medical practice to the local hospital in return for the timely receipt of hospital discharge summaries. Lastly, PHI recipients need a benefit that outweighs their costs/risks in obtaining the PHI. An example of this is a hospital concluding that the expense and risk of an HIN connection would be worthwhile if it could lower administrative costs at patient registration by obtaining the patient demographic data from the HIN.

Finding an acceptable distribution of risks and benefits with confidentiality risks is only a start. The same types of distribution issues arise in the areas of risk management for PHI integrity and availability. For example, every recipient wants PHI to be current and correct (i.e., to have integrity). PHI providers naturally bear a burden in providing dependable PHI. Will the risk/cost tradeoff that seems acceptable to the PHI provider also be acceptable to the PHI receiver? As another example, it would be great to have a patient registration process that gathers the patient demographics from the HIN when the patient is admitted. But, what if the HIN is not up at that time? How small must the risk of an HIN outage be? How much are the various parties willing to pay for increasing levels of HIN availability? How will these costs be distributed so as to be agreeable to each party? An HIN information security risk analysis must manage these types of issues to every party's satisfaction.

There are groups that have presented various aids for security risk management in HINs. The Markle Foundation, Interconnecting the Health Enterprise (IHE), the HIMSS Privacy and Security Toolkit, the eHealthInitiative, Health Level 7, and projects under the Office of the National Coordinator of Health Information Technology, the HHS Office of Civil Rights (OCR), and the Center for Medicare and Medicaid Services (CMS) offer support to the practitioner. These organizations provide structures in which to analyze some security issues in an HIN. The IHE structure,[1] the HITSP structure,[2] OCR's Privacy and Security Framework,[3] and the HL7 EHR structure[4] are examples. There are also some "early adopter" models of an operating HIN (e.g., the Indiana HIE, the iHealthRecord). The California Healthcare Foundation published a study in June 2007, entitled "Privacy, Security, and the Regional Health Information Organization."[5] It summarizes privacy and security challenges and practices for current RHIOs/HIEs.

These structures and early adopter models can be used as aids by the practitioner. But, each one is limited in some way. None address the full range of information security risks in an HIN. Where risks are addressed, there is not sufficient detail for these structures to be directly applied. More importantly, making choices about risk in an HIN is partially driven by the level of trust among the parties. This is inherently subjective, and therefore, varies from one HIN to the next and also varies over time. So, practitioners who are building or connecting to an HIN can expect to have to do some individual work in addition to using these aids.

Large Sharing Community

If the typical HIN is to succeed, the PHI must be shared by a large community of PHI providers and recipients. The HIN must make PHI easily available for appropriate access and adequately protected otherwise. An HIN is a large and fluid community, so managing access is not easy. Keeping PHI access privileges current is challenging for a single institution (e.g., a hospital). And monitoring for misuse of access at a single hospital is difficult. The burden of managing the access in an HIN's large community of institutions, individuals, and systems can rapidly become a nightmare! Not only is the community large, but it changes quickly, making access management even more difficult. The size, dynamism, and access audit challenges of the community lead to a kind of anonymity that raises the risk of misuse of access. The problem of identifying patients for access to an HIN and within records in an HIN is a significant challenge. This challenge is intensified by the concern that using a universal health identifier would itself create serious confidentiality risks.

Data integrity and availability also take on new levels of risk (and benefit) in an HIN. Data come from more sources, are available to more users, and provide more functionality than data in a single institution. People create data that is used beyond the checks and balances of their small work group. This creates added risk that the data may not be available and in the correct form when a recipient needs them. If the recipient knows that the data are inadequate, then only efficiency is injured. However, if the recipient uses inadequate or outdated information, the patient may be injured.

Comprehensive Longitudinal Records

Many HINs include among their services the idea of maintaining comprehensive longitudinal health records (CLRs) of individuals' health information. These CLRs are used to support continuity of care and to provide data for use in personal health applications (e.g., in PHRs). Managing the information security risks associated with the storage and use of these CLRs is a very demanding task. More PHI is at risk in the HIN's CLR and PHI co-location adds to the risk. Further, the number of individuals who access the PHI is higher. Yet, the practical ability to monitor for inappropriate access is lower in most HIN models. This is an important hot-button issue that provokes an emotional reaction in both patients and providers. A "trust me, I'll look out for your data" model may be adequate in a single hospital's HIS, but many participants are likely to demand more transparency, accountability, and control for an HIN's practices in this area.

An HIN may fail to continue operations due to financial shortcomings. The prospect of such a failure raises the question of how security risks will be managed under such circumstances. Can they be transferred to another HIN? Will they just cease to be available? Will the HIN have the resources under these circumstances to assure that the CLRs are at least protected from exposure? These and other issues related to the HIN failure should be considered during the HIN risk-analysis.

Erroneous PHI

An HIN's operational model focuses on making valuable PHI available at the point of care in a timely way on a regular basis. But, what if that information is incorrect? It will happen; it happens in today's typical healthcare enterprise institution on a regular basis. HINs have the inherent potential to spread this false information. In an HIN setting, this element can potentially do far more damage as a consequence of sharing the data than would occur if the PHI was not shared. Incorrect PHI arises from two main sources:

Accident. Paper records, of course, depend on manual entry and all of the inevitable errors that come with that process. Even when EHRs are used, much PHI is captured today by manual entry carried out under great time pressure with few checks and balances. This leads to unintended errors in the records. Accidental patient misidentification (or selection) when PHI is recorded is a special case of accidental

PHI corruption that is commonplace in healthcare. The usage pattern of PHI within a single, small medical practice helps to prevent injury based on these errors. In that scenario, the physician provider who enters the data is likely to be the same person who later accesses the record. At worst, the user of the PHI can confer with the person who entered it. Further, this physician also has other experiences with the patient to aid in corroborating and correcting the record. However, the remote recipients of PHI delivered by an HIN do not have these advantages in detecting or avoiding use of erroneous PHI and are therefore at greater risk of using erroneous data in a way that causes injury (e.g., giving penicillin to a person whose record [incorrectly] says that he or she is not allergic to it).

Fraud, medical ID theft. Sometimes medical records have intentional errors, which can also be spread via an HIN. These errors occur in cases of medical identity theft wherein the thief misuses the victim's identity in various ways, often to gain access to medical services or products. Falsifying records to obtain reimbursement for non-provided medical services or products also occurs. In either case, the victim ends up with information in his or her medical record that is incorrect and may be spread via an HIN. Typically the incorrect data are diagnoses, drug history, and procedure history, the very critical data healthcare providers depend on for further diagnosis and treatment. To the extent that an HIN offers PHI access to individuals who would not have had it otherwise, that HIN also creates a new risk of medical identify theft.

There are resources for managing risk in this area. The Office of the National Coordinator for Health Information Technology (ONCHIT) recently commissioned an initial environmental scan for medical identity theft (see http://www.hhs.gov/healthit/resources/reports.html) and AHIMA has published a general treatment of the topic in a book called *Medical Identity Theft* (2008 edition available at http://imis.ahima.org/orders/). Overall, the medical community has only begun to understand the extent of existing levels of medical identity theft and methods to control the risks associated with this activity.

In addition to the problem of detecting these types of errors, an HIN-risk model must resolve how amendments are to be made to all of the HIN recipients' in-house records. Care providers may have acted on the false information in a way that requires remedial care (e.g., canceling a prescription). Therefore, a process to review the changes in each care setting will need to be in place. This is not just a technical problem; managing the risks associated with erroneous PHI flow using an HIN will reach into clinical operations, liability concerns, accreditation status, and regulatory compliance. The OCR's Privacy and Security Framework has a treatment of HIPAA Privacy Rule obligations related to correcting records used in an HIE. [6]

Law, Regulation, and Standards

There are federal and state laws and regulations related to managing PHI. HIPAA's Privacy and Security Rules are the most well-known federal regulations. There are also:

- Special regulations covering drug and alcohol treatment records, and mental health records (42 CFR, part 2).

- Regulations related to information management in medical research (21 CFR, part 11).
- State-specific medical practice laws.
- State identity theft protection statutes.
- Accreditation standards related to information security and privacy.

In February 2009, the American Recovery and Reinvestment Act[7] (ARRA) became law. It contains incentives for meaningful EHR adoption. This includes HIE and PHR usage requirements. There are also many new privacy/security safeguards and enforcement measures in the law. Most notable among these new provisions is a requirement for HINs that operate as Business Associates of HIPAA-covered entities to be subject to the core provisions of the HIPAA Security Rule. Most of these safeguards were intended to take effect before the end of 2009. It will take some time for practitioners and regulators to form a usable understanding of the precise obligations of this law, but several elements of it are intended to affect how security and privacy in HINs will be managed.

Some of these laws and regulations have direct security requirements in one or all three of the CIA areas. Others have only privacy requirements that carry with them implied security needs. These laws typically focus on process requirements for one healthcare provider to share PHI with a third party (e.g., another physician) without the patient as an intermediary. For this reason, these laws are frequently called third-party disclosure laws.

Many HINs focus their sharing activities on PHI disclosures among healthcare providers and, thus, are subject to all of the third-party disclosure law and regulation elements noted previously. Other HIN models treat the HIN as an agent of the patient (e.g., Web-based PHRs). With the HIN as a patient's agent, all PHI disclosures are made *to* the patient or *by* the patient. These "person-oriented" HIN models have very little law or regulation coverage today. What law and regulation coverage there is seems to support the rights of patients to have access to their records and to provide their records to whomever they choose. These types of HINs are not generally reputed to be qualified as covered entities under HIPAA; they are not generally considered medical providers as specified in most state laws. If operated as a business (e.g., Google Health and Microsoft's HealthVault might qualify), these HINs would likely be covered by state identity-theft protection laws and Federal Trade Commission regulations.

The HHS Office of Civil Rights recently published a large collection of guidance as to how the HIPAA Privacy Rule applies to HINs.[3] This guidance gives the HIN developer and HIN participant a great deal of guidance about which operations will be required and permitted in pursuit of supporting privacy in the context of an HIN.

Some recommendations for information security practices related to PHRs exist. The NCVHS has a recommendation on PHRs.[8] HL7 has a PHR functional model in trial that has security elements.[9] And there is draft legislation associated with assuring security in person-oriented HINs: H.R. 7038 – "Independent Health Record Trust Act (IHRT) (Title V)."

Other draft legislation is focused in areas that affect HIN security and privacy: S.1693 - "Wired for Health Act;" H.R.6357 - "PRO (TECH) T Act;" and H.R.6898 - "Health-e IT" are examples. But, no national legislation has yet passed that squarely targets HIN security and privacy issues.

Standards for HIT that contain some security-related elements are in the early stages of development. The Certification Commission for HIT[10] now certifies the security-related features of inpatient EHRs, ambulatory EHRs, and HIEs. The HIE certification is just now in its first generation. It covers only limited aspects of information security. CCHIT certification of PHRs is on the drawing boards. The Healthcare Information Technology Standards Panel (HITSP)[2] was formed in 2005 as a general means for creating and selecting standards relevant to interoperable health information services. HITSP uses a model in which "use cases" of health information (e.g., bio-surveillance) are examined as a way of capturing the essential information management needs involved in some specific activity. Relevant HIT standards are highlighted in each use case. Many of these use cases generate security-related activities and specify the associated standards (e.g., HITSP Collect and Communicate Security Audit Trail Transaction).

The Office of the National Coordinator for HIT and the Agency for Healthcare Research and Quality (AHRQ) sponsored a line of work starting in 2006 called the Health Information Security and Privacy Collaborative (HISPC). The project was accomplished by various teams around the United States. The focus of the initial work was to explore the current variations in business practices, policies, and laws related to privacy and security of health information, with an eye toward developing a comprehensive plan for protecting health information and locating barriers and solutions related to appropriate health information exchange.

The Solutions Group in HISPC worked in five major domains: legislation, executive orders, leadership and governance, stakeholder education and knowledge, and support for HIEs. In each domain, the work sought to develop ways to build policies and practices that would support privacy, security, and appropriate HIE. The materials from the project[11] may be of use to the reader who wishes to become involved with the parties in his or her state who played a formative role in this work.

Lastly, Integrating the Healthcare Enterprise (IHE)[1] is a consortium composed of major provider associations, government agencies, education associations, standards organizations, consulting companies, and health-related commercial enterprises. IHE focuses on developing, describing, and testing IT standards' *use* in the context of various types of healthcare-related work. These standards are called "profiles" (e.g., Cardiac Cath Workflow). The information-sharing work in the IHE model is embedded in a set of "transactions" for each workflow profile. The interoperation of systems that use IHE standards are tested at periodic "Connectathons."

IHE provides standards for some of the security-related operations that an HIN would need to implement. These standards are found in a collection of profiles called "IT Infrastructure." For example, an Enterprise User Authentication profile is in the IT Infrastructure. These IT Infrastructure profiles typically show how a security-related operation can be carried out, but in a general way (e.g., identifying users, creating audit trails, keeping a common timestamp). In doing this, the IHE leverages existing standards from sources such as Health Level 7 (HL7), American Society for Testing and Materials (ASTM), Digital Imaging and Communications in Medicine (DICOM), Clinical Context Object Workgroup (CCOW), and the Internet Engineering Task Force (IETF).

The typical reported usage of the IHE framework is to support a project involving a single institution integrating clinical operations internally. There are also some early reports of HINs with a stated commitment to the IHE framework (e.g., CareSpark[12]). An HIN development group could use IHE as a framework for developing the operational details of security operations for the HIN. It would also have to develop detailed approaches to the security issues and operations not covered by the IHE framework in its current form today. For example, security risk assessment, security program audit processes, and managing security breaches.

Practitioners involved in an HIN may take this early legislative and standards activity as a sign of interest in developing aids and constraints that may affect their information security management activities. But, the details of the effects are not certain today. So, this is another factor that increases the risk management load in the area of HIN usage.

Other Parties/Uses

In the discussion of HINs, we have focused on professional care providers and patients, which seems to infer they are the only participants in an HIN. But, there are many other parties who have an interest in gaining value from HINs. Pharmaceutical companies could find great value in improving drug development and performing postmarketing surveillance using HIN data flow. Medical researchers may find a bounty of data that can aid in forming ideas for controlled studies or in following the care of clinical trial participants. Those who allocate funds to health research could use HIN-based PHI as a way of studying which research efforts to support. Insurers may seek to use HIN-based activities to reduce costs for themselves and to support more preventive self-management measures among their plan members. Public health agencies could use access to data to detect outbreaks and learn how to best distribute their resources. Disaster response would be greatly aided by knowledge of the health needs of those members of the public involved in the disaster. Lay caregivers for adults can use HIN-based processes to aid in care provision and the coordination of professional care. This is a large group of about 47 million lay caregivers (e.g., an adult helping to assure that his or her elderly parent is getting the right care at the right time). Taken together, these additional potentials for HINs produce another level of complexity in managing information security risk.

All Together Now!

Each of the six key HIN environmental factors previously listed brings its own challenge to managing security risk. All of the factors must be managed if the HIN is to be successful. Organizing this collection of activities and interactions is itself a challenge to the practitioner.

The next two sections will provide background information and guidance for these practitioners (e.g., ISOs [Information Security Officers], CPOs [Chief Privacy Officers] as they consider engaging in an HIN. The first section is devoted to HINs that focus on interinstitutional data-sharing (i.e., an entity-oriented HIN). The remaining section is devoted to HINs that focus on using the patient as the key party through which data flow (i.e., a person-oriented HIN). Of course, any given HIN would likely be a type of hybrid of these approaches; the separation of these two types in this discussion is intended to help the reader see the security-related differences in these two HIN models.

INTEGRATING WITH AN ENTITY-ORIENTED HIN—SETTING THE STAGE FOR HIN PRIVACY AND SECURITY

HIN privacy and security model development is rooted in the idea that healthcare providers will share PHI about patients that they have in common. Further, this will be done in a way that others cannot readily access the shared PHI. This orientation to sharing PHI among healthcare entities in an HIN defines an entity-oriented HIN (EO-HIN).

PHI on paper was shared between providers long before the idea of electronic-sharing of PHI emerged. Much of health privacy law (and related security measures) was established in this period and is oriented toward sharing information on paper. Even more recent laws cover paper-based sharing due to the low rate of electronic sharing today. This area of state and federal law and regulation generally requires that each provider obtain some form of permission from the patient before the provider can legally disclose the patient's information with a third party outside the boundaries of the care-providing entity. These laws are often referred to as third-party disclosure laws (TPD laws).

In the typical TPD law, disclosures are allowed under broad permissions granted as part of the consents gathered when becoming a patient at a healthcare facility. The required "security" in carrying out these disclosures is typically limited to a broad obligation to keep patient information confidential. There are also special TPD laws that require added confidentiality measures; for example, laws related to drug-abuse treatment.

The HIPAA Privacy and Security Rules require significant attention to security at each facility covered by HIPAA. This includes attention to securing disclosures of PHI. The Privacy Rule does not require permission from the patient to disclose PHI for "treatment, payment, or healthcare operations." The Privacy Rule has only a broad obligation to protect confidentiality of PHI in any form of media.

The HIPAA Security Rule includes many requirements related to the confidentiality, integrity, and availability of *electronic* PHI. This includes requirements for electronic third-party disclosures. Many HIPAA "covered entities" contract with commercial enterprises to carry out covered activities that include PHI use. In these cases, HIPAA requires covered entities to create a Business Associate agreement (BAA). The BAA passes along many security obligations to business partners. Many covered entities further reduce security risk by contractually requiring added protections.

EO-HIN Structure

The typical EO-HIN, as depicted in Figure 6-1 is structured as an organization running a health information-sharing service as a Business Associate to all of the HIPAA-covered entities that subscribe to the EO-HIN. There also may be non-HIPAA-covered entities involved (e.g., medical practices that don't take insurance). This structure is the basis for legal PHI flow among the participating entities who disclose PHI in support of treatment, payment, and healthcare operation of *only* those patients that they have in common. At a minimum, the entities use HIPAA Security Rule standards, and the EO-HIN uses the Business Associate requirements as the basis for information security risk management. An HIN participant agreement (a.k.a., a Data Use Agreement) may also spell out additional terms needed to assure each participant that the others will cooperate and have adequate security practices. Some EO-HINs may retain PHI for later provision to participants. Other EO-HINs may support only PHI transport with no long-term retention. The PHI-retaining model, of course, has more security challenges than the transport model.

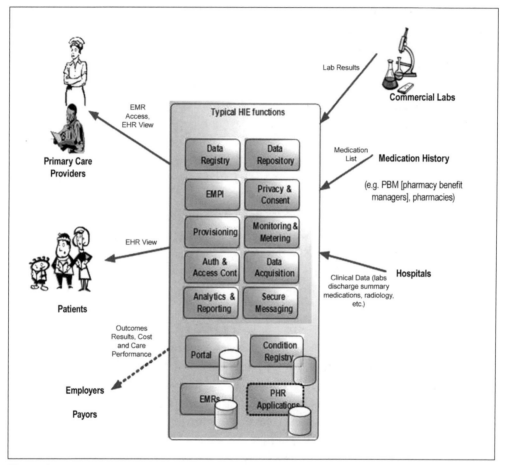

Figure 6-1: Typical EO-HIN Structure.

The structure just described grounds most healthcare entities in a familiar environment. It does not directly address the special risk management issues raised by HIN that were described in section one. That is where all of the new work is required to adequately secure the EO-HIN.

Several state and national organizations are developing ideas related to meeting the extra challenges in security management for EO-HINs. Notable among these organizations are the Office of the National Coordinator for Health Information Technology (ONC), American Health Information Community (AHIC), Markle Foundation, e-Health Initiative, PrivacyRights.org, HIMSS, State Alliance for e-Health,

Certification Commission for Health Information Technology (CCHIT), OCR, IHE, AHIMA, and HITSP. A Web page with links to these organizations and related projects can be found at http://www.hhs.gov/healthit/privacy/state.html.

A key project that involves these organizations is the development of the Nationwide Health Information Network (NHIN). ONC created this project as a way of developing an architecture for connecting HINs. NHIN is not intended to be a single HIN for the United States; it is only intended to serve as a tested framework for interconnecting HINs (e.g., RHIOs, HIEs). The NHIN development process is focused on exploring use cases associated with health information-sharing. For each use case supportive policy, technology, and operations are defined, prototyped, and implemented in a trial form. The NHIN focuses on the confidentiality aspect of security as it arises within the context of a healthcare operation. For example, the Patient-Provider Secure Messaging Use Case supports the operation called "Patient sends secure message to provider." This approach offers the practitioner some orientation as to which operations need securing. It does not offer all of the guidance needed as to how confidentiality can be secured and does not provide significant insight into integrity or availability needs.

In addition to covering some aspects of security for operations within an HIN, the NHIN project has also taken up the task of developing the model for connecting HINs to each other. This work includes attention to confidentiality protections. As part of this work, the NHIN project is developing a model agreement for EO-HINs called a Data Use and Reciprocal Support Agreement (DURSA). ONC also hopes to have a similar model agreement for production NHIN member use.

There are many examples of operational EO-HINs that have developed an approach to security and privacy. The e-Health Initiative performs an annual survey that explores that state of HIE development.[13] Each of these operational EO-HINs has settled on some way to manage security, but the details are not generally made public. For an example of a developing EO-HIN framework, see the North Carolina HIE description at http://www.nchica.org/NCHIE/intro.htm.

Managing Risk When Participating in an EO-HIN

With this as the state-of-the-art, what is a security risk manager to do when faced with the prospect of connecting his or her institution to an EO-HIN? One way to proceed is to develop a risk assessment focused on the EO-HIN along with strategies for risk management. Consider risk in the following areas:

Confidentiality

- How will you ensure that the PHI is being delivered to an authorized party?
- How will you ensure that the disclosure is permissible—by law and institutional policy?
- When in the HIN process does your legal/regulatory/accreditation responsibility to protect PHI begin and end?
- When in the HIN process does your need to protect your reputation with the public, as related to your protection of patient data, begin and end?
- What will it cost to reduce confidentiality risk to a level that is acceptable?

- What are the benefits to HIN for your organization?
- Is the cost/benefit ratio favorable?
- How will patients be reliably identified?

Integrity

- When you deliver PHI that is acted on by others, what is the extent of your obligation (legal, public) to assure that the data are correct, current, and delivered in a timely way?
- When you accept PHI for others, how would integrity risk limit your use of the data?
- When you or another party discovers that delivered PHI is incorrect, how will correction to the data and potential remedial care be managed?
- Is the cost/benefit for these operations favorable?

Availability

- How does the EO-HIN model affect your obligation to have information systems and clinical/business services up and operating to obtain and release PHI?
- Are the other EO-HIN participants able to meet your availability needs in delivering PHI?
- What uptime requirements are there for the EO-HIN itself?

    Once your connection to a viable EO-HIN is initiated, you will likely see the advent of more services that leverage the EO-HIN. As these new services are considered, it is very important to revisit the risk assessment and management framework. Even if you don't add new services, underlying risk will shift and new laws will likely affect your security posture. For example, practitioners taking up this activity in the 2009 and 2010 timeframe should be especially attentive to the new safeguards and enforcement measures of the American Recovery and Reinvestment Act of 2009. So, it is important to revisit your risk management program periodically. When you do, the same questions previously posed can be asked again in the context of the totality of the new service set, shifted risks, and new laws and regulations.

INTEGRATING WITH A PERSON-ORIENTED HIN—SETTING THE STAGE FOR A PO-HIN

The right of a patient to have access to his or her PHI held by a provider is well-established today. The HIPAA Privacy Rule, in particular, provides a fairly broad requirement for covered entities to disclose to the patient all of the PHI in the "designated record set." More recently, ARRA has even established a legal right for a patient to have the PHI in this designated record set "transmitted" in electronic form if the covered entity maintains the PHI in electronic form (Sec 13405(e)). This designated record set consists of the PHI used to make medical decisions about the patient or to seek payment for services. The Privacy Rule has time limits for response to such a request and a few exceptions that would allow or prevent providers from supplying the PHI. There is even a broad requirement in the Privacy Rule that the PHI be provided in the form that the patient requests. These provisions all supercede any more stringent state law requirements that might inhibit a patient's access to his or her PHI.

Generally, the right of a person to disclose her PHI to whomever she wishes is not limited by law or regulation. A patient may want to disclose her PHI to others for a variety of reasons: to better manage her health, to seek second opinions, as part of seeking legal counsel related to care, to aid her lay caregivers, or to assure continuity of care among providers who may not communicate among themselves.

Proponents of patients having ready access to their PHI point to several key benefits to using this access:

- Patients can use the PHI (together with some other resources) to better manage their health, be involved with their care, and coordinate their care. This will support improved health.

- Patients can more readily seek the best price for health services and products. This may reduce out-of-pocket costs and, in the long-term, insurance premiums.

- Patients can spot errors in health records and can act to prevent the errors and limit damage (e.g., denial of insurance, fraud including medical identity theft).

- Patients can spot facts in lab/procedure reports that affect diagnosis and care that busy clinicians may overlook.

- Patients can help detect (and prevent) inappropriate PHI access when the records include logs of access by others.

- Patients can share records with their lay caregivers to help them in providing care.

There are 47 million lay caregivers for adults in the United States today—an exceedingly large group. These lay caregivers can aid in achieving all of the advantages of the other points listed above, as well as reduce their own burden in caring for the individual.

There are also concerns about patients using their own PHI including:

- Patients have limited ability to usefully interpret the records. This may result in confusion, distress, and inappropriate action by patients. Workloads for healthcare providers may also increase.

- Providers may be less willing to accurately chart concerns knowing that the patient may be offended or distressed when reading such notes. This may endanger proper care.

- As patients are more easily able to seek care as a result of having their PHI, there may be a loss of provider business to competitors.

A collection of personal medical records in the hands of the subject of the records has come to be known as a personal health record (PHR). Electronic PHRs have evolved over the last few years to take on abilities that paper PHRs could not practically acquire. These new abilities include being integrated with the EHR systems in healthcare providers' medical offices in ways that allow for easy two-way PHI flow. More recently, it has become possible to acquire an electronic PHR that can gather data from and share data with multiple providers' EHRs. This last arrangement amounts to the e-PHR acting as a pivot point for health data exchange and sets the stage for a person-oriented

HIN (a PO-HIN). Managing the risks involved with the hopes and concerns of the PO-HIN model is a serious task with different problems and opportunities than the EO-HIN model.

PO-HIN Structure

The typical e-PHR with EHR integration features (hereafter called an iPHR) is structured as a product or service provided to patients and to healthcare providers. Typically, the iPHR is vended by a commercial enterprise. Depending on the business model, the patient and provider may or may not pay for the use of the iPHR. Frequently, the funding model calls for the use of targeted advertising and sale of anonymized data to others. Popular buyers of anonymized data are medical researchers, health services planners, and commercial health product providers. The data in a PO-HIN are organized around a person, not around a set of regional HINs that must be interconnected to achieve national scope. (See Figure 6-2.) So, the PO-HIN model does not contain an NHIN-like facility.

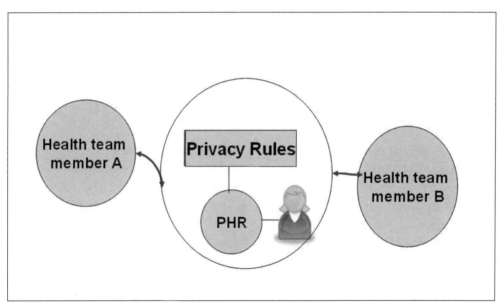

Figure 6-2: Typical PO-HIN Structure.

Several groups have focused on promoting the development of PO-HIN models. The AHIMA, the Markle Foundation, the Robert Wood Johnson Foundation (especially through its Project HealthDesign), the eHealthTrust, the IHE, and the ONC/AHIC (through consumer empowerment use-case development) are key among groups supporting a consumer empowerment orientation to HIE. AHIMA's Web site (see http://www.myphr.org) has a set of resources, including a list of links to many iPHR Web sites, as well as Web site references for other types of PHRs. The iHealthRecord by Medem is a good example of this sort of structure and has been in service for several years. There are "early adopters" for the PO-HIN model, including the iHealthRecord and eHealthTrust. There are several groups in the planning/research stage for a PO-HIN, including the NC Southern Piedmont HIE,[14] the Louisville HIE,[15] and the Washington State Health Record Bank.[16] (See Figure 6-3.)

Recently, a new "layer" of integration engines has emerged that allow PHRs and EHRs to attach to them for the purpose of conveying information between PHRs and EHRs. Microsoft's HealthVault and Google's Google Health are the most high profile examples of these integration engines today. In addition to interfacing with PHRs and EHRs, these integration engines include the storage of PHI, the logic for permitting the flow of PHI or access to it, and basic PHR capabilities. The security arrangements for both the PHRs and the integration engines are made by the vendors.

- LouHIE – Louisville Health Information Exchange.
- Washington State (its state-wide RHIO principle base)
- Health Record Bank of Oregon
- CareEntrust – of Kansas City, MO
- Healthy Ocala – of Ocala, Florida
- State of Kentucky – statewide health information exchange
- Duke Heart Center's Health Record Network
- Northrop Grumman's NHIN prototype
- Dossia (a joint project with Intel, Wal-Mart. AT&T, Cardinal Health, New Orleans Health Dept, and others)
- NC Southern Piedmont Health Information Exchange (SoPHIE)
- SharedCarePlan.org – an RWJ project in Whatcom County, Washington
- The latest round of implementation grants for the National Health Information Infrastructure (for projects like this) require significant consumer information flow controls
- HRN (the Health Record Network). http://www.healthrecord.org/
- Vendor Examples: YouTakeControl, Patient Command, eHealthTrust, Microsoft HealthVault, SharedCarePlan, Google Health, Dossia, iHealthRecord

Figure 6-3: PO-HIN Examples.

Some security elements for these services are described in their terms of use and privacy policies. Some claim a significant responsibility for security. Others make it clear that they have no contractual obligation to users to protect the PHI. Terms of use and privacy policies typically include language that allows the vendor to change the terms whenever desired, frequently without notice to the users. Terms of use that provide for independent audits of security operations with results going to users are uncommon.

Seen from an information risk-management perspective, this structure is very different from the EO-HIN structure in several key ways:

Confidentiality. All of the disclosures from the covered entities are made *to* the patient rather than to a third party. Disclosures to covered entities are made by the patient who is the subject of the disclosure. The OCR Privacy and Security Framework indicates that, under certain conditions, a HIPAA-covered entity would be required to disclose PHI to a PO-HIN when it is acting as the patient's agent.[3] This implies that the provider would be required to take this risk and to manage it well. This drastically changes the portion of the risk distribution model that concerns itself with the risk of inappropriate disclosure from that of the EO-HIN model. In the PO-HIN model, if you are disclosing PHI for a patient *to* that patient then it is not an inappropriate disclosure. This applies regardless of the state in which the covered entity operates or the state in which the patient lives. This arrangement implies that assuring that the disclosure is being made to the right patient and that PHI is accepted from a properly authenticated patient are the key confidentiality management issues in a PO-HIN.

Concerns about state and federal third-party disclosure laws and their requirements are not present in this model as they were in the EO-HIN model. An advantage that affects risk management of the PO-HIN approach is that the patient can decide whether to send PHI that was received from one provider to another provider. This is done using a set of automated rules backed up by specific permission from the person for cases not managed by the rules. This person-powered approach to permitting disclosures relieves the PHI source provider of determining whether the law and the patient approve of the PHI flow to another party.

Most PO-HIN model implementations include a logging facility that will allow a consumer to see who has actually been accessing her PHI from among those individuals and categories of individuals who have been given access capability. For example, the patient may have allowed access from anyone in the local emergency department; the log would show actual access from the individuals in the ED.

This logging feature protects confidentiality by alerting those who might misuse their access to PHI that the subject of the record can detect the misuse. Further, the patient will have strong evidence of the misuse that can be used in sanctioning the misuse. This is an improved protection over the typical periodic audits carried out by in-house auditors. The probability of a misuse being audited is greater and the insight brought to the audit by the patient is greater. For example, the patient knows that the person working in the ER is the estranged spouse with whom the patient is having a contentious divorce, but the in-house auditor would not know this.

Integrity. Accidental and fraudulent corruption of the data communicated through a PO-HIN model is still a risk as it was in the EO-HIN model, but with some important changes. In the PO-HIN model, a patient can act to see that the data are both about him/her and are reasonable. This capability inserts a potentially strong new security control (patient review) that can keep incorrect data from spreading; this potential for spreading false PHI is a key risk with the EO-HIN model. Healthcare professionals who work in the area of detecting and correcting errors of this type estimate the patient misidentification error rate to be between 0.1 percent and 1 percent of transactions in which humans "select a patient." Given the number of selection events that a typical person's record is subject to, this form of error alone is a significant integrity risk. Record corruption caused by fraud (e.g., medical identity theft) is a risk in the PO-HIN model as it was in the EO-HIN model. Again, the PO-HIN provides a risk reducer in the form of patient review. One integrity risk in a PO-HIN often raised by healthcare providers is that consumers will change copies of PHI obtained from one provider before presenting it to another provider (e.g., changing HIV-status). This could result in care that might be inappropriately provided based on this false information, and providers considering some PO-HIN information as being less credible and therefore less useful. This problem could be averted with the use of technical safeguards (e.g., digital signatures provided by the source healthcare provider's EHR). Features such as this one are currently not required for EHR certification or are common in EHRs.

The EO-HIN model and the PO-HIN model both need to consider how patients are going to be reliably identified. The use of universal patient identifiers in the context of third-party disclosures has been controversial. Most EO-HIN models depend on probabilistic matching for identifying patients. PO-HIN models have more flexibility in this area. Each subject of information exchange has an account in the PO-HIN and thus has an identifier. This identifier will be unique (within a given PO-HIN) and could be shared with contributing systems to better assure long-term positive matching.

Availability. A PO-HIN model implementation typically delivers data over the Internet from servers. The availability of the Internet at the point of access and the availability of the servers are required for PHI access. The typical EHR will make local copies of these data for its own use. Patients can make copies of data on their own PCs. These steps may mitigate the need for PO-HIN availability in many cases. Many PO-HIN model services advertise the availability of PHI in a medical emergency as an advantage. It is not clear that these services have availability that is greater than the average Internet-based service. This availability risk may be lower in EO-HIN designs that include "hardened" links and server farms operated along with other medical-grade information services.

Transparency and choice. The OCR Privacy and Security Framework notes that "Trust in evolving health information technologies can best be established with openness and transparency about the policies, procedures, and technologies that affect how individuals' health information is used."[3] In the EO-HIN model, security arrangements are managed with agreements among the EO-HIN participants. Patients whose PHI flows in an EO-HIN have little knowledge of the quality of the security arrangements and have no viable choice about the ongoing security arrangements. Most PO-HINs primarily depend on market forces to assure security. First, PO-HINs depend on consumers making choices about who they should trust with their PHI. Second, they depend on healthcare providers who may resist offering PHI to patients if they believe that the connecting service is inadequately secured. Last, PO-HINs are at risk of having to advise customers of security breaches under most state identity theft protection acts. These market-driven PO-HIN models have some transparency through the visibility of the terms of use, word of mouth, and online reviews that can help consumers choose which PO-HIN to use.

In addition to the commercial PO-HIN, there is another PO-HIN model frequently described as an independent health record trust (IHRT) that with it brings different transparency features. An IHRT is an HIN that is structured as a trust and is run for the benefit of the IHRT members. The membership is entirely composed of individuals whose PHI flows through or is stored in this HIN. This IHRT organizational model improves the potential that security arrangements will favor consumers because of the nature of the responsibilities of the trustees. Pending federal legislation (H.R. 7038 – "Independent Health Record Trust (IHRT) [Title V]) would create a set of broad responsibilities for information privacy and security for IHRT trustees with certification requirements, required audits of security measures and public reports of the results. This legislation also includes a provision that would limit consumer changes to data to clearly marked amendments; this would be another way to reduce the integrity risk of concern to healthcare providers noted in the previous section.

How could a consumer judge the actual security performance of an HIN, and what can a consumer do if unsatisfied? Consumers can directly experience many forms of security failures in their use of both EO-HINs and PO-HINs. In addition, state identity theft protection laws assure that confidentiality failures become known by requiring notice to the affected consumers. The laws apply to typical businesses, including healthcare providers and HIN service vendors. They frequently apply to state and local government agencies. Breaches also frequently become public. When a PO-HIN has this kind of confidentiality failure, consumers can make choices about who to use in the future. By comparison, when EO-HINs have this type of failure, there are fewer consumer choices, short of perhaps opting out entirely and thereby also missing out on HIN benefits.

Taken together, the four factors I have discussed (confidentiality, integrity, availability, and transparency/choice) describe a security risk management environment for a PO-HIN that has significant differences with an EO-HIN model. The differences in the security approach arise mostly from the shift toward increased patient responsibilities and choices (and fewer provider responsibilities) in the PO-HIN model, as compared with the EO-HIN model.

Managing Risk When Participating in a PO-HIN

Information security risk managers should apply the same process for managing risk for PO-HIN participation as was recommended in the "Managing Risk When Participating in an EO-HIN" section. But, they should expect different answers to the information risk questions for the PO-HIN model. This is due to the differences in structure of the models noted previously. For example, consider the risk management question "How will you assure that a disclosure is permissible—by law and institutional policy?" In an EO-HIN, answering this question involves significant work. Indeed, the labor involved in taking up this complex issue combined with low benefits to the disclosing party for getting it right and high costs for getting it wrong is frequently listed as an important inhibitor to third-party disclosures. In a PO-HIN the answer is virtually always that providing the PHI to the patient is not just permitted, it is required.

SUMMARY

Routine electronic PHI flow shows great promise to improve healthcare. Doing so is on virtually everyone's short list of key ways to defeat many of the dysfunctions that have come to characterize systems of health and care. Operating these systems with proper regard for the security of PHI is more than just a tactical feature of an HIN. It is essential to creating the conditions that will allow the desired benefits to emerge from HIN use while avoiding harm to individuals and institutions.

The entity-oriented and person-oriented approaches to PHI-sharing and storage provide models in which risk management activities can be carried out. The balance of responsibility falls more to healthcare providers in the entity-oriented models and more to patients in the person-oriented model.

Many groups are now working on setting standards for these models and how they should be implemented. Practitioners in hospitals and medical practices are likely to be considering participation in at least one of these new HINs over the next few years. Those considerations must include a thoughtful review and adjustment of information security policy to accommodate the risks involved. This chapter has provided background and guidance in support of that review and adjustment.

Discussion Questions

1. Which national laws and regulations structure the exchange of PHI to third parties? Which of your state laws address PHI exchange?
2. What are the key differences in the structure of the entity-oriented approach to an HIN and the person-oriented approach to an HIN? How might a hybrid model take advantage of the best features of each approach?
3. Compare and contrast the ability of consumers to influence the security arrangements in the PO-HIN model and the EO-HIN model.
4. List the key functions of a DURSA.
5. How would a consumer become aware of the terms of use and privacy policy associated with a commercial PO-HIN?
6. How would a healthcare provider advise/educate patients about the use of an HIN?
7. Describe several ways in which the typical medical practice could benefit (i.e., improve care, reduce costs, enlarge market share) from acquiring PHI via an HIN.
8. Argue for whether a healthcare provider's risk/benefit ratio in being involved with an HIN is greater in a PO-HIN or EO-HIN.
9. How can access to PHI for lay caregivers be best managed in the EO-HIN and PO-HIN models?
10. A new Massachusetts law requires a long list of security measures to protect certain personal information held by any "person" who is a citizen of Massachusetts (e.g., a company, hospital, HIN, individual). Review these measures and the situations to which they apply. Describe how the law would affect an HIN's security program. Would the personal information of a citizen of Massachusetts be covered by this law if the HIN itself was not in Massachusetts? Would the law's applicability vary, depending on whether the data of the citizen of Massachusetts came from a care episode in Massachusetts or not? The law can be found by searching for "201 CMR 17.00" under www.mass.gov.

References

1. Integrating the Healthcare Enterprise. IHE profiles. Available at: http://www.ihe.net.
2. Healthcare Information Technology Standards Panel. HITSP standards. Accessed April 24, 2009. Available at: www.hitsp.org.
3. U.S. Department of Health & Human Services. OCR privacy and security framework. Accessed April 24, 2009. Available at: www.hhs.gov/ocr/privacy/hipaa/understanding/special/healthit/.
4. Health Level Seven Inc. HL7 EHR functional model. Accessed April 24, 2009. Available at: www.hl7.org/ehr/downloads/index_2007.asp.
5. Rosenfeld S, Koss S, Siler S. Privacy, security, and the regional health information organization. California Healthcare Foundation. Accessed April 24, 2009. Available at: www.chcf.org/documents/chronicdisease/RHIOPrivacySecurity.pdf.
6. U.S. Department of Health & Human Services. HIPAA correction guidance. Accessed April 24, 2009. Available at: www.hhs.gov/ocr/privacy/hipaa/understanding/special/healthit/correction.pdf.

7. American Recovery and Reinvestment Act. The Library of Congress. Public law 111-5. Accessed April 24, 2009. Available at: http://thomas.loc.gov/cgi-bin/query/z?c111:H.R.1.enr.

8. U.S. Department of Health & Human Services. Personal health records and personal health record systems: a report and recommendations from the National Committee of Vital and Health Statistics. February 2006. Accessed April 24, 2009. Available at: http://www.ncvhs.hhs.gov/0602nhiirpt.pdf.

9. HL7 PHR-S Functional Model. Available at: http://h17.org/ehr/.

10. Certification Commission for Health Information Technology. [Web site]. Accessed April 24, 2009. Available at: http://CCHIT.org.

11. RTI International. Health Information Security and Privacy Collaboration (HISPC). [Web site]. Accessed April 24, 2009. Available at: www.rti.org/page.cfm?objectid=09E8D494-C491-42FC-BA13EAD1217245C0.

12. CareSpark Consortium. [Web site]. Accessed April 24, 2009. Available at: www.carespark.com/index.php?option=com_content&task=view&id=55&Itemid=55.

13. eHealth Initiative. National health information exchange survey shows increased activity, cost savings, positive impact on physician practices. Accessed April 24, 2009. Available at: www.ehealthinitiative.org/HIESurvey/.

14. Duke Translational Medicine Institute. Southern Piedmont Health Information Exchange (SoPHIE) Planning Group wiki. Available at www.dtmi.duke.edu/wiki/display/pohie/Home.

15. Louisville Health Information Exchange Inc. Available at: www.louhie.org.

16. Washington State Health Record Bank. Available at: http://www.hca.wa.gov/hit.

Chapter 7

Portable Devices

Terrell W. Herzig, MSHI, CISSP

RISKS ASSOCIATED WITH USE OF MOBILE AND STORAGE DEVICES

Couple ultraportable computing devices with advances in the availability of communications such as Wi-Fi networks, and you have the makings of an infrastructure to access information from any place at any time. Allowing healthcare professionals to remotely access clinical information can greatly improve efficiencies. No longer "tethered" to physical workstations located at the end of a hallway, the physician can as easily access clinical data from the point of care as from the concourse of a busy airport. Physicians can now use portable devices to prescribe medications, order lab reports, create orders, and check for drug interactions. Using locally installed applications, clinicians can also access medical and pharmaceutical reference books. Gone are the days when devices served one function; no longer does a cell phone function only as a cell phone, for example. Smart phones bring with them the functions of a cell phone, a personal information manager, and a personal assistant, capable of running office applications.

While advances in mobile computing have facilitated the exchange and management of patient information, the security risk associated with accessing healthcare information "outside" the bounds of the healthcare organization is considerable. The increased access to medical information could lead to the misuse and abuse of patient information. In 2006, the Centers for Medicare and Medicaid Services (CMS) issued guidance on the use of portable devices within a healthcare environment.

This chapter will examine the risks associated with the use of mobile computing devices, including laptops, PDAs, and mobile smart phones, as well as the use of portable storage devices and their related hazards.

CMS Guidance on Portable Devices

Citing a number of security incidents related to the use of laptops and other portable devices, CMS issued a seven-page guidance related to the use of such devices when working with ePHI. The guidance encourages covered entities to be extremely cautious about allowing offsite use of and access to ePHI. Access should be based on business need and allowed only when the organization has evaluated the risk. According to CMS:

> "A covered entity's analysis of the risks associated with accessing, storing, and transmitting ePHI will form the basis for the policies and procedures designed to protect this sensitive information."[1]

What Are the Risks?

We spend a lot of time, especially when traveling, using mobile devices to answer e-mail and work from our phones. We create, edit, and store Word documents and spreadsheets, read PDF files, and access other organizational files. We exchange e-mail messages containing sensitive information and maintain confidential documents on the device. In some cases, we may store passwords used to login to Web sites or the hospital network. While the greater accessibility these allow is established, mobile devices also present unique security threats. The following are some of the threats:

- Loss or theft of the mobile device.

- Exposure of sensitive data.

- Interception of data over unsecured networks.

- Viruses particular to mobile devices (including e-mail-related viruses).

Before an organization can develop a sensible policy related to the use of portable devices, it has to understand the risks associated with their use. Frequently, organizations will only consider the risk incurred with use of the device itself, similar to those included on the previous list. They fail to analyze the risks to the organization and the resulting damages from a subsequent data breach. To fully comprehend all possible risks associated with these devices, healthcare organizations should consider these additional risks and other parties that may also incur the risk:

- **Individuals whose PHI is compromised.** A data breach could result in embarrassment for the individual, misuse of his or her personal data, fraud, or identity theft.

- **Hospital or healthcare facility associated with the incident.** The facility could risk the loss of trust on the part of patients and constituencies, loss of reputation, loss of competitive position, negative publicity, and possible fines and litigation.

- **Employees involved in the incident.** Employees implicated in the breach can suffer embarrassment, loss of wages, disciplinary action, fines, and penalties.

In addition, healthcare institutions may find themselves in situations of regulatory noncompliance. Investigations may be conducted by the OCR, CMS, the Justice Department, or the Federal Bureau of Investigation (FBI).

Almost daily the news media broadcast stories of individuals losing a portable computing or data storage device containing thousands of records with very sensitive personal information. A recent survey conducted by the Ponemon Institute[2] reviewed 31 security breaches, ranging in size from 2,500 records to 263,000 records. They found that, on average, organizations spent $182 per record lost and a total cost of $4.8 million per breach. Considering risk in terms of the storage size of portable media available today, a USB drive no bigger than a human thumb could result in the loss of millions of records. An office supply store recently advertised a 4-gigabyte USB drive for under $9. Such devices will often attach to a keychain, a fact that should make you shudder!

HIPAA regulations and subsequent CMS Guidance state that each covered entity will maintain an accurate and up-to-date inventory of all of its devices, including portable devices. Considering that anyone can walk into a store and purchase a USB device, what is a healthcare organization to do to control and inventory the use of these devices? The first step after understanding the threat is to develop the appropriate policies.

DEVELOPING PORTABLE DEVICE POLICY

A comprehensive set of policies should encompass the device's complete life cycle, from purchase through the operational lifetime to end-of-life and physical destruction. Developing such a policy set is an enterprisewide effort and will depend on the dedication of senior management. Effective mobile device policies cannot be created in isolation. The policies must address the continual creep of consumer technologies into enterprise-wide IT operations. Everyday, affordable and portable smart phones enter the market. This advance in technology results in a continuous influx of privately owned mobile devices with demands to interface with the corporate IT infrastructure. End users choose to adopt devices that meet their workflow and personal needs, often without consideration to facility workflows and platform stability. Attempts to ban devices or discourage their use most often fail. Ironically, it is not uncommon for the first offenders to be the executives to which the IT organization reports.

Mobile policies should be explicit about user responsibility and how user's actions impact mobile security. Key policy elements must include:

- What is allowed?
- What is supported and at what level?
- Who will pay for the support?
- Who buys and owns the device?
- What voice and data services will be covered, and who will pay for them?
- How will the device interface with the network infrastructure?
- User responsibilities.

The terms "mobile computing" and "portable devices" mean different things to different organizations. Some healthcare organizations may consider a laptop to be a mobile device, while another may consider it a desktop device. Some organizations may discredit the smart phone as a practical mobile device. However, they need to be aware that it can execute programs and store massive amounts of information.

When creating your portable device policies, consider the technologies that are available, those that are active in your inventory, and other portable devices that may have a consumer focus, such as USB drives, DVD writers, and portable hard drives.

When you have developed your policies, be sure to then develop appropriate educational materials for the workforce. Do not assume that posting it on the corporate intranet will effectively inform everyone of the policy's contents. Actively and openly discuss the policy through meetings, e-mails, workshops, and other means of organizational communications.

A successful portable device policy should include the following topics:

- **Acceptable use.** Define appropriate user behavior by specifying the devices and applications that meet the organization's policies. Include e-mail, Web usage, and Internet access with mobile device use. Be sure users understand appropriate methods for access to the corporate infrastructure.

- **Product standards.** What devices, peripherals, external storage, and additional technologies are to be supported? Will exceptions be allowed? If so, how will they be addressed? By whom? What is the level of support? If multiple products are listed, what are the criteria for deciding the appropriate device?

- **Security procedures.** This section must specify the minimal installed security software, controls, and device settings. If the device is lost or stolen, how must it be reported? To whom? What are the expectations for backups and software patches?

- **Data restrictions.** What type of data is allowed to be stored on a device? Where is it allowed to be stored? Who is allowed to authorize the use of sensitive information on a portable device?

- **Ownership.** Who owns the device? Who owns the data? Allowing users to purchase and use their own devices for healthcare operations increases the risk to the organization and the user. If the device is owned by the individual, the healthcare facility will have limited control of the device and the consequent security. Furthermore, both the facility and the individual may be increasing their legal liabilities in cases in which a personal portable device is misused. For healthcare organizations, I do not recommend individuals be allowed to purchase their own portable equipment for corporate use. I witnessed an investigation regarding the theft of information on a portable device. During the scope of the investigation, investigators seized a number of physician-owned laptops. The authorities kept the devices for almost 90 days before returning the property. In healthcare organizations, it may be necessary to remind the workforce who owns clinical data.

- **Enforcement and sanctions.** How will the policy be monitored for compliance? What are the ramifications for a violation? Who will enforce the policy?

- **Network access.** All portable devices must be screened prior to reconnection with the corporate network. When a user removes a device, a period of time may pass prior to it being returned. In such cases, the organization no longer knows the condition of the device and its security state. Therefore, a method of re-establishing the trusted device must be in place. Appropriate tools include Network Access Control (NAC) to validate the device's security state prior to allowing it back on the network (see Chapter 9 for more information on remote access).

- **Liability.** Liability determines responsibility if a device is lost or stolen, if data are leaked, or even, perhaps, if an employee is injured or caused an accident while using the device when driving or operating equipment.

- **Appropriate purchasing strategies.** How is the workforce member allowed to purchase the portable device? What are the requirements?

- **Budgets and reimbursements.** What are the monthly operational costs and who pays these charges? Will reimbursements be required for personal use?

MANAGING PORTABLE DEVICE AND STORAGE MEDIA ASSETS

IT struggles with managing hardware and software assets. With the increase in the acquisition of mobile assets, such as laptops, PDAs, cell phones, portable drives, and memory cards, the difficulties of tracking assets is compounded.

In the past, most large corporations would only track capital assets. Today, the costs of most IT devices fall below corporate capital cost guidelines. This often leads to gaps in an organization's IT inventory, particularly in the area of mobile devices.

Memory cards and thumb drives are cheap and abundant. They are small enough to fit in a pocket or handbag without detection. It is not the physical cost of the asset that makes it a suitable target for tracking, but the information it may contain. If a device has the capability of storing sensitive information, it should be tracked in the same way as other IT assets. The major problem to focus on is the possibility of losing portable devices, which is enormous. Scan the Internet for recent articles about lost devices, and you will quickly understand the damage these small devices can bring to an organization.

The loss of sensitive data is not the only security threat a thumb drive can pose. Consider that the intent of the device is to move data from computer to computer. This very quality, that these devices can interface with other machines, makes it easy for them to transport malware. Such devices are increasingly being linked to the propagation of computer viruses and worms (e.g., conflicker worm).[3]

So how do you inventory and track such small, cheap devices? In keeping with the theme of this book, the task must involve layers of multiple security controls to lead to an effective device-management strategy. First, make sure your portable device policy clearly states that personal devices should not be used for corporate business. Given the sensitive nature of health information, neither the organization nor the individual need to encumber additional risk by using personal devices to transport or access ePHI.

Second, your policy should explain the appropriate use of portable devices, including when and in what cases it is permissible to use them, and how to properly acquire them. Management must be involved and understand the risks associated with the use of portable devices and, consequently, should play an active role in accepting responsibility for issuing devices for employee use. Once you have clearly defined expectations and the conditions for obtaining and using portable devices, avenues for purchasing these devices must be clearly defined.

The IT department will need to work closely with purchasing and acquisition to ensure that portable devices are purchased and configured appropriately. By establishing exact procedures, configuration burdens can be minimized in ways similar to desktop equipment management. This concept is key. Harkening back to my earlier statements about not developing policy in a vacuum, when developing policies for portable devices, the users' needs and the organization's need to deliver patient care must be considered. New devices are introduced into the consumer electronics market daily. Such devices continue to get smaller, more portable, and enriched with features that consumers don't want to be without. Portable devices, especially smart phones, come and go almost on a monthly basis. Devices in use today will disappear tomorrow. New devices appearing in the market today may not play well in the current enterprise environment but may work well in a future version. While the typical business may be able to use managed diversity to support mobile/portable devices, the sensitivity of the information involved in healthcare demands tighter controls.

To reduce the risk of workforce members using cheap portable drives or unauthorized devices, consider deploying end-point management tools. End-point management tools work by locking down user workstations to prevent the unauthorized use of USB devices, CD and DVD burners, and external devices such as portable hard drives. Realize, however, that this technique assumes the organization has sufficient security policy controlling the use of personal workstations within the healthcare delivery organization. These workstation controls are mandated by HIPAA and should be in force.

End-point security tools can tie to active directory and lightweight directory schemes, enabling easy management and transparency to the user. These security tools should be centrally managed, and the security policies they enforce should be active independent of the PC's connectivity state. By using these tools, the organization can establish policies about limiting use to certain types of devices; allow use of a device as long as it is encrypted with a sufficient encryption technology, shadow the data moved to and from the device, securely erase data no longer needed, and inventory and track each device.

Depending on the size of the entity, additional management tools may be needed to effectively manage portable devices. The following is a list of some management tools available:

- **Software distribution and management tools.** Application provisioning and device management suites allow for the remote management and provisioning of devices.

- **Asset-tracking tools.** Depending on the types of mobile devices, it may be necessary to maintain additional asset-tracking tools or deploy device-specific agents to adequately inventory and track a device.

- **Device management tools.** These tools include utilities to monitor and update device configurations and apply updates, such as OS updates.

Finally, consider the use of recovery tools, which are available not only for laptops, but for higher-end smart phones. The tools usually install an agent in the device's bios or a similar area that makes it difficult for a thief to erase or reformat. When an organization installs the product, it will establish a quick connection to a central monitoring facility and check its status. If the device has been reported lost or stolen, the tool can provide tracking information to law enforcement for recovery and activate appropriate countermeasures to permanently destroy any data it may contain. Using tools such as end-point management and recovery software can greatly reduce the risk of information being disclosed if a device is lost or stolen. If a workforce member loses a laptop with sensitive information on the hard drive, would it not be far better to be able tell your patients that their information was not only encrypted, but the information was destroyed and the equipment recovered?

SECURITY CONTROLS FOR PORTABLE DEVICES

As we work our way from portable device policy to security controls, it is important starting out to have a firm commitment to a minimal set of security controls for all portable devices. If the organization considers implementing a portable device within its infrastructure, then settings or controls commensurate with policy must be provided. Healthcare organizations should consider the following security controls for all of its portable devices:

- **Password protection.** Mobile devices should be protected by strong passwords. If the device is capable of deleting sensitive information or clearing the device after a number of failed login attempts, it should be configured to allow such action. For devices such as USB drives, select those devices that have on-board encryption and prompt the user to enter his or her key when activating the drive. A number of devices are available that offer central key management. This is important for any device that utilizes encryption technologies. Users forget passwords and the organization may need to gain access to the device in the absence of an individual.

- **Storage card protection.** Many mobile devices utilize SD cards (secure digital cards), or mini-SD or flash memory to hold gigabytes of data and images. Such cards are portable and can be removed from the device. If the card is removed, it could be accessed by inserting it into another drive or device. If sensitive information is stored on the card, it should be encrypted. Pay close attention to biomed devices that use this technology as a means to transport medical data.

- **Encryption.** Data files should be encrypted to protect their contents. Consider whole disk encryption products in which the entire hard drive is encrypted and do not depend on the user to understand how to manually encrypt and decrypt files. Several products are available to encrypt the drives of laptops and other portable devices.

- **Backups.** To protect against the loss of sensitive data, portable devices must be backed up to a secure location. Your portable device policy should address this requirement, and IT should offer sufficient support to aid mobile workers in backing up their devices. Users should not be allowed to back up unencrypted sensitive data to their home PCs.

- **Software restrictions.** Policies should address what software users will be allowed to operate on the mobile device. As with PCs, refrain from allowing users to operate under administrative rights.

- **Acceptable use policy.** Define the acceptable methods of connecting to the corporate network. Will a VPN client be required? Can a user connect via terminal services or a remote desktop? Can the user synchronize to the network via a workstation cradle or Bluetooth device? Will NAC controls be employed to verify security settings prior to connecting?

- **Antivirus and malware software.** Does the mobile device require the installation of personal firewall software and antimalware software? An array of software is available to manage malicious code threats on laptops and other portable computing devices. Smart phones with limited functionality may not need these controls. An evaluation of risk, based on the type of device, is necessary.

- **Personal firewalls.** Does the portable device support personal firewall products? If the answer is yes, a personal firewall should be used.

- **Physical security.** Train and remind users about appropriate physical security measures when using a portable device. If traveling by car, remember to secure the device in the trunk if it must be left in the automobile. Educate the user on how to properly secure removable media when they are not needed. Remind the user about his or her responsibility to avoid allowing the unauthorized viewing of sensitive information in public and common areas.

- **Screen lockouts and timeouts.** Portable devices with display screens should enforce screen lockout and timeout policies. These precautions are often overlooked in relation to portable devices. Forgetting to set these controls can leave the device open for misuse if lost or stolen.

- **Audits and configuration checks.** Portable devices can be off the corporate network for long periods of time. Therefore, routine audits and configuration checks of all portable devices should be conducted.

- **Incident reporting.** Each user must be trained on what to do if a device is lost or stolen. The user must understand the importance of timely reporting and the appropriate parties to contact.

- **Wireless access and the use of public Wi-Fi.** All remote users should be educated on the hazards of using public wireless access. Your policies should also address using wireless technologies when transferring sensitive information.

An abundance of information sources to help readers develop appropriate policy and procedures related to the management of portable devices can be found on the Internet. Appendix A contains a wealth of links that can provide guidance and resources for meeting best-practice standards. A good starting point is NIST.

THE IMPACT OF VIRTUAL MACHINES ON PORTABLE DEVICES

Just as the last few years have shown explosive growth of portable devices and mobile computing, so too has another technology gained strength. The development and deployment of virtual computing environments have boomed as a result of increases in hardware performance, security risks to PCs, concern for the environment, and the need to maximize datacenter resources. Many organizations have discovered they can obtain greater performance from their server environments by virtualizing the hosts. The use and deployment of virtual workstations can reduce the need to utilize personal computers and allow the use of thin clients or terminal desktop environments.

The deployment of thin clients can keep data resources in a secure datacenter environment instead of on a remote desktop. By eliminating a full personal computer desktop and its vulnerability intensive operating system, certain security risks can be reduced. Thin clients typically do not have operating systems or hard drives, and therefore, do not require frequent OS updates or patches. The device can be configured not to operate if it is removed from the organization.

Virtualization decouples the software from the hardware device. By combining thin-client technology with virtualization technology, users connect to network resources and are instantly presented with virtual PC capabilities within the thin-client environment. When provisioned, the user can access the same Windows' resources and applications as if using an actual PC. The difference is the PC is running as a software application on a server in the remote datacenter. Only screen updates and keyboard activities are being transmitted across the network.

Additional security benefits are recognized when using thin-client technologies and two-factor authentication. Smart-card technology can be used on the thin client to provide two-factor authentication and help maintain state information. This is particularly attractive in healthcare environments, such as hospitals, in which the workforce is continuously mobile. A clinician can insert his or her smart card into a thin-client device and key a pincode, logging into the clinical systems. When the task is completed, removing the smart card from the device can put the user's session into hibernation. When the user inserts his smart card at another location and enters his pin number, the previous session state is immediately restored. Productivity is increased by reducing sign-in times.

The use of thin-client technologies and virtual environments are not limited to PCs and are becoming more common in the mobile device market. Thin-client mobile application servers deliver Web content and application support to browsers and content-rendering engines on mobile devices. Mobile thin-client application servers are capable of supporting hundreds of mobile devices.

Contractors and Unmanaged Personal Computers

As previously discussed, the use of unmanaged PCs within the corporate setting is a substantial security risk. Many healthcare facilities have contract workers entering and exiting the facility on a daily basis. Most contract staff are equipped with laptops and mobile devices configured for their company's connectivity and security standards. When they arrive at your workplace, they immediately want network connectivity. Unless you have them shadowed by a PC technician, you have little control over the use (or misuse) of their devices. I recently had a contractor on site who attempted to start-up BitTorrent so she could download music while she worked (our security controls blocked the access and logged the information).

To provide adequate protection in this environment, the organization must have clearly defined policies that outline the expectations of contract employees and other third-party workers. Deploying NACs would be an appropriate control to consider. Virtual machines (VM) can also provide security. Contract employees could be given access to the applications and data needed by way of a virtual workstation, which would greatly reduce the risk of data leakage and issues with unmanaged PCs. Some advantages to using VM workstations for unmanaged laptops and portable devices are outlined next:

- Corporate data and applications are effectively isolated from software installed and running on the remote device.

- The VM is running within the corporate data center, independent of the hardware configurations of the laptop or portable device.

- The VM environment can offer security from basic security breaches in the host remote device file system.

- Data are encrypted and retained within the data center and will not be lost if the contractor's device is lost or stolen.

- The remote sessions can be terminated via managed intervention.

The Use and Deployment of Wireless in Healthcare Operations

One of the largest data breaches in the history of the United States was discovered and reported in 2007. TJX, the parent company of TJ Maxx and a line of other department stores, became the victim of wireless hackers and weak wireless security controls.[4] According to news reports, hackers used equipment to intercept and decode traffic between hand-held payment scanners, allowing them to steal credit and debit card information.

Wireless networks offer convenience and access to network resources, which are especially beneficial in healthcare. Patients and patient families can use wireless networks to connect with family and friends while their loved ones are in the hospital. Mobile biomed devices require wireless access as part of their mobile capability. But implementing appropriate wireless access is not without risk and involves careful planning before committing to an installation. A cabled network infrastructure connects two end-points with physical cable. Intercepting a communication over a wired network requires a deliberate intrusion into the cable or switch connection.

With wireless, the connections are established by beaming radio waves through the air to connect the end-points. Radio waves can propagate for long distances. Since wireless equipment requires radio waves to connect, anyone with the appropriate wireless equipment can connect if appropriate security measures are not taken. The following are specific threats and vulnerabilities of wireless networks:

- Malicious users could gain access through wireless connections and bypass perimeter firewalls.

- Sensitive information that is not encrypted could be intercepted.

- Denial of service attacks could be carried out against wireless access points and other devices.

- Handheld wireless devices can be easily stolen.

- Data could be compromised without detection.

- Individuals gaining access from the inside could use your network to launch attacks.

- Individuals gaining access could masquerade as legitimate hosts and compromise account information.

As you can tell from this list, managing wireless networks requires greater effort than managing wired networks. Many organizations underestimate the costs associated with properly deploying a wireless network. Wireless routers from local department stores, built for the home market, give users the false impression that wireless networks are simple to set up. The first step in deploying a wireless infrastructure is to conduct a thorough risk assessment and develop appropriate security policies. These policies should include the minimum required security configurations for access points and the devices that will connect to them. It should also take into consideration the minimal requirements for devices that will attach to the wireless network. The policies must consider the use of the wireless network for care delivery, biomed equipment, patient access, and perhaps even the use of public components.

Organizations planning wireless networks must take into account the physical controls in place within the facility. Physical security measures are the first line of defense against the theft of equipment and insertion of rogue access points. Prior to the deployment of a wireless network, healthcare organizations may want to consider the use of wireless security solutions specifically designed to isolate rogue-monitoring equipment.

A SHORT PRIMER ON WIRELESS

Wireless LANS. Wireless LANs (local area network) offer greater flexibility and portability than their traditional wired counterparts. In a wireless LAN, network cards use radio frequencies to connect computers to the network through what is known as an access point (AP). The access point, in turn, connects to the wired LAN via cables. Users can move about within range of a wireless access point and remain connected to the network infrastructure. A wireless LAN device can reconfigure while on the move.

Ad-hoc networks. Ad-hoc networks include technologies such as Bluetooth, and are designed to dynamically connect portable devices, such as cell phones, laptops, and PDAs. Whereas a wireless LAN uses a fixed network infrastructure, an ad-hoc system relies on a master-slave device communication principle to communicate.

Wireless standards. Wireless LANs are based on the Institute of Electrical and Electronic Engineers (IEEE) 802.11 standard. The 802.11 standard was developed to support medium-range, high data-rate applications that are compatible with network technologies, such as Ethernet networks. The 802.11 standard is the original WLAN standard and was designed to support 1- to 2-megabit per second (Mbps) throughput. In 1999, the 802.11a standard was published and provided for communications within the 5-gigahertz (GHz) band and supported speeds up to 54 Mbps. During the same time period, IEEE completed work on the 802.11b standard, which operates in the 2.4-2.48 GHz band and supports speeds up to 11 Mbps. Finally, to round out the popular wireless standards in use, is the 802.11g standard. The 802.11g standard operates in the 2.4-GHz bandwidth.

Other standards have emerged that are important to consider. The 802.1X standard provides a security framework for networks, including Ethernet and wireless networks. The 802.11i standard defines specific wireless security functions that operate with 802.1X.

Keep in mind that the 802.11 standard permits devices to establish either a peer-to-peer (p2p) network or a network based on fixed APs. Thus, the standard defines two basic network topologies: the infrastructure network and the ad-hoc network. Devices in an ad-hoc configuration can share files and communicate with the use of an AP. This is an important feature in light of possible security issues.

Security of 802.11 Wireless LANs

Because of how radio devices operate, security services had to be incorporated to provide a secure operating environment. The early wireless standards provided the Wired-Equivalent Privacy (WEP) protocol to protect transmissions between clients and access points. WEP does not provide end-to-end security, but security for the wireless portion of the traffic. WEP provides three basic security services for the WLAN environment.

- **Authentication.** A primary goal of WEP is to provide a security service that can verify the identity of client stations. This provides access control to the network by denying access to client stations that can not authenticate properly.

- **Confidentiality.** Privacy is a second goal of WEP (or least in common with that of a wired network). The objective is to prevent casual eavesdropping of material being transferred.

- **Integrity.** Another goal of WEP is to ensure that messages are not modified in transit.

Authentication. 802.11 provided two means to authenticate wireless users attempting to gain access to the wired network: open-system authentication and shared-key authentication. The open-system model accepts mobile stations without verifying the identity of the station. The open-system method is one-way—only the mobile station is authenticated. The client must trust that the communication is with a real AP. Open system authentication is the only required form of authentication by the 802.11 standard.[5]

Shared key authentication is a cryptographic technique for authentication. It is based on a challenge-response scheme that a client has knowledge of a shared secret key. The client using a cryptographic key that is shared with the access point encrypts the challenge from the AP and returns the result back to the AP. The AP decrypts the result from the client and allows access only if the challenge matches. Such challenge and response techniques have been known to be weak and suffer from attacks like the "man-in-the-middle" attack.

Privacy. The 802.11 standard supports privacy via the use of cryptographic techniques, specifically WEP utilizing the RC4 symmetric key cipher algorithm. This technique encrypts the data to protect traffic such as TCP/IP, IPX, and HTTP. The main issue with this portion of WEP is it only uses a 40-bit key for the shared key. Some vendors have offered non-standard extensions that support larger keys.

Integrity. The 802.11 specification outlines a method to provide data integrity for messages sent between clients and access points. This technique uses simple Cyclic Redundancy Checks (CRC). A CRC-32 frame check sequence is calculated on each data payload prior to transmission and is encrypted. When the message is received, decryption is performed, and the CRC is recomputed. If the CRCs are not the same, an integrity violation occurred, and the packet is discarded.

The 802.11 specification does not identify any means of key management. Therefore, generating, distributing, storing, loading, and so on are all left to the individuals in charge of administrating the WLAN. As a result, substantial vulnerabilities could be introduced into the WLAN environment, including non-unique, zero-based, factory default, or other form of weak keys.

WEP Weaknesses

Because of the inherent weaknesses in the WEP protocols, numerous methods of attack have been developed. Tools, such as AirSnort and WEPcrack, are readily available on the Internet and do not require a lot of skill to operate. In some cases, a complete, live CD image can be downloaded and burned to a blank CD. The distributions can then be booted on any workstation that has a CD-ROM as a bootable device. Once the system is booted, the operator selects the attack and executes a few scripts. Utilizing these tools, I have personally seen WEP keys cracked and access to data gained in less than an hour.

Wi-Fi

The 802.11 standard for wireless networking is also known as Wi-Fi. The IEEE, realizing the shortcomings of 802.11 security, began developing the 802.11i standard. A non-profit industry consortium of WLAN equipment and software vendors, called the Wi-Fi Alliance, developed an interoperability certification program for WLAN products. The Wi-Fi Alliance created an interim solution to the security issues while the IEEE worked on finalizing 802.11i. Accordingly, the Alliance created Wi-Fi Protected Access (WPA) which was published in 2002.[5]

WPA, designed to work with pre-WPA wireless network cards through firmware, upgrades and implements most of the security enhancements in the IEEE 802.11i standard. The alliance's WPA2 certification indicates compliance with the full standard. In particular, WPA2 introduces an Advanced Encryption Standard (AES)-based encryption algorithm.

Additional Wireless Risks

Users often want to communicate back to the corporate network when traveling. As a result, they are often seeking public wireless access in conference centers, airports, hotels, and restaurants. These networks are untrusted and introduce additional risk. Because they are public, they can be accessed by anyone, including malicious users. If a user connects to a free public Wi-Fi service and then connects to their corporate internal network, they become a bridge for the public traffic. This could potentially allow anyone on the public network to gain access to the bridged corporate network.

Securing the Wireless Infrastructure

As you plan to deploy a wireless infrastructure, consider the following guidelines:

- **Update the wireless devices default passwords.** Each WLAN device comes with default settings. These settings may include administrative passwords that may not be activated or are blank. Change the default passwords and, if necessary and supported, use two-factor authentication techniques.

- **Activate the appropriate encryption settings.** Set the encryption settings to the strongest encryption strength available in the product. Avoid WEP and implement WPA2 or better technologies.

- **Provide for resets.** When purchasing access points, purchase equipment that will not negate security settings if the equipment is reset to its factory defaults.

- **Consider using MAC ACL filtering.** A MAC address is the hardware address that uniquely identifies a network-attached device. Several 802.11 products provide capabilities to designate permissions based on a device's MAC address.

- **Change the Service Set Identifier (SSID),** which is the name you assign to a wireless Wi-Fi network. All devices that participate in a particular WLAN must use this same, case-sensitive name to communicate. These names can consist of strings up to 32-bytes long. The SSID of the AP should be changed from the factory default. The default values of SSID used by many vendors have been published and are well-known.

- **If possible, disable the SSID broadcast feature.** A wireless client can determine all of the available networks in a given area by actively scanning for APs. This is accomplished using a special type of messaging called a broadcast probe message. This probe triggers a response from all 802.11 networks in the area. Disabling the broadcast SSID feature causes the AP to ignore the probe message from the client. This will force the client to perform active scanning with a specific SSID.

- **Change default cryptographic keys.** Always change the default keys and change them often. Consider the use of RADIUS server technology and dynamic keys for this task.

- **Disable Simple Network Management Protocol (SNMP).** Some wireless APs may be configured to use an SNMP agent as a network management tool to monitor the status of the APs. The SNMP protocols contain well-known and exploitable vulnerabilities. Due to these vulnerabilities, disable SNMP, if at all possible.

- **Change the default channel.** Vendors will commonly use a default channel in all of their APs. If two or more APs are located near each other, but are on different networks, interference issues can arise and, in some cases, cause a denial of service.

- **Employ an effective Intrusion Detection System (IDS).** IDSs allow the monitoring of network traffic and can spot intruders or attacks on the system.

- **Check the Patch Status.** Wireless vendors supply updates to their products' firmware similarly to that which software manufacturers use to release to correct problems and add functionality. Keep abreast of new firmware upgrades and apply them as deemed appropriate.

- **Virtual Private Networks (VPN).** Consider VPN deployment within the wireless environment as an additional layer of security, especially if you have mobile employees who may be using public access points that may be open or only employing WEP encryption.

- **Public Key Infrastructure (PKI).** PKI provides an infrastructure for public key certificates and, as a result, provides applications with secure encryption and authentication. WLANs can integrate PKI for authentication and secure network transactions.

- **Create dedicated Virtual Local Area Networks (VLAN).** A VLAN is a logical conjugation of devices within a LAN that is created via software rather than manually moving cables in a wiring closet. It combines the user workstations and associated network devices into a single unit, regardless of the physical LAN segments to which they are attached. Using dedicated VLANs in a wireless environment can segregate traffic. Dedicated VLANs facilitate the use of network access control lists. Different VLANs can be defined with the wireless connections to further separate security policies. This approach can be used to provide both wireless guest access and secure clinical operations across the same APs. Dedicate a VLAN to management consoles and systems to help secure the WLAN wireless management.

- **Public WLAN support.** If a WLAN will be supporting unauthenticated users, install a firewall between each WLAN and its distribution system. This functionality may also be available by utilizing VLANs. Consider authentication systems that will allow easy public access but which are geared toward temporary authentication. This will allow for trace-back capabilities when dealing with potential breaches.

- **Firewalls.** Install firewalls on client devices participating in a WLAN.

- **Auditing.** Develop audit processes and logging procedures. Logging should be routed to a central server, analyzed, and stored securely.

- **Purchase APs** that terminate associations after a configurable time period, requiring stations to re-authenticate after a specific length of idle time.

- **Disable ad-hoc mode.** Unless your organization has specific business requirements (watch out for certain biomed devices) for peer-to-peer networking, disable this mode in favor of an infrastructure mode.

- **Perform** wireless assessments on a frequent basis.

- **Securely dispose of WLAN components.** When disposing of WLAN equipment, be sure to clear all sensitive information (for example, shared keys).

Wireless Guest Access

Let's face it: Healthcare organizations have a great need to provide guest access to their network infrastructures. Healthcare employs an increasing number of consultants, contractors, and remote workers. Patients are accustomed to Internet access, and bed-bound patients want to stay connected to the workplace, family, and friends.

The defacto standard in connectivity for consultants and contractors is the laptop computer. The divergent roles and needs of these individuals often require access to more resources than traditional, single VLAN portals. Combining the need for multiple roles with access to differing resources, healthcare organizations are looking to role-based provisioning of the wireless infrastructure so that guest access is assigned a role that will provide that guest with specific functionality.

A WLAN-specific guest access role-provisioning solution has the benefit of controlling access points and the added advantage of being able to control bandwidth. By defining roles, network administrators can define roles for different groups. Policies can be associated to groups. Remote employees, contractors, and vendors can have specific policies applied to their group and assigned to different VLANs dependent on these policies. Customized captive portal sign-on pages for each role can identify the resources available to the user.

SUMMARY

The technologic lines between our personal and professional lives continue to blur. Tools such as PDAs, laptops, and smart phones, which were once widespread only among business executives, have found their way into the average employee's lifestyle. Employees are encouraged to work at home with high-speed cable modems and their own personal computers, often with wireless connections they have configured themselves. From home, they move large amounts of data between work and home within spreadsheets, Word documents, and Access tables. Transcriptionists also work from the comfort of their homes, whether they are independent, contracted to a hospital, or associated with a transcription company. Voice files are moved down to the transcriptionist's home computer and transcribed. The resulting document is then uploaded to the healthcare facility.

More and more employees transfer corporate e-mail to private systems, such as Gmail, Hotmail, and Yahoo, preferring to consolidate their messaging services to provide a central one-stop message center for their own convenience.

The entrance of consumer technologies into the enterprise is challenging traditional security models. New tools to manage the risks from consumer devices are expensive and sometimes immature. Enterprises are adopting tools such as NAC to help manage the threats.

In addition to the use of portable devices is the growth in social networks and Web 2.0 technologies. Some of these services can create a risk of information leaks; others can open new channels for the spread of malicious programs. One incident resulted in the termination of two workforce members because they uploaded a patient's photo to a social network site.

As more workforce members come to depend on home PCs to connect to the organization's network, corporate infrastructure must take into account the connection of this unmanaged and likely insecure PC. VPN access with NAC support is needed to adequately protect this remote connection. Consider deploying end-point management tools to control the leakage of sensitive information via external hard-drives and portable USB keys. Finally, educate employees on the proper use of wireless technologies and how to properly configure their own equipment.

Organizations should review their legal obligations and estimate in advance their potential liability from the use of portable devices, particularly if personally owned devices are allowed for corporate work. Data kept on home systems and other private devices can be seized by court order.

Employees should receive a yearly briefing of appropriate use of and liability associated with corporate resources. Workforce members should sign an annual consent and responsibility statement.

Organizations should be cautious about providing antivirus, firewall, and security software for home use and voluntary installation on home systems. By participating in these activities, the organizations could be taking direct responsibility for the integrity of these systems. Connections to corporate networks should be made through VPN connections with NAC and firewall monitoring that can scan a user's system before the connection is completed. Rather than waste funds bringing unmanaged PCs up to the corporate standard, deny connections to equipment that fail to conform to the corporate standard. It then becomes the user's responsibility to get his or her system in proper working order.

Discussion Questions

1. Discuss the risks associated with portable devices and media.
2. Discuss the difficulties when attempting to inventory portable devices.
3. Discuss who is responsible for the use of portable devices and media within an organization.
4. Discuss the advantages and disadvantages of using wireless within a healthcare organization.

References

1. Centers for Medicare & Medicaid Services. CMS HIPAA Security Guidance. Available at: http://www.cms.hhs.gov/SecurityStandard/.

2. 2006 Annual Study: Cost of a Data Breach. Page 2. Accessed December 16, 2008. http://download.pgp.com/pdfs/Ponemon2-Breach-Survey_061020_F.pdf.

3. Messmer E. Downadup/conflicker worm: when will the next shoe fall? Networkworld.com. January 23, 2009. Accessed December 16, 2008. Available at: www.networkworld.com/news/2009/012309-downadup-conflicker-worm.html.

4. Bosworth MH. Wireless hackers suspected in TJ Maxx breach. Consumeraffairs.com. May 7, 2007. Accessed December 16, 2008. Available at: http://www.consumeraffairs.com/news04/2007/05/tjx_wireless.html.

5. Guide to Securing Legacy IEEE 82.11 Wireless Networks. Accessed December 15, 2008. http://csrc.nist.gov/publications/nistpubs/800-48-rev1/SP800-48r1.pdf.

CHAPTER 8

Medical Device Security Implications

Leanne Cordisco, BMET

SPECIAL CONSIDERATIONS OF NETWORKED MEDICAL DEVICES

Any exploration of security within the world of healthcare IT would be incomplete without a thorough examination of the networked medical devices performing diagnostic tests and treatment therapies on patients. Many similarities exist between the security needs of medical devices and other devices on the healthcare enterprise network; however, important differences also exist, and ignoring them may cause significant patient injury.

This chapter will focus on special considerations of networked medical devices in the area of security, including the life-critical nature of medical devices, common architectures of clinical networks, the blurred line between medical devices and the IT system, the roles of biomedical engineering and IT, operating system support including patches and upgrades, MDS^2 documents, HIPAA audit implications, and wireless issues.

Medical Devices—Integrating Medical Technologies

Hospitals have a staggering array of diagnostic and treatment tools at their disposal today. Medical devices, as the link between the patient and the HIS in particular, play a crucial role in the digitization of healthcare. Installing, maintaining, and decommissioning medical devices is a profession with many specialty areas, and security of these devices is a common thread running through each of the specialties. To best understand this complex world, it is necessary to first understand the definition of a medical device.

According to the FDA, a medical device is "an instrument, apparatus, implement, machine, contrivance, implant, in vitro reagent, or other similar or related article, including a component part, or accessory which is:

- "Recognized in the official National Formulary, or the United States Pharmacopoeia, or any supplement to them;

- "Intended for use in the diagnosis of disease or other conditions, or in the cure, mitigation, treatment, or prevention of disease, in man or other animals; or

- "Intended to affect the structure or any function of the body of man or other animals, and which does not achieve any of its primary intended purposes through chemical action within or on the body of man or other animals and which is not dependent upon being metabolized for the achievement of any of its primary intended purposes."[1]

This vague definition allows for unlimited complexity in purpose and form factor, and causes confusion within the world of healthcare, specifically in biomedical engineering and IT.

As early as the 1960s, medical devices were merely manual machines, unchanging in design and use for many decades. But the transistor ushered in an evolution in medical device design, bringing electronic control and precision to formerly manual processes. In the 1970s, electronic medical devices became commonplace; however, these electronic devices were not computerized. Although electronic medical devices contained power supplies, circuit boards, and microchips, they contained no operating systems as we know them today. Rather, they relied solely on vendor-generated software.

Today, medical device manufacturers rely on the PC industry to supply the hardware and operating system platforms on which their proprietary healthcare applications run. This difference is significant, and the result is that many medical devices deployed in healthcare today are essentially that of a Windows-based PC with a purpose-specific form factor around it, a healthcare application installed on it, and clinical accessories attached to it. The benefits are plentiful. Medical device "sticker prices" can be kept low by the use of PC industry-standard components. Raw processing power and speed allow for complex diagnostic, therapeutic, and life-support devices to transform healthcare and patient safety. Repair parts including power supplies, hard drives, and displays are globally available.

However, these advances do not come without a cost of ownership. As a Windows-based system, they can be vulnerable to any attack that can be performed against a home computer. The implications to patient safety are frightening. Both medical device manufacturers and hospital personnel have taken steps to provide the highest levels of security to sensitive medical devices.

NETWORKED MEDICAL DEVICES—
LIFE-CRITICAL VS. MISSION-CRITICAL NETWORKS

One benefit of constructing medical devices on PC platforms is using off-the-shelf networking components and TCP/IP to allow the movement of patient data between systems. This collection of devices moving clinical patient data over an isolated or shared infrastructure comprises a clinical network. Clinical networks carry real-time patient data, which if compromised, may cause significant patient injury or death.

For example, a patient in an ICU bed will have his cardiac activity monitored by at least one cardiovascular monitoring system. The patient's ECG waveforms are transmitted to a central monitor at the nurse's station for continuous monitoring. Consider also that a patient in an ICU bed may be connected to twelve or more clinical devices, many requiring network connections, all with unique alarm tones and patient connectors. If any of these data were compromised or lost, responding to the patient's life-threatening emergency could be significantly delayed. Not surprisingly, for this reason the urgent and important nature of data moved across clinical networks is known as life-critical data. Compare life-critical data to mission-critical data within a hospital. E-mail and payroll data move across the healthcare enterprise constantly. If these functions were to crash, the ability of the healthcare organization to complete its mission would be significantly compromised, but it would not stop. The same is not the case with life-critical networks. The potential for loss of life demands assigning the highest priority to the uptime of these networks and the timely movement of information across them.

Bandwidth is an issue. Life-critical alarms reaching their intended destination must not be at the mercy of a slow network. For this reason, some facilities choose to have isolated clinical networks installed for life support and other high-risk monitoring systems. Understanding clinical network architecture is crucial in developing a robust healthcare IT security program.

There are three common iterations of clinical network design in healthcare today. They are listed in order of their relative security risk:

- **Physically isolated using proprietary protocols**. These networks are commonly built to support monitoring functions within a single department. Device manufacturers sold connectivity between their products as a benefit and built proprietary protocols similar to TCP/IP that allows communication between their devices, but prevented communication to other vendors' systems. Frequently, these systems were installed with their infrastructure and cabling physically isolated from the hospital's enterprise network. These systems are the lowest security risk because of their inability to communicate using TCP/IP and their lack of access to the Internet.

- **Physically isolated using TCP/IP protocol**. These networks can be found in radiology or in other areas in which significant amounts of clinical data from varying manufacturers may need to move across a network of devices for very specific purposes. The sheer volume of data moved demands that the clinical network be isolated from the enterprise, or both the clinical and enterprise systems would be greatly strained. TCP/IP is used to ensure basic connectivity between the systems. It should be noted that other protocols, including DICOM and HL7, will often be utilized to move the vast amounts of clinical data generated within a radiology department. Devices on this type of network can access the Internet through a gateway, allowing remote clinicians access to the patient data and manufacturers access to support and troubleshooting functionality.

- **Logically isolated using TCP/IP.** Ubiquitous infusion pumps and vital sign monitors may be used throughout the entire hospital. Their information payload is relatively small when compared to digital imaging systems found in Radiology. For this reason, many hospitals choose to carve out VLANs within their existing enterprise for these and many other networked medical devices. Some facilities choose to call this the "medical VLAN" or the "clinical VLAN." Another option for these devices is to simply exist as part of the hospital enterprise. The devices on these clinical networks—with their PC-based platforms and relatively easy access to the Internet, their close proximity to the public, and their sheer number—make them great security risks.

Medical Device vs. Information System

The components of a clinical network may not always be obvious. The all-encompassing definition of a medical device has caused the line between medical device and enterprise device to blur. Walk into any server farm and study the racks. You would be hard-pressed to distinguish between the e-mail server and the server containing patient ECG trending data. The two might use the exact same hardware, but should they be supported in the same way by the same team?

Also consider the possibility that a clinical application may reside on a server that hosts many administrative functions. Some medical manufacturers sell software-only versions of their products, allowing maximum flexibility for deployment to best fit customer needs.

Servers are not the only devices in question. Recently smart phones and PDAs have been used clinically to provide near real-time data and alarm functionality to mobile clinicians. According to the FDA, a medical device is considered to be an apparatus intended to mitigate or treat a disease. A smart phone capable of providing asystole detection certainly meets the definition of a medical device.

Unfortunately, there is no clear-cut guidance for managing these "blended" clinical/IT devices.

IT can easily make the argument that they should manage the server. They have experience with the hardware and physical access to the server room. They have a schedule for routine vulnerability and malware scans and can push an image to the server for ease of support. However, IT may also periodically take down the server for routine maintenance and push OS patches to the server in response to a new and public threat.

Biomedical engineering can also easily make an argument to manage the server. Biomed has control over the rest of the clinical network that uses the server for data storage. And biomed has a thorough understanding of the complex configurations within the clinical application running on the server. And, it is biomed that will get the call if clinical network is down.

An additional element of complexity to consider is the risk class of the device. The FDA assigns a risk category of Class I, II, or III to all medical devices as part of its approval process. Class III is considered the highest risk as evidenced by assigning life-support systems to the class. Class I is considered lowest risk. Recently, the FDA reclassified certain types of data storage systems from the highest risk class, Class III, to the lowest risk class, Class I. The storage devices are known as Medical Device Data Storage (MDDS). By design, they warehouse patient data to be retrieved at some point in the future. The FDA published a full definition of an MDDS and its rationale for lowering the risk class of these kinds of systems:

> "An MDDS is a device that electronically stores, transfers, displays, or reformats patient medical data. It does not provide any diagnostic or clinical decision making functions. An MDDS could, for example, store alarm data

being generated by a connected medical device, but would not be able to generate alarms on its own. The MDDS device is currently classified into class III, the highest level of regulatory oversight. The MDDS was initially placed in this classification by default.

FDA is proposing to reclassify MDDS devices from class III to class I. Based on the history of use of this type of device in clinical practice and on the experience of FDA reviewers, the agency concludes that in the hands of a healthcare professional, an MDDS is safe and effective under general controls. The application of general controls, including the software design controls in part 820, would be consistent with the principle of applying the least degree of regulatory control necessary to provide reasonable assurance of safety and effectiveness. The application of this lowest level of regulatory oversight would be consistent with the treatment of other devices with similar risk profiles. Software used to store, transmit, and communicate patient medical data, such as Laboratory Information Systems and Medical Image Communication Systems, is typically classified into class I."[2]

This ruling is significant because it provides documentation for considering any device that can manipulate clinical data a medical device. This may provide some guidance for hospitals as they seek to develop a comprehensive support policy for all networked medical devices, including blended devices.

Clear ownership of blended clinical/IT devices and detailed planning are the keys to managing and securing the device. The plan should always include the input and sign off of both IT and Biomedical Engineering, for both are major stakeholders in the correct operation of the hardware and software running on it.

Elements to consider in a support plan of a blended clinical/IT device include:

- Departmental ownership.
- Complete pre-installation security disclosure.
- Troubleshooting tree.
    - First call ownership.
    - On-site time guarantee.
    - Clinician alert plan for repairs requiring system to be taken down.
    - Verification of repair completion and system functionality before call closure.
- Periodic vulnerability scans.
- Periodic OS patches and upgrades.
- Installation and use of antivirus software.
- Device decommissioning and the removal of PHI.

Operating System Support for a Medical Device

Medical device manufacturers take every precaution to develop safe products. This applies to the device's actual functionality as well as its ongoing security. Knowing how an off-the-shelf version of Windows has been modified greatly assists in developing a security policy for OS-based medical devices.

The challenge of a medical device manufacturer is to allow connectivity between authorized elements of the healthcare IT world, while disallowing connectivity to anyone else. They accomplish this through hardening the OS.

- All unnecessary parts of the operating system are removed. For example, if the device will never need Internet connectivity, the manufacturer will remove Internet Explorer.

- Any unused ports are shutdown.

- The passwords of the default user accounts are modified. This provides only limited protection, as every machine is shipped with the same, newly-changed passwords. A quick Google search will provide the default passwords for Windows OS as well as medical devices. It is a best practice for a hospital to change all default passwords once they install a new medical device. When this is done, it is critically important to inform all service personnel, including manufacturers' representatives, of the password changes.

- The OS is embedded on a separate partition of the device's hard drive and that drive is made read-only. All patient data and device configuration is then stored on a separate drive for extra security.

Every device manufacturer publicly provides a listing of relevant security information for a medical device. The Manufacturer Disclosure Statement for Medical Device Security, or MDS,[1] is a document in an industry-recognized format developed in conjunction with HIMSS to respond to customer requests regarding security features and functionality of medical devices. A template for this document can be found on the HIMSS Web site.[3] MDS[2] documents may be located on a manufacturer's Web site.

Hardening occurs at the manufacturer and user level and is a never-ending process. Real-world examples tell us that systems deemed secure today may be exploited by new vulnerabilities tomorrow. The standard IT industry response to defend against new exploits is OS patching and upgrades. However, it is not as simple as immediately applying every patch and upgrade to every OS-based medical device.

The reason patches and upgrades are not immediately applied to medical devices has to do with the intercession of FDA policy. Although some confusion exists as to the determining reason, in actuality it stems from a straightforward process.

A manufacturer submits a device to the FDA for 510(k) pre-market approval, which is based on concrete hardware, OS, and medical device application specifications. Having obtained approval, the manufacturer may then sell the medical device as long as it meets those defined technical specifications. If the manufacturer changes the device's form, fit, or function, or applies changes that could affect the safety of the device, then the manufacturer must again return to the FDA for approval. Generally, patches and upgrades do not change the form, fit, or function of a device nor do they affect the safety of a device. Therefore 510(k) approval is not needed.

However, even when the manufacturer is not required by the FDA to resubmit for 510(k) approval, they are required to perform verification and validation tests of any patch or upgrade that may be applied to a medical device. The scope of the patch or upgrade will determine the scope of the verification and validation testing performed.

Some patches may only require minimal testing, while some OS upgrades may require all device functionality to be retested.

Manufacturers do perform verification and validation testing as quickly as they can. However, it may seem interminably long when a known vulnerability is exploited and a hospital's medical devices may be at risk. Manufacturers publicly post the findings of these vulnerability tests on their Web sites through the same security portal used to post MDS[2] documents.

Maintaining accurate security documentation for OS-based medical devices is no trivial matter. Consider the average three- to five-year lifespan of a Windows server in the healthcare environment. Now consider that the useful life of a medical device may be five times greater, up to 15 years. A good security plan should always include supporting networked medical devices, even if the underlying OS is obsolete.

Wireless Medical Devices

Wireless medical devices require further attention, for it is more than a Wi-Fi issue. Radio frequency usage for medical devices spans a host of frequency ranges. Table 8-1 lists the frequencies used in a US hospital in 2005.[4]

It is important to remember that life-critical data are moving across the wireless network and that a drop out or downtime of just two minutes can significantly affect patient safety. Therefore every possible wireless failure should be considered and defended against. Consider the following list of wireless safety breaches.

- Unauthorized client authenticates to your network and can participate as an authorized user.
- Unauthorized client captures other clients' network traffic and can decrypt and analyze it.
- Unauthorized access point can spoof your client into thinking it is communicating with your infrastructure.
- Unauthorized user physically steals an AP from your infrastructure.
- Unauthorized user connects to the configuration port of an AP and can modify configuration.
- Rogue, insecure access point is connected directly to the network.

Consider the following actions to prevent wireless breaches:

- Build redundancy into the wired network with available ports in areas that commonly use wireless medical devices, in case of loss of wireless signal.
- Always configure the highest level of encryption on all wireless medical devices; do not use WEP.
- Turn off SSID broadcast, if possible.
- Deploy controlled-based wireless networks to detect and lock out any rogue AP activity.
- Always password-protect the console port of an access point.
- Use tools to detect changed AP configurations.

- Use tools to detect significant numbers of authentication attempts with different keys/passwords from a single MAC address.[5]

- Perform periodic site surveys to detect and mitigate any changes in the RF environment.

- Develop and maintain an RF-usage database and appoint a frequency coordinator to oversee it.

Table 8-1: Common Radio Frequencies Observed (Found) in Hospitals.

FREQUENCY	USE
100–150 kHz	RFID[1], less than 2 m
500 kHz to 165 MHz	AM radio
13.56 MHz	RFID[1], less than 2 m
35 MHz	pager
43 MHz	pager
54–88 MHz	TV channels 2–6
88–107 MHZ	FM radio
137 MHz	pager
138 MHz	pager
152 MHz	pager
153 MHz	pager
158 MHZ	pager
174–216 MHz	biomedical, TV channels 7–13
220 MHz	biomedical, telemetry by Eaton
406–512 MHz	biomedical, business band
433 MHz	RFID[1], less than 600 ft
435 MHz	walkie-talkie 0.5 W
450 MHz	cell phone, 0.5 W or less
454 MHz	pager
462–467 MHz	CB radio
470–608 MHz	TV channels
608–614 MHz	**biomedical, not shared**
614–668 MHz	TV channels
814 MHz	cell phone, GSM
835 MHz	cell phone, GSM
847 MHz	cell phone, GSM
869–893 MHz	cell phone
900 MHz	cell phone, 2 W or less
902 MHz	cell phone, GSM
902–927 MHz	Sony microphones, FM
902–928 MHz	RFID[1], 5 m or less, ISM
915 MHz	Mortara biomedical, mobile phone
1395–1400 MHz	**biomedical, government radar**
1427–1432 MHz	**biomedical, not shared**
1.800 GHz	cell phone, GSM
2.4 GHz	WAN[2]
2.4–2.5 GHz	ISM, STL, microwave ovens, cordless phones
	Bluetooth devices?
2.45 GHz	RFID, less than 30 meters
5.725–5.875 GHz	ISM, point to point, microwave ovens
6.800 GHz	cell phone, 1 W

In January 2007, the FDA released a guidance document on the use of RF technologies in medical devices. Although the document is not solely focused on security issues, the FDA makes clear their expectations for wireless medical devices:

Security of data transmitted wirelessly and wireless network access

Security is a concern in the use of RF-wireless technology because it can be easier for unauthorized eavesdropping on patient data or unauthorized access to hospital networks to occur.[6]

The Role of Biomedical Engineering in Medical Device Security

Prompt and thorough support of networked medical devices requires cooperation between Biomedical Engineering and IT, since the two groups and their respective skill sets fit hand and glove.

In recent years biomedical engineers have made tremendous progress in earning IT certifications to better interact with their IT counterparts. It is now common to see the Net+ certification as a requirement for employment. Medical device manufacturers seek out biomedical engineers with Microsoft and Cisco certifications to employ in their field service teams. Networking skills are a requirement for it is the biomedical engineer who will be responsible for the installation and maintenance of most medical devices in a healthcare facility, including TCP/IP and DICOM configurations, and in some cases, HL7 configurations.

Biomedical engineering has strong relationships with medical device manufacturer representatives, resulting from long-standing service contracts. These relationships may be leveraged to provide rapid results when searching for MDS[2] documentation; OS-patch information, replacement parts, and configuration data.

Biomedical engineering is also a valuable resource for HIPAA audits. For the first time since the introduction of the HIPAA Title II Security Rule, the US government is performing compliance audits. As part of the HIPAA readiness, Biomedical Engineering can provide security information on the medical devices within a healthcare facility. In 2004, the American College of Clinical Engineering and ECRI produced a CD designed to provide technology managers the tools needed for preparing for HIPAA compliance. The CD contains many templates including the Biomedical Equipment Survey Form. This template may be used by a biomedical engineer to capture relevant security data from an MDS[2] form for every medical device within the hospital.[7]

Most importantly, biomedical engineers know how to minimize downtime for networked medical devices. Many network configuration settings can be modified within the medical device application. Configuration data and patient trending data may be downloaded and stored before service work or upgrades are performed. Biomeds have access to service modes that allow for thorough device testing before they are placed on the network and used on a patient. Lastly, biomeds have the ability to correctly decommission a device from the network by removing all traces of ePHI from its memory.

SUMMARY

It has been seen that securing networked medical devices is similar to securing other types of networked equipment. However, as the line between medical device and IT infrastructure continues to blend, the issues of ownership and maintenance increase in complexity. Any security plan for networked medical devices should include sign off by IT and Biomedical Engineering, at a minimum. Elements to consider in the security plan should be device ownership, first-call response, periodic vulnerability testing, periodic patching and updating of embedded OSs, and approval by clinical teams to perform maintenance functions on these life-critical devices. Only through cooperation of these major stakeholders can the risk of significant patient injury be mitigated.

Security considerations must be examined throughout each stage of the life of a medical device, from pre-purchase to decommissioning. Medical device manufacturers play an important role in disseminating relevant security information to their customers. MDS[2] documents posted on manufacturers' Web sites can provide security information critical in the evaluation and purchase of networked medical devices. These security portals are also where OS patch and update vulnerability testing results can be found. It is therefore beneficial to schedule recurring inspections of manufacturers' security portals for relevant device data.

Table 8-2 summarizes the security activities required for support of networked medical device throughout their useful life.

Table 8-2: Medical Device Life Cycle Security Tasks.

Product Cycle	Activity
Pre-Purchase	MDS[2] acquisition
	Frequency coordination activities
	Biomedical Equipment Survey Form
	Encryption options
	Bandwidth considerations
	Network design: isolated or shared infrastructure
	Consider software-only versions of medical devices
	Device ownership: Biomed or IT
Installation	Initial configurations
	Start-up safety testing
	Change default passwords and inform all service personnel
	OS revision inventory
	Network diagrams
	Establish first-call ownership vs departments and include response time
	Determine FDA risk class and build appropriate support plan
Ongoing Support	Periodic review of manufacturer security portals
	OS patch deployment
	OS upgrade deployment
	Ongoing vulnerability tests
	Device software upgrade deployment
	Hardware replacement
	Rogue AP detection
Decommissioning	ePHI removal
	Hardware destruction

Discussion Questions

1. How does a life-critical device differ from a mission-critical device, and how would a security plan be amended to mitigate risk to patient safety?
2. Why is the inclusion of Biomedical Engineering so important in the development of a security plan for networked medical devices, and how should ownership of security tasks be distributed between Biomedical Engineering and IT?
3. How does OS support of networked medical devices differ from other elements in a health IT infrastructure?
4. How do medical device manufacturers keep customers informed of important security-related issues, and how often should that information be reviewed?
5. What are the major security breaches when using wireless technologies for networked medical devices, and how can those risks be mitigated?

References

1. Is the Product a Medical Device. Accessed January 22, 2008.
   Available at: http://www.fda.gov/MedicalDevices/DeviceRegulationandGuidance/Overview/ClassifyYourDevice/ucm051512.htm.

2. Federal Register. Proposed rules. February 8, 2008;73(27):7501. Accessed January 22, 2009. Available at www.fda.gov/OHRMS/DOCKETS/98fr/E8-2325.pdf.

3. Healthcare Information and Management Systems Society. Manufacturer disclosure statement for medical device security. Accessed January 22, 2009. Available at: www.himss.org/asp/topics_focusdynamic.asp?faid=99.

4. Harrington D, Carney T. ICC prep. 24x7 Magazine. Accessed January 22, 2009. Available at: www.24x7mag.com/issues/articles/2005-01_08.asp.

5. Grubis M. Concepts in Wireless LANS for Healthcare Facilities. 16.

6. Date accessed – January 22, 2009. http://www.fda.gov/downloads/MedicalDevices/DeviceRegulationandGuidance/GuidanceDocuments/ucm077272.pdf.

7. ECRI Staff. «Information Security for Biomedical technology, A HIPAA Compliance Guide: A HIPAA Compliance Guide.» *9-2-3 Biomedical Equipment Survey Form.doc* June 2004. Multimedia DVD.

CHAPTER 9

Remote Access

Terrell W. Herzig, MSHI, CISSP

SAFE REMOTE ACCESS TO MEDICAL INFORMATION

Healthcare organizations today face huge challenges. They must strive to improve patient care, streamline operations, reduce errors, maintain patient confidentiality, and accomplish these things while reducing cost. Many large care delivery organizations have moved to providing outsourced diagnostic services and remote x-ray image consults. Whereas in the recent past, physicians and clinical staff would be paged at all hours and have to travel to the hospital to care for patients, drivers now enable and support remote access to clinical information, thereby making patient care operations more efficient.

Remote access to medical information can help healthcare providers reduce administrative costs, reduce errors, and expand accessibility. Clearly, physicians need rapid access to clinical data for proper patient care. With remote access, data from medical imaging equipment, as well as a patient history, lab values, radiology images, vital signs, and other information can be sent electronically in real-time directly to the physician who needs it, even if that physician is located at home, in another facility, or at another remote location. The physician can then provide immediate feedback to other clinical staff located on site. And patients can more readily communicate with their physicians, schedule appointments, and in some cases access their own records.

With remote access, healthcare organizations can connect to remote branch clinics, insurance companies, laboratories, transcriptionists and additional organizations. Vendors can get real-time feedback on the operations of expensive medical equipment and save costs through remote support operations. Multiple healthcare organizations may form regional information exchanges or networks to improve patient care and business opportunities. Finally, don't lose sight of the importance remote access will have when dealing with disaster recovery and/or the importance it will play in issues related to natural disaster and possible pandemics.

As healthcare organizations continue to leverage the Internet and Web-based applications as a communications channel among medical staff, patients, regional exchanges, and external corporations; privacy and security are absolutely critical. This chapter will examine the technology and techniques required to provide safe remote access to the use cases described.

THE IMPACT OF HIPAA ON REMOTE ACCESS

On December 28, 2006, CMS issued security guidance for the remote use of ePHI. CMS issued the guidance in response to a number of security incidents related to the use of laptops, portable and mobile devices, and remote access to ePHI. The guidance document recommended that covered entities place emphasis on the following:

- Risk analysis and risk management.
- Appropriate policies and procedures for the safeguarding of ePHI.
- Security and awareness training on the policies and procedures.

Before any healthcare organization pursues a remote access solution, be it with vendors, patients, or by clinical staff, the appropriate policies and procedures must be in place and a thorough risk assessment should be conducted.

The risk assessment should take into account the following:

- What business functions are driving the need to provide access (the use cases for remote access)? Who will have access—employees, vendors/contractors, clinical staff, external compliance and auditors, business partners, and patients?
- Will you issue custom equipment or allow the use of external workstations and personally owned equipment (the type of device used for remote access)?
- What security controls will be required on the end device? Has your policy documented the requirements for encryption, antispyware, antivirus software, terminal services, remote control, and firewall support on the end device? How will you confirm these settings during connection?
- What type and depth of logging activities should be enacted?
- Who supports the remote user and to what degree?
- Will remote storage of ePHI be allowed? Under what circumstances? How will ePHI stored remotely be destroyed when its use is no longer required?

As you can quickly see, the risks associated with remote access fall into three areas[1]: access, transmission, and storage. All three areas must be considered over the entire remote access application. Too often, individuals will assess only the vulnerabilities related to the particular end-point device and forget about the vulnerabilities that lie along the operational path.

The results of the risk assessment will form the basis for the subsequent policies and procedures the entity will design to protect access to ePHI during remote access operations. This chapter will focus on providing guidance related to the integrity and safety of ePHI as it is transmitted over networks and the provisioning of remote access. The reader should consult the chapter on portable device security for a better understanding of security concerns with portable devices, laptops, and media.

Policies and Procedures

As the CMS guidance points out, policies and procedures cannot be effective without sufficient dissemination and workforce education. A sound security awareness and training program must provide for the education of an entity's workforce each time a policy is created or significantly modified. Never assume your workforce will read a policy because it was signed and posted on your internal Web site. Make sure your policy addresses your standards for connectivity and the security controls that must be in place. Do not forget how critical it is that access be restricted to the amount of information necessary to complete the task at hand and based on a need-to-know. An effective policy should cover all of the expected business use cases, with specific procedures to document how each business case will function. Be sure to address security-related incidents and how to respond to them. Before using remote access technologies, the workforce should understand how to report such incidents and the ramifications for noncompliance. I would particularly like to see a procedure that actively documents the request for remote access, be it from an employee, physician, or vendor. This type of procedure provides an opportunity to better assess the risk and allows me to reinforce our policies and procedures by educating the user, then having them attest to the requirements by signature.

As an entity granting remote access to ePHI, a number of issues will quickly surface. If you are granting access to vendors, community physicians, and other individuals who may not be your entity's workforce members, your policies and procedures must address how these users will be provisioned. This may require implementation of processes to create unique user-IDs and authentication functions for these external users, as well as for your internal workforce members. You may need to consider implementing tools, such as Remote Authentication Dial-In User Service (RADIUS) or similar technology (more on this later).

Workforce clearance procedures will need to be examined before granting access to assure the remote access use cases are covered. When a workforce member leaves your organization, make sure the workforce member's access rights are removed at the same time other system clearance functions are undertaken. Implement two-factor authentication techniques (see Chapter 5) when granting remote access to systems that contain ePHI.

Establish remote access roles specific to applications. Remote users may require different levels of access based on job function. If you are employing VPNs, the use of such roles can provide additional security.

Establish logging capabilities that update to a central server. When considering audit log components and events to monitor, consider the information you may need to reconstruct what occurred over the link in the event a breach occurs. I have worked incidents for which having additional data in the audit logs would have proven beneficial.

Use secure connections and protocols for the transmission of ePHI over networks, and ePHI sent over the Internet must always be encrypted. If utilizing internal wireless access within your organization, make sure sufficient wireless security is in place and encryption is in use. For remote users, prohibit the use of offsite wireless APs to transmit ePHI (such as coffee shops and other public Wi-Fi areas).

METHODS FOR REMOTE ACCESS

Dial-In Access

Although this is considered old technology, it is still in use today. However, with the data loads demanded by healthcare, dial-in access would be time-consuming and frustrating to use for the transmission of clinical data. Dial-in works by providing a dial-up or remote access connection to the organization's network. Dial-in solutions do not tend to scale well and become more expensive and difficult to manage as the solution increases in size. With dial-in access, the remote PC requires a modem, communication software, and appropriate access to telephone network connectivity. The healthcare facility would be required to host a pool of modems and appropriate server technology to handle incoming calls.

While this technology is rapidly giving way to faster technologies, such as cable modems and DSL, organizations should not entirely disregard the technology. As the technology has been in existence for some time, it is not difficult for users to establish their own remote access farm using their PC and a modem. Some vendors still utilize modems to remotely connect to their servers for support applications.

Never assume you have no unauthorized APs within your organization. Proper remote access should funnel all remote use into a single control area, but never underestimate the ability of a user to establish a remote dial-in connection and open a hole in your defense perimeter. I have discovered users who have "hijacked" fax lines to access their personal computers after hours. Consider and establish a plan to periodically scan for phone circuits and verify they are being used for their intended business function.

Integrated Services Digital Network

Integrated Services Digital Network (ISDN) is a network service that can provide end-to-end digital communications and fully integrate technologies, such as circuit switching, private line, and packet switching with applications such as voice, data, and imaging all over existing public twisted-pair cable.

While ISDN began life as a WAN technology to connect remote facilities, it has dropped substantially in cost as newer, faster technologies develop. With this drop in cost, ISDN services may provide a suitable private connection to physician residences and small clinics. While still being available as a remote access technology, its slow speed has rendered it obsolete in favor of faster technologies, such as DSL and cable modems.

Point-to-Point Links

A point-to-point link provides a single, pre-established path from one location to another. Point-to-point lines, also referred to as "leased lines," are usually leased from a carrier. For a point-to-point connection, the carrier allocates pairs of wire and hardware to your line only. This type of circuit is based on bandwidth requirements and the distance between the two connected points.

Digital Subscriber Lines

Digital Subscriber Line (DSL) utilizes the existing telephone-cabling infrastructure and provides high bandwidth services to the home or organization. DSL uses a greater range of frequencies than ordinary dial-up services and, as a result, allow for a fast connection and higher bandwidth. Only a fraction of the telephone line capacity is being used when a normal phone call takes place (the lower frequencies). By transporting data in the higher frequencies, DSL can leverage the idle bandwidth for data. This results in it being possible to access the office or Internet while simultaneously making a phone call.

Cable Modems

A cable modem enables a PC to access the Internet via the local cable television (CATV) network. CATV coaxial cable can operate at speeds up to tens of millions of bits per second. Using traditional coaxial cable installed by CATV operators, these modems can access speeds up to 1,000 times faster than analog modems.

Cable modems are not real modems in the conventional sense. They modulate and demodulate a signal like a real modem but operate more like routers and operate much like Ethernet LANs.

Cable modems allow high-speed shared access over the same media used for cable TV delivery. Cable modems simply use the narrow band of frequencies unused for TV channels. A standard cable modem is essentially a two-way repeater connected between a user's PC (or LAN) and the cable segment. As such, everything sent through the cable modem is repeated along the segment to your local PC and everything on your network back out to the segment. Thus, the private conversations you are having with your network-attached devices may not be all that private. Every TCP/IP packet that goes out between the PC and the Internet is available for eavesdropping along the way. Therefore, another layer of security is needed to keep this sensitive information out of the hands of your neighbors.

Users within the walls of their private organizational network are accustomed to the speed and ease of access to internal resources. Today's users expect the same access to these resources through Internet connectivity, regardless of their location. The wide array of user needs makes the design of remote access harder. Indeed, one design will not meet all needs. This is even more apparent in healthcare. On the inside of the organizational firewall, access to resources is typically unrestricted except for restricting some applications or systems, whereas the firewall imposes access restrictions outside the organization. Consequently, allowing remote access often requires entry through the firewall perimeter, which must be controlled and monitored to prevent unauthorized access.

Access control mechanisms (see Chapter 5) must be able to provide granular access control—down to the application on a system if deemed necessary. Work with the assumption that a remote user can access only the components of the infrastructure he or she has been authorized to use. The security manager must establish and approve the configured access.

Unless your organization owns the physical wire itself, remote access will depend upon a service provider to provide connectivity to the user and the organization. This may come by any of the access methodologies we have just examined. Remember that regardless of the method of connectivity, the pathways by which your data travel will probably move across shared network connections. Care must always be taken to protect your data while they are in transit. Tools abound (many of them free on the Internet) to enable even the novice user to download and eavesdrop on communications traffic. The principal countermeasure in use to protect information over a data circuit is encryption.

VIRTUAL PRIVATE NETWORKS

With the availability of high-speed Internet access, more and more individuals and organizations are turning to the Internet for their communications needs. Healthcare organizations are using Internet connections as an alternative to higher-priced services, such as point-to-point links. These changes have spurred the growth of the Internet to directly compete with traditional network services. All Internet connectivity is accomplished via a standard TCP/IP suite of protocols, and any device supporting IP can connect to any other device.

The Internet is a publically shared network, and this has several disadvantages. First, by the nature of its openness, the protocols used for communication also subject the information transfer to eavesdropping, packet manipulation, and spoofing. Using a virtual private network (VPN) can address these concerns by implementing encryption, authentication, and data integrity. Second, there is no guarantee of quality on the Internet, meaning packets can arrive in any order—if they arrive at all. Internet connections are also vulnerable to traffic congestion, node and link failures, and unresponsive hosts.

The VPN standards define how the data are to be encapsulated at the source, how tunneling will occur through the protocols, and how the information will be de-encapsulated at the destination. VPNs allow the remote user to function in a network that is as secure as the local user. VPNs provide transparent transport services without requiring that applications be rewritten or redesigned. This is a benefit over Secure Sockets Layer and Transport Layer Security (TLS), which require that the application be rewritten and compiled with the support of the application.

Site-to-Site VPN

When an organization has sufficient business use cases and needs to exchange data, it may decide to establish dedicated connections between the facilities. As we have just learned, such solutions can be expensive. The organization must pay for its connection each month, regardless whether or not it is used. Typically, the organization must accurately "guess" its bandwidth requirements or face having to increase the bandwidth during its contract cycle. Healthcare organizations can connect multiple facilities, each with its own network over the public Internet by using dedicated equipment and strong encryption standards. This greatly reduces cost due to not having to lease circuits but instead using the publicly available infrastructure. When an organization chooses to connect one or more remote locations into a single private network using the Internet, we refer to this as a site-to-site VPN. Vendors of imaging and biomed equipment would often maintain expensive brick-and-mortar facilities near large medical centers to support their equipment or require expensive leased circuits to provide remote support. Today, we see more vendors requesting site-to-site VPNs using the public Internet. A VPN can grow to accommodate more users and different locations than dedicated, leased circuits.

A well-designed VPN uses several methods for keeping your data secure. Let's start by considering firewalls. You should already have a good firewall in place before you implement a VPN, but a firewall can also be used to terminate the VPN sessions. Firewalls can restrict the number of open ports, what type of packets are passed through, and which protocols are allowed through.

Another protective benefit of VPN connections is the use of encryption. Most modern VPN systems use public key encryption, which we have examined in previous chapters. This prevents individuals who may successfully compromise the physical data link somewhere within the Internet from obtaining data or eavesdropping on communications.

IPSec VPNs

Remember when we mentioned earlier that Internet communication is based on a TCP/IP suite of protocols, and this raises a series of issues? One of the issues related to the suite of IP protocols is the lack of native encryption within the protocol suite. As an answer to this shortcoming in the protocol design, Internet Engineering Task Force's (IETF) solution was to extend the IP protocol suite. This extension is known as Internet Protocol Security (IPSec) and is a collection of protocols that provides authentication and encryption at layer three of the Open Systems Interconnect (OSI) network model. IPSec has been included by the IETF in the specifications for IP version 6 (IPv6). IPSec VPNs provide enhanced security features, such as better encryption algorithms and comprehensive authentication. (See Figure 9-1.) IPSec has two key encryption modes: tunnel and transport. Tunneling encrypts the header and payload of each packet, while transport only encrypts the payload.

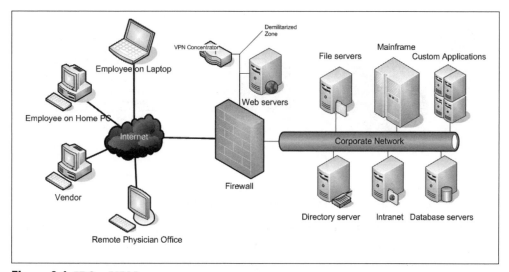

Figure 9-1: IPSec VPN.

Most VPNs rely on tunneling to create a private network that reaches across the Internet. Essentially, tunneling is the process of placing an entire packet within another packet and sending it over the net. The protocol of the outer packet is understood by the network and both end points. These end points are called tunnel interfaces.

With tunneling, you can place a packet that uses a protocol not supported on the Internet (such as Microsoft's NetBeui) inside an IP packet and send it across the Internet. You can also take a packet that uses a non-routable private address and place it in a globally addressed public packet to extend the private network over the Internet.

Secure Socket Layer VPNs

IPSec VPNs have long been the standard for VPN deployment. However, IPSec is complex. The more sites that connect to each other, the more links and secure tunnels need to be maintained. If IPSec is being utilized to provide remote access, it requires special client software to be loaded on each remote machine. This can be problematic for inexperienced computer users.

Secure Socket Layer (SSL) VPNs offer application-layer secure access using capabilities found in Web browsers. No custom clients are required; only an Internet browser, standard equipment on all personal computers. The idea behind the SSL VPN is directed at remote users. The limitation of SSL was that browsers could only access Web-based applications. SSL VPNs continue to make advances by attempting to Webify non-Web applications or by pushing Java or Active X SSL VPN agents to the remote machine on the fly. These plug-ins gave the remote computer the ability to create network layer connections comparable to IPSec, without having to distribute dedicated client software. (See Figure 9-2).

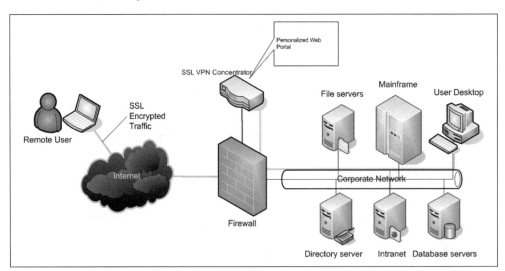

Figure 9-2: An Example of an SSL-Based VPN Solution.

IPSec VPNs are still the preferred method of site-to-site VPNs because a gateway is required with either technology, and currently IPSec is stronger within this area. Many SSL vendors don't offer site-to-site connectivity. Please note an interesting recent development with Internet Service Provider (ISP): With the increase of residential broadband services (DSL and Cable Modem) most telecommuters use IPSec-based

VPN clients. Some ISPs have started blocking IPSec traffic from residential accounts unless the customer upgrades to a business account (as opposed to residential rates). Note that these providers are not likely to block SSL-based VPNs, since SSL is used routinely for access to bank accounts and online shopping sites.

Authentication, Authorization, and Accounting Servers

Authentication, Authorization, and Accounting (AAA) servers are used for more secure access in a remote-access VPN environment. When a request to establish a connection comes in from a dial-up client, the request is proxied to the AAA server. The AAA server then checks to determine:

- Who you are (authentication).
- What you are allowed to do (authorization).
- What you actually do (accounting).

The accounting information is especially useful for tracking client use for security auditing, billing, or reporting purposes.

Authentication and Administration Servers for Remote Access

Centralized authentication systems can provide significant benefits to security administrators. They permit easier user administration for adding, modifying, and deleting users because the account management processes can be executed in one place.

RADIUS is one of the most popular authentication systems today, and its source code is readily available on the Internet. Because of its distribution via open source channels, it is available for multiple OS platforms. A RADIUS server requires two configurations—one specifying a client and one for users. The client configuration file contains the IP addresses of the clients, and a shared secret key is used to authenticate the connections. The user file contains the user ID, password, and specific authorization parameters. Parameters are passed between the client and the server using a multifield message encapsulated in a UDP packet. By utilizing the UDP protocol, a RADIUS server can process a large number of incoming connections. When a user logs into a device, an access-request message is sent to the server and is encrypted with the secret shared key. When the RADIUS server receives the request it authenticates the client by decrypting the packet using the shared secret key for the client as configured in the client configuration file. If the packet can be decrypted, the user information is validated against the user configuration file and a response is returned. If the user credentials match those stored in the RADIUS database, the server responds with an access-accept message.

Because RADIUS is open and can be extended, there are variations in how the proxy and database functionality is implemented among variants. When planning to implement RADIUS, it is best to determine functional requirements and then choose an implementation that best meets the requirements. Some factors to consider include:

- What devices will be authenticated—modems, VPNs, firewalls?
- What protocols will be supported?

- What services will be required? Will you require services such as telnet or third-party authentication?

   Terminal Access Controller Access Control System (TACACS). Cisco systems adopted the TACACS protocol to provide service for its products and then enhanced the protocols by separating authentication and accounting. Cisco also added encryption to all TACACS transmissions. Unlike RADIUS, TACACS uses a single file to store all server options and user authentication information. The configuration file specifies the shared secret key and the accounting information. When a TACACS client requests authentication of a user, it sends a request to the server during a TCP session. The request type can be an authentication, authorization, or accounting. Due to the fact that TACACS uses the higher overhead TCP protocol, it might impact server performance during peak authentication cycles.

   Which VPN should my organization use?

   The answer to this question will depend on a number of factors. Some of the factors to consider include:

- **The types of remote access needed**. Typically, care delivery organizations find themselves needing to communicate remotely with their own clinical staff, community physicians, support vendors and business partners, and patients. It is likely that one method of remote access will not satisfy all of these requirements.

- **The stage of remote access deployment**. Facilities that have a high concentration of Web-based applications and a young remote access program may be able to implement an SSL VPN-only solution. Healthcare organizations that have established long-term remote access programs will likely have a mix of different remote access technologies and are probably established with IPSec-based VPN connectivity.

- **Number of applications and application type**. Older legacy applications may not function well in the SSL VPN environment and therefore lean toward the IPSec approach.

- **Workflow needs**. The role of the connecting user will help the organization plan its remote access needs. For example, a support vendor may need to be able to take full control of a server to determine issues related to a support call.

- **Future plans**. Will the organization need to provide access to additional healthcare organizations, providers, and patients? Does the organization have plans to implement portal services?

Common Remote Access Needs Based on User Role

A recurring theme from the chapter on Identity and Access Management (Chapter 5) is that of defining roles with the care delivery organization to facilitate user provisioning and management. The continuation of the role-based principal will be a necessity when implementing remote access strategies. Let's examine some of the different roles and responsibilities related to remote access.

   Access for medical staff. Physicians and caregivers have a number of needs for remote access. Nurses, physicians, and clinical staff need access to schedules and patient appointment calendars. To provide a continuum of care, physicians need access to clinical information for decision making and support, as well as order entry. Radiologists need to remotely view diagnostic images. It can take a number of systems to support these roles and the bandwidth requirements of the connection may be high.

Access for administrative staff. Administrative staff typically wants access to specific applications, file shares, and e-mail. This workforce tends to be extremely mobile and wants to take their work with them. Moving data to portable devices to facilitate this workflow would introduce a number of high-risk security threats (see Chapter 7). The better approach is to examine the workforce needs and offer a VPN solution that can afford access to network file shares, leaving the data in the datacenter.

Administrative staff often requires continuous access to e-mail, and as a result, does not like Web-based e-mail interfaces. This situation requires the selection of a VPN solution that will allow the e-mail client to connect to the organization's e-mail server using internal "fat client" protocols. In some cases, the administrative user may request remote control of his or her desktop. If the organization receives a substantial number of such requests, it may wish to consider virtual technologies (discussed later in this chapter).

Researchers. Although research may not be much of an issue in most healthcare organizations, it is a sensitive subject at academic medical centers. Clinical research is typically performed by clinicians with academic appointments. In this environment, it is not uncommon for a clinician to have an academic office, as well as an office within the care environment. This can lead to a lot of issues when providing access. Typically, within the healthcare facilities and inside the health system firewall, access is routine. When the physician moves to his academic office, he may find himself a remote user to the organization's firewall. Often, in response to this issue, the clinical researcher will want to copy research data to a laptop or a portable device, such as a thumb drive. This introduces additional security risk (see Chapter 7). Academic research centers may benefit from virtual machines (VM) to help alleviate these types of issues. (See Figure 9-3.)

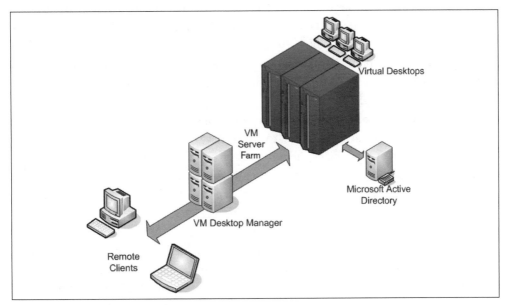

Figure 9-3: **Virtual Desktop for Remote Access.**

Vendors. Providing access to vendors and contractors can include all of the preceding use cases. It is not unlike a vendor or partner to want real-time bi-direction data feeds (such as the case with reference laboratories), remote control of servers (for diagnosis and correction of system maintenance problems), real-time telemetry (for monitoring the health of diagnostic equipment), and installation (patching and upgrade installations). Such needs often require a diverse availability of remote access tools and methodologies.

It is impossible to support all of the various remote access methodologies out there. It is up to each healthcare organization to evaluate their needs and infrastructure to develop policies and strategies for providing remote access. It is critical during the contract negotiations and purchase evaluation stages of product selection to make sure the vendor can support the product within your current remote access infrastructure. Over the past 20 years, I have had vendors request remote access with tools such as Web-based desktop sharing and Internet chat conferencing software. By examining your infrastructure and developing policies related to practices you are comfortable in supporting, providing remote access becomes more manageable.

A final word of caution about remote vendor support and vendor-provided support solutions. Be wary of placing remote managed devices behind your firewall. Such requests are becoming more frequent. I have seen this predominately in the imaging sector. An imaging vendor will want to install their own switches, routers, and firewalls within your network infrastructure. Vendors will often claim they have "certified" such components as part of their systems and cannot unbundle them without having to resubmit for FDA approval. An honest dialogue and inquiry prior to the decision to make a purchase can save hours of work and possible misunderstandings.

Contractor support. Most healthcare organizations use external contractors and consultants in some capacity. Providing access to your internal resources may require only a few hours or many months of onsite and remote connectivity. Contract workers nearly always travel with laptops, which means a foreign device connecting to your internal infrastructure that is outside your control. You must still protect your resources while providing connectivity to allow the contractor to complete his job function. When the assignment is complete, you must also make sure your organization's information stays internal to your organization and doesn't end up on a Google search engine somewhere (don't laugh…it can happen).

Network Access Control. Network Access Control (NAC) systems can prevent foreign systems from gaining access to your network until they align with your organization's security policies, thereby preventing corruption of your corporate information assets. NAC works by evaluating the security state of a system or user as it connects to the network and monitors the state of systems that are already connected. If NAC detects a system that fails an integrity check, it is capable of remediating the system or quarantining the system based on established security policy.

To benefit from NAC, an organization must define security configuration requirements, identity and access rules, and of course, actions for remediation and network control policy. Each device type will require its own set of policies that define the desired state of its operations. For example, on a laptop, it may be mandated they meet the following criteria:

- The device must be up-to-date on antivirus engine and signatures.

- The device must have the most recent security patches for its OS.

- A personal firewall must be installed and running.

- The laptop must have antispyware installed and be free of malicious software.

Identity and access policies are used to provide granularity to network access based on the user's role. When network access of a noncompliant system is constrained, policy can provide a varying degree of application access from a quarantine state, based on the identity of the user.

NAC policy will need to access current asset inventories and can help maintain an accurate database of asset information. The asset inventory will be required to handle organizational devices in which the security state cannot be baselined but must still be allowed on the network.

THE RISE OF THE PORTAL

Enterprise portals are becoming an integrated component of healthcare organizations. An enterprise portal can provide access to content, applications, information, and human resources. Established with care and planning, the portal can improve workflow, collaboration, and remote access to resources necessary to accomplish their job and take care of patients. Portals can also improve competitiveness and name branding, as well as consumer awareness.

Strong customer service and consumer awareness are created by providing client services, such as online registration and appointment scheduling, secure patient/ physician communications, online bill payment and account status, electronic prescriptions, and possible e-visits.

Portals do not come devoid of obstacles. The amount of integration with legacy applications and provision of privacy and security are two key concerns. User enrollment, maturity of portal vendor solutions, and identification challenges can all be perceived as barriers to portal deployment.

Physician portals. Many hospitals have invested heavily in clinical automation and EHRs. This brings the prospect of offering Web integration with the abundance of clinical data to extend the reach of these systems to not only internal physicians but also to affiliated physicians. Once clinical activities such as order entry, results viewing, scheduling, and clinical documentation have been made available in an online repository, the hospital can provide access and value to its remote access program.

Patient portals. Patient management and business activities, such as admitting, discharge, appointment scheduling, electronic prescriptions, and confidential communications between patient and physician, not only enhance care but provide brand recognition among the community. The current generation of consumer is spending significant amounts of time online and often obtains electronic banking services, shopping, and entertainment via the Web. It is likely the consumer will want components of healthcare accessible via Web technologies as well.

Payor functionality. Provider-payor portal services could provide cost-savings and revenue-enhancing functionality. Linkages integrated into the portal can enable providers, payors, and plan members to communicate, collaborate, and exchange information for processes such as patient eligibility, claims processing, benefits coordination, and claim status.

Supplier services. By connecting business partners and suppliers' online catalog connectivity, employees can obtain pricing information or access online requisitioning.

Things to Consider When Implementing a Portal

Implementing portals will require the commitment of resources and senior management support to be successful. The healthcare organization must have a clear and consistent vision of what it wants to accomplish with the portal. Project management will be critical and will require strong planning. Do not rely on vendors to supply this skill set. It will require the involvement of stakeholders, including administration, physicians, nursing, HR, and IT personnel.

Pilot the portal internally before deployment. This should include stress testing and vulnerability penetration testing to insure security. Do not push the product to service if problems are encountered in testing. Premature deployment can damage the project if the community cannot access the site or perceives it to be substandard. Early deployment without sufficient testing may open security vulnerabilities.

Finally, make sure your patient, physician, and employee enrollment processes are well documented, tested, and convenient. Users and patients will be reluctant to participate if they perceive the sign-up process to be difficult.

SUMMARY

Remote users frequently work without supervision and without direct access to technical support. They travel through and work in remote locations where no physical security or system monitoring is available and in direct view of persons who may wish to damage, copy, or steal their systems. Coupled with uncooperative and/or unprepared users and the recipe is ripe for disaster. No amount of technology can compensate for users who do not support the attitude of privacy and security. Therefore, healthcare organizations must make security processes mandatory and tie them to the business practices.

Security practitioners must incorporate security policy and toolsets that are not perceived as annoyances by the users. If users have sufficient permission and perceive a control to be annoying they will deactivate or circumvent the control. Security must function as an enabler to the business objectives of the organization. Security should be as transparent as possible.

Healthcare cannot depend on technology to create a strong security posture. Only by developing policies, security awareness and training, and appropriate sanction policies can an organization hope to achieve a safe operating environment. Develop policies that users can understand, and take the time to explain them. Do not expect users to understand the technologies provided to enforce security policy.

Security personnel cannot forget or become complacent toward old security exploits that may leave systems vulnerable. Old exploits and malicious code continue to circulate. If you ignore the threat, you will likely encounter it again. Remote users and foreign connected systems can provide fresh opportunities for old exploits. Remote users can fall out of date on patches and virus signatures. When they attach to the organizations' network infrastructure, infections can propagate. Internal systems can fail because they were not patched under the assumption they could not be exposed to the Internet. Biomed devices may be behind in patches due to their vendor having issue with the deployment of a patch. As more biomed equipment incorporates common off-the-shelf components such as the Windows OS, vulnerabilities within directly connected patient care devices will increase. No system should ever be allowed to connect to the network without a safety check. Healthcare organizations must consider controls such as NAC.

The lack of a comprehensive or weak encryption policy can lead to data leakage (and legal disclosure), data loss, theft, and possibly, improper access. Data that are not protected when a device is powered off, or when the user is logged off, is a severe security risk. A large number of portable devices are lost or stolen each year. Organizations must accept that remote and mobile devices will disappear and budget for the appropriate data protection.

Users must be educated on the proper use of devices outside the organization's control, such as public Wi-Fi stations and kiosk computers. This problem must be addressed with the use of VPN technologies, such as SSL-based VPNs that encrypt virtual sessions and reduce the likelihood that residual data will be left on these external devices.

Finally, weak user authentication can lead to stolen credentials. Authentication is a legacy problem that keeps causing challenges for remote access. Remote and traveling users want quick access, not complex login challenges. Working remotely and on the run will cause workers to forget to log off systems, leave equipment behind, and be unable to remain aware of their surroundings. Such situations can lead to a security challenge. Some healthcare organizations don't like the cost associated with strong authentication and multifactor solutions and may continue to use simple passwords. Examples of weak authentication can include:

- User IDs and static passwords recorded by malicious keystroke software. Such software is widely available on the Internet, and malware applications can open access to remote Web sites—uploading the stolen credentials. Most users will select one password and use it for access to all of their electronic access.

- Users who write down their passwords. The only resolution to this issue is to replace passwords with stronger methods.

This chapter has strived to make the reader aware of remote access opportunities, technical solutions, and considerations to reduce risk for remote operations. Opportunities abound for healthcare organizations that can implement safe and effective remote computing strategies.

Discussion Questions
1. Describe the risk associated with remote access to ePHI.
2. Explain the differences between IPSec, VPNs, and SSL VPNs.
3. What are the issues that must be considered when implementing a portal?

Reference

1. Excerpt from http://www.cms.hhs.gov/SecurityStandard/Downloads/SecurityGuidanceforRemote UseFinal122806rev.pdf.

CHAPTER 10

Training the Workforce

Terrell W. Herzig, MSHI, CISSP

GETTING THE WORKFORCE ON BOARD WITH SECURITY

They are your most important asset. They are also one of your highest security risks. Every day, you trust your organization's reputation, financial, and customer well-being to the hundreds of individuals that comprise your workforce. The human element is what makes your organization unique. It is also the one element that no amount of technology or policy can control. Therefore, the implementation of any successful security program depends on a sound security awareness and training program.

The entire workforce must accept accountability for your organization's security policies and controls. This includes all full-time and part-time employees, contractors, volunteers, temporary workers, and consultants. However, to gain such support, healthcare organizations must undergo changes in culture. Security awareness must focus on being an agent of such change, deeply embedding a security consciousness organizationwide, instead of making security a one-time training event that is quickly obsolete and forgotten.

Your Most Dangerous Asset: The Human Resource

A comprehensive security awareness program is mission critical for all healthcare organizations. Employees and workforce members lack the skills and experience to recognize and report security problems, take appropriate actions, and behave in a manner that complies with organization policies and practices.

A security awareness program gives the employee the knowledge to deal with actual and potential security threats that can be encountered on a daily basis, helping to create and foster a climate in which all employees are accountable for information security. The primary purpose of an information security and awareness program should be to shift the organization's culture away from a negative view of information security, often characterized by forceful, restrictive, and burdensome policies, to a positive view in which employees understand the importance of protecting information assets.

This mindset enables workforce members to understand the rationale underlying the policies and adapt to new circumstances. When faced with various security concerns, including physical access, e-mail, social engineering ploys (i.e., posing as an employee out of the office in an attempt to get an account reset) password management, and phishing schemes, workforce members will be able to make the right decisions.

To be effective, security awareness programs should focus on topics relevant to the employee's work. Time should be spent addressing the plausible threats to information assets, and delivery should be on an education level commensurate with the employee. Training should avoid technical jargon and IT details that alienate or fail to hold employees' interest. The core training program should also address issues involving how to identify and protect sensitive information, as well as how to store, transport, and dispose of the information correctly.

A few years ago (2006), I worked on an incident that involved a clinical staff person with PHI incorrectly stored in an Excel spreadsheet. During the interview, the individual told me the spreadsheet did not contain PHI. When I asked the individual to recall the fields of data in the spreadsheet, that person began listing patient name, address, medical record number, date of birth, gender, and certain diagnostic codes. After a moment, I asked why the individual told me the spreadsheet did not contain PHI when the elements that were cited were all considered PHI. The answer I received was appalling but serious: "Oh…that's not the individual's electronic record; it was just certain elements that had been extracted from the paper chart!" The nurse seriously thought that PHI was the entire medical record and not individual elements. Of significance is the fact that this individual had undergone our organization's HIPAA training program, which included a section dedicated to the 18 elements that are explicitly referenced in the regulations!

Workforce members become desensitized to the information with which they work on a daily basis. When individuals regularly see the same information, albeit for different individuals, they tend to "tune it out," a process known as *acclimation*. We all become acclimated to the data with which we work, minimizing their content sensitivity and use within our work environment.

Employee Responsibilities

An effective security training and awareness program will hold employees accountable for their actions. Whereas, in a criminal court, a defense citing ignorance of the law is not considered a sufficient defense, it sometimes will protect an employee who is fighting a policy violation. The key to avoiding such "ignorance" is to provide comprehensive policies that are properly disseminated, enabling the healthcare organization to enforce employee compliance. Awareness and training programs are a critical part of the dissemination process and must be adequately tracked. Detailed records of employee training will make the enforcement of policy easier.

Organizations must demonstrate due diligence; they must warn the employee that misconduct, abuse, and misuse of information will not be tolerated. Employees must understand that the organization will not defend any employee engaging in inappropriate behavior. Documentation showing that this understanding was made clear, in turn, can help reduce the organization's legal liability, as a defense counselor will seek to prove that an employee's alleged misconduct was not adequately defined or prohibited by the organization.

Achieving success in your security awareness program means that everyone in the organization recognizes the basic security realities. The fact is that certain people, both inside and outside the organization, may deliberately threaten information assets by tricking the employee into bypassing security procedures. Workforce members must understand that security threats are sometimes neither deliberate nor malicious and are often the result of simple error or negligence, or the result of not adhering to security policies. Employees must have a clear understanding that policies, procedures, laws, and regulations are necessary to prevent damage to the organization's reputation, financial well-being, and the safety of its employees and patients.

Contractors, Consultants, and Vendors

Contractors, consultants, and vendors are a faction of the healthcare workforce often overlooked in an organization's training efforts. Onsite consultants and contractors nearly always bring their own portable devices and require connections to your infrastructure. More likely than not, they have been trained according to their company's policies, procedures, and acceptable use. In healthcare, I have encountered many vendor contractors who did not possess a basic background in HIPAA regulations. Therefore, you can assume these workforce members need the same training as permanent workforce members. Your IT policies and procedures must be made clear, and the contractors must be monitored for policy compliance.

What are effective ways to monitor for contractor and consultant adherence to an organization's policy? For implementation of technical controls, such as antivirus, patching updates, and endpoint monitoring, consider the use of NAC tools. These tools are capable of verifying compliance with policy down to the technical component level, including the use of encryption technologies.

Additionally, contractors, consultants, and vendors, should be directed and educated (and their access monitored) to not remove data from the organization's premises without senior management or contract approval. Any moving of data should be defined, arranged, and documented in work contracts. Acknowledgement of such training and training records can be maintained just the same as documentation of training in the records of the regular workforce. Disciplinary options, which should be clearly stated in the contract, should be appropriate for contract workforce members and should include conclusive statements that define the possible legal actions that your organization may use in response to an incident.

Temporary Workers and Volunteers

Temporary workers and volunteers should undergo the same training as any other new hire. They are typically brought into the work environment and put to work immediately. This line of action can be a huge risk to the organization in terms of IT policy and procedures. First, most organizations experience a huge turnover in temporary employees. Most large organizations have their own temporary employee services, but some use an agency to locate replacement and temporary workers on limited notice. Temporary workers often have no knowledge of the environment into which they are walking, much less the policies and procedures the organization has in place. Companies with their own internal temporary pool are struggling with filling available slots and do not want to invest in the time required to train a temporary employee.

Putting a training plan in place for volunteers and temporary workers is critical however. These employee groups must focus immediately on the privacy and security compliance requirements of their new job roles. With the successful completion of training, they can both begin adjusting to the organization and learning about the organization's policies and procedures.

Organizations often do not subject contractors, consultants, and temporary workers to the same screening and background checks as other internal workforce members. If outside temporary services are being employed, the organization has no control over the pre-employment screening procedures, background checks, and hiring practices. Yet, contractors and consultants (and sometimes temporaries) often will be given highly privileged access to the organization's information assets.

The contracting organization is within its rights to require contractors to screen employees who will be working with corporate data. However, such steps are rarely taken, putting the healthcare organization at risk. The same issue applies to consultants and temporary employees, though the transient nature of the working relationship presents practical barriers to a rigid screening process. Employers consistently underestimate the ability of contractors and consultants to take advantage of even limited access to important information systems.

Former Employees

Former employees comprise individuals who no longer work at an organization. In some cases, the employee may re-enter the organization as a consultant or a contractor. In this situation, if the organization's account management practices are weak, the employee may have retained access to information resources. It is also possible for a former employee to gain access to the organization's information assets directly through "back doors," or indirectly through former associates. Workforce members anticipating conflict with an employer, or even termination, may prepare back door access to the computer system, create alternative passwords, or simply stockpile proprietary data for later use or blackmail. The Internet is ripe with cases in which separated employees have returned to exact vengeance on their former employers. Consider the recent case of the network administrator who held an entire San Francisco network system hostage by locking out the administrator accounts and not surrendering the passwords.[1] Such stories indicate a need for improved account management and better termination processes. This situation is particularly true when it involves large numbers of layoffs. Layoffs can result in a pool of disgruntled employees and former employees with access and motivation for vengeance.

COMPONENTS OF EFFECTIVE SECURITY AWARENESS PROGRAMS

For a security awareness program to be effective, it must contain certain elements. First, all new workforce members should undergo an organizational orientation. During this orientation, the employee should be educated on the organization's security and privacy policies and risk management culture. This security and privacy training should include policies on appropriate/acceptable use of information resources, such as access control procedures, e-mail use and etiquette, Internet access, social networking, portable devices, media disposal, and the handling of personal and proprietary data.

Second, educate workforce members on how to report incidents. This training would include the process to report an incident, who should be contacted, as well as who should *not* be contacted (e.g., employees should not contact the media directly), and the timeliness of reporting the incident.

Third, reminders containing basic instruction in policies, issues, and expected behaviors should be sent to all employees on a routine basis. Consider adding an annual refresh to corporate training and ongoing compliance programs. Develop and demonstrate the training efforts for distribution and understanding of new policies and changes to policy that may occur. Every new policy developed within the organization should be accompanied with an introduction and word of support from management and some form of training to educate employees.

Develop and distribute frequent updates and awareness in the threats and vulnerabilities faced on a daily basis. Too frequently, this simple task is ignored. Keep the workforce population informed about phishing scams, viruses, social engineering schemes, and other security events. Eventually the workforce knowledge and understanding of security issues will increase, and your overall security program will benefit.

Lastly, periodically conduct assessments of your training programs and awareness activities to demonstrate program effectiveness. I have experienced an increase in incident reporting following every training event. Two awareness events I find particularly effective are the "town hall meeting" and "lunch and learn" programs. If after effective training, you note an increase in incidents, realize it can't be that an organization experiences more incidents as a result of educating the workforce, so it's a situation in which training has produced an increase in the attentiveness of the workforce to security principles and privacy and security issues. However, if the number of reported incidents continues to increase without decline, then I would tend to think the program is not meeting its progress goals.

I like to use actual incident data (sanitized) in awareness and training materials. People like to be entertained and are more focused on material when it is presented in an interesting way and when a direct correlation to their particular work environment is established. I was recently invited to present a series of town hall awareness campaigns. My opening presentation began with headlines copied directly from national news stories. After briefly detailing the national incidents, I drilled down on similar incidents within our organization. Careful not to make critical remarks, I used the opportunity to explain why a particular control or safeguard works to reduce the risk of the negative event occurring again. The effectiveness of such a presentation can be measured immediately by the amount of audience participation that is generated.

Program progress and effectiveness go hand-in-hand. If your program is not demonstrating noticeable changes in attitudes and behaviors, then consider more effective means of developing, structuring, and presenting materials. Periodic assessments depend on identification of metrics that can be associated with behavior. The metrics must be developed during the design of the program to indicate whether the program is achieving the desired results. Look at numbers associated with help desk calls, incident reports, and employee evaluations.

Your program assessment must include confirmation that the training program is being conducted and has been successfully completed by each employee. Sanctions may be needed to enforce training requirements, such as the suspension of network access until the training requirements have been met. I recently encountered a medical student so belligerent to training that his clinical privileges had to be suspended until he complied with his new resident training program.

Training Methods and Technologies

Many techniques and technologies exist to deliver the security awareness message. Given that people respond better when something is presented multiple times and in different formats, I encourage the use of a variety of techniques and multiple messages. Security awareness techniques should be creative, changed frequently, and diversified across the awareness program.

After the initial training, several methods and techniques can be used to sustain awareness or launch new awareness campaigns. Among the more popular techniques are the use of newsletters, posters, Web sites, e-mail distribution lists, live events, paraphernalia, and the distribution of branded merchandise.

Newsletters. A security newsletter can be an effective tool to keep information security topics at the forefront of employees' minds. Consider using a combination of print and electronic distribution techniques. One exciting approach with which I have been involved is the use of electronic newsletters with embedded multimedia content. Electronically distributed newsletters can report back when they are downloaded and reviewed, providing feedback and metrics. Another advantage of electronic newsletters is the capability to expand the content with embedded audio, video, and hyperlinks. The newsletter can be structured to present brief, but intelligible topics that communicate an awareness fact that is expanded by the reader to pursue more in-depth information.

Don't abandon printed material. Although it is costly to print and distribute hard-copy newsletters, there is a population and market that can be reached when they pick up a conveniently placed paper newsletter and take it with them. Printed and electronic matter should contain the customary volume and issue-tracking features. These features provide for archiving and referencing past materials, and can provide proof of security awareness efforts in case of legal issues. Use graphics to brand the material with the organization's standard look and feel, which will subconsciously motivate users to review the material, as it is perceived to be endorsed by the organization's management, another awareness success factor. While each issue will be distinct, the form and layout should be consistent across issues.

Newsletters (print and electronic) should offer a consistent mix of content. The newsletter should include the following subject areas:

- How-to related articles and content.

- New security threats to the organization's assets.

- Schedules for upcoming classes, seminars, and special events.

- Planned installations and upgrades.

- Updates and refreshers on policies (especially changes). Keep it "lightweight" in this area.

Posters. Posters that impart security awareness concepts should be displayed in high-traffic and common areas, especially in spots where IT technology is heavily employed. Posters should be visually attractive to quickly catch employees' attention. The poster content must be brief and well-designed to communicate the concepts in short space requirements. Posters quickly fade into the surroundings, so frequently replacing them with new, professional designs and content is necessary. Do not print a bulk of a few poster designs with the thought of rotating the posters or reusing them after time has passed. Once a particular poster has become familiar to the workforce, it will thereafter go unnoticed, even when the poster is removed and brought back after a time.

Organizations will often supplement the use of posters by creating an electronic desktop equivalent as a screensaver slide show, which can be managed by central policy within the IT support area. However, use this practice judiciously as people will tire quickly of the slides.

Web sites. Web sites specializing in security awareness and information are great ways to keep content fresh and employees informed. The key to an effective Web site is to keep the content fresh and to get the workforce to visit the site regularly. When new information is made available on the site, use e-mail to alert the workforce. Do not hesitate to explore additional Web technologies, such as blogging and RSS feeds to help call attention to content and help workforce members disseminate the material. The site can also maintain awareness archives, multimedia support, and how-to videos, links to print articles, links to reference materials such as disaster recovery plans and downtime procedures, and live policy links.

Before creating and maintaining an internal Web site, investigate tools and programs that are already available. Reinventing a training program that may exist commercially is not an efficient use of internal resources. Examine what other healthcare organizations are doing and whether their programs are successful before deciding on an approach.

Security, management and the Web development team should work together with design and educational specialists to develop a Web site that is informative and practical. Too often, security professionals attempt to develop and implement Web projects from their isolated vacuums. The result is a Web site that appeals only to the security team. Keep items such as page load times to a minimum. Consider the constituency and where the site will be used. (I have witnessed awareness programs presented on beautiful Web sites that were not available at the organization's remote clinical sites.) Keep the technical jargon to a minimum. Never overestimate the computer literacy of the workforce. While many of the younger "digital native" citizens speak fluent computer, the middle and older generations may still not be comfortable with a keyboard and a mouse.

As with all training and awareness techniques, get feedback on the Web site. Do not be afraid to ask about what the employee liked or did not like about any feature of the awareness program. Remember that the goal of awareness programs is to make the workforce aware of the organization's security policies and practices.

Merchandise. A merchandizing program is a more expensive form of implementing awareness and training. While merchandise may not cost much on a per unit basis, storage and distribution can be expensive. Common items used in merchandising campaigns include t-shirts, coffee mugs, pens, badge holders, mouse pads, and items that I like to refer to as "attention deficit toys." The idea behind merchandising is that the items are printed with awareness messages as constant reminders of information security compliance.

The effectiveness of merchandising is questionable. These programs get the immediate and short-term attention of the workforce, but the message content is often lost unless it is reinforced through the use of other technique.

Town hall meetings, lunch-and-learns, and discussion groups. All of the ideas discussed so far are built on the same concept: live interaction with a group of individuals. One of the most effective methods to reach people is to talk to them. Much is gained in awareness programs by having an individual present at the activities. This presence not only communicates the importance of the material, but it demonstrates that management is dedicated to the program. One of the most successful awareness programs in which I participated involved small departmental meetings to discuss security awareness. These meetings are especially effective when food is served. However, beware that when you invite an audience to lunch while you attempt to entice them with the latest Internet phishing scam, you will be competing for their attention. The presentation will need to be clear, concise, well-delivered, and engaging. Otherwise, the only thing you may accomplish is leaving your employees with a case of indigestion!

SUMMARY

Security awareness and training must be an integral part of your security program. Your hospital's workforce is the first line of defense your organization has to protect its information assets.

An effective security awareness and training program must have the support of senior management. If executive management doesn't show much interest in the program, then it's unlikely that employees will take it seriously. However, if your organization can create and implement even a simple program and update it consistently, the heightened awareness may save you from an expensive and high-profile disaster.

Your security awareness and training program is a proactive control to protect the confidentiality, integrity, and availability of your IT assets. When designing your organization's security awareness and training program, senior management must set the expectations for employee behavior and what will constitute acceptable behavior.

While there are many controls that can be put into place to safeguard information, your security awareness and training program should take into consideration the practical limitations to the number and type of safeguards you can implement, and how much of your employees' time you can consume in the education process. Therefore, your security awareness and training program needs to be focused. Do not hesitate to involve representatives from all aspects of the workforce in the development and implementation of the program.

Remember, the goal of any good security awareness-training program is to get the biggest return on security for the time invested in training. To obtain a large return on security, you should plan your program to focus on the low-hanging fruit—the areas that could potentially mitigate the highest risks.

Discussion Questions
1. Discuss the information security risks posed by workforce members.
2. Describe the elements of an effective data security training program.
3. Explain the methods of sustaining awareness of data security policies.

Reference
1. Maxcer C. Jailed SF sysadmin holds parts of city net hostage. TechNewsWorld. Accessed April 17, 2009. Available at: www.technewsworld.com/rsstory/63813.html?wlc=1229448662.

CHAPTER 11

The Importance of Incident Response

Brian Evans, CISSP, CISM

HOW IMPORTANT IS INCIDENT RESPONSE?

Today's healthcare environment is competitive enough without an incident interrupting your organization's operations. However, adverse events, such as system crashes or unauthorized access to confidential data, do occur and result in negative consequences to your organization, employees, and patients. Incidents can be expensive to organizations in terms of system downtime, labor costs, fines and penalties, or loss of reputation. Patients can be adversely affected as well, with an incident resulting in delayed or interrupted healthcare delivery, identity theft, or embarrassment from a breach with their patient data. When these events happen, organizations are often faced not only with having to inform their patients of the incident—most states have enacted regulations requiring organizations to notify individuals affected by unauthorized access of their information—but with the great difficulty of keeping out of the public eye.

On top of this, organizations are required to observe the regulatory standards affecting the healthcare industry that essentially mandate an incident response program to comply with their requirements. These standards include the HIPAA Security Rule, CMS Core Security Requirements, Federal Rules of Civil Procedure-Electronic Discovery, Payment Card Industry-Data Security Standard, and the SOX Act. In reference to the SOX requirements, former Securities and Exchange Commission Chairman Christopher Cox stated: "Congress never intended that the 404 process should become inflexible, burdensome, and wasteful."[1] In other words, the intent of these laws and regulations is not to break your organization's budget but to establish a functional information security program, which includes incident response capabilities. Since some form of regulatory requirement affects your organization, it is not only good business practice to have incident response capabilities, but it is also a compliance issue.

The Health Information Technology for Economic and Clinical Health (HITECH) Act contained within the American Recovery and Reinvestment Act of 2009 (ARRA) and signed into law February 17, 2009, sets new standards for EHR programs and requires healthcare organizations to comply with new IT security-breach notification rules. The act essentially establishes a federal breach notification requirement for unencrypted health information. This means, after discovering a breach, covered entities, Business Associates, and vendors who handle PHI are required to:

1. Notify each individual whose unsecured PHI was obtained.
2. Notify the FTC.

Business Associates must notify the covered entity of any breach. Breaches affecting fewer than 500 individuals in one state must be logged and submitted annually to the secretary of Health & Human Services (HHS). If more than 500 individuals of a state are affected by a breach, notice must also be provided to prominent media outlets following the breach's discovery. Notifications required under this section must be made without unreasonable delay.[2]

Failure to bring programs into compliance since September 18, 2009, could subject organizations to fines and other penalties in the event of a breach. If HIPAA or the HITECH Act is violated due to willful neglect, HHS may be required to assess a penalty in the amount of $50,000 per violation, with no maximum penalty for multiple violations. The term "willful neglect" is not defined, but arguably that standard will apply whenever there is a failure to adopt safeguards and procedures required by law. Lesser penalties may be imposed where the violation does not result from willful neglect, or is corrected within 30 days of the date it is discovered or should have been discovered.

The secretary of HHS is required to fully investigate cases when an initial investigation of a complaint indicates possible willful neglect. Regulations projected to be enacted by 2012, will allow harmed individuals to share in penalties collected under the act, which should increase the likelihood and frequency of complaints. State attorneys general may also sue under the HITECH Act to obtain an injunction or damages of up to $25,000, increasing the likelihood of uneven interpretation of the law.

Another reason your organization should focus on incident response is that regardless of how diligently information assets are safeguarded, issues or events will inevitably occur. Organizations are in a better position now than in the past when it comes to determining the cost of an incident by calculating the labor dollars involved with response and mitigation, legal expenses, help desk calls, lost employee productivity, regulatory fines, breach notifications and so on. But even in an increased regulatory environment, there are organizations, large and small, that still react to each incident with undocumented ad hoc procedures, which ultimately wastes time and money. This lack of due diligence is a result of inexperience and a lack of fully understanding what it takes to effectively respond to and manage an incident from senior management on down. When a trained incident response team is deployed into action, it reduces the time it takes to triage the event, identify the incident, scope and contain the incident, and ultimately mitigate the issue. These actions alone can reduce costs and monetary loss along with a potential loss of reputation to the organization.

When organizations put forth the effort, they quickly find there are low-cost, high-impact incident response solutions available to them. Most of these solutions are administrative in nature, requiring a policy and an incident response plan, both of which include documented procedures and defined roles and responsibilities. More on these follows. Training and testing are other parts to the overall solution. This investment in time spent implementing and maintaining an incident response program can ultimately provide consistency and efficiency to an ad hoc, undefined process. Bottom line: incident costs are reduced with proper preparation.

Consider incident response, the process and action an organization takes in responding to an incident, as a core element to the overall information security program. An important part of the incident response program includes a policy and an incident response plan, referred to previously, which provide strategic direction, as well as detailing the actions to be taken when an incident occurs, such as who performs these actions, what reports get generated, and who reviews the findings. Implementing an incident response policy and plan provide organizations with the ability to adequately and effectively address events as they occur.

DEFINING WHAT CONSTITUTES AN INCIDENT

An incident can be defined as any event, actual or suspected to have occurred, which destroys or degrades the availability, integrity, and confidentiality of information system resources, computer-based systems, computer-maintained data files, documents or procedures. There are too many types of incidents to provide an exhaustive list, but the following are some examples:

- Multiple failed login attempts.
- A worm-infected host.
- A crashed Web server.
- A stolen laptop.
- An unusual deviation from typical network traffic flows.
- Slow access to hosts on the Internet.
- A filename with unusual characters.
- A threatening e-mail message.
- An auditing configuration change in its log.
- E-mails bounce with suspicious content.
- A confidentiality breach.

ARRA defines a breach as "the unauthorized acquisition, access, use, or disclosure of protected health information that compromises the security or privacy of such information, except where the person to whom the information is disclosed would not reasonably have been able to retain such information or in certain specified circumstances of inadvertent disclosure or unintentional acquisition of the information." Among the act's provisions is defining the date a breach is "discovered" as the "first day on which such breach is known to such entity or associate, respectively, or should reasonably have been known to such entity or associate to have occurred."[3] Those entities that must comply with notification requirements are also required to maintain reasonable security and breach detection measures that would assist them in discovering breaches in a timely manner. Violations of the Health Breach Notification Rule will be treated as unfair or deceptive acts or practices and will carry the same enforcement and penalty provisions as violations under the FTC Act.

If your organization is a covered entity already subject to HIPAA regulations; was not previously subject to HIPAA compliance, but is subject to ARRA's HITECH Act provisions; or will become subject to the FTC's Health Breach Notification Rule, then you should begin a dialogue with your legal counsel and other entities with which your organization shares PHI to be sure they are meeting the act's requirements.

Any compliance strategy under the HITECH Act should include the following initiatives:

- Take inventory of your current Business Associates and vendors.

- Identify entities with which you share PHI that may be subject to the same privacy and security rules as covered entities and carefully manage data exchanges with them.

- Update your HIPAA privacy and security policies and procedures.

- Develop or modify your existing Breach Notification Policy to comply with state and federal breach notification provisions. This may also be a good time to bring your Incident Management policies and procedures into line with Payment Card Industry (PCI) standards and other regulatory requirements and industry standards.

- Map PHI data to critical systems and assess whether the systems can meet the new standards.

- Review existing and planned systems to ensure you can fulfill the new standards' reporting requirements.

PREPARATION

To build an effective incident response program, you need to first review what is currently in place. Therefore, it is important to assess your organization's current incident response capabilities; identify opportunities for integration, redundancies, and areas of improvement; and execute a plan to mitigate those gaps. An assessment can help determine whether a centralized or decentralized model works best for your organization and what kinds of integration are necessary. There is ample literature and documentation available to provide guidance in building an incident response program. The National Institute of Standards and Technology's (NIST) Computer Security Incident Handling Guide[4] is an excellent benchmark to measure against because it is an up-to-date, relevant best practice reference.

This is all part of the Initial Phase in the Incident Response Life Cycle, as illustrated in Figure 11-1.

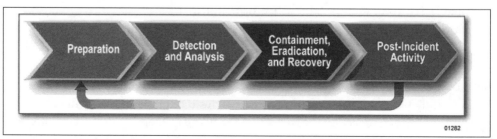

Figure 11-1: Incident Response Life Cycle.[3]

Consider the preparation phase as pouring the foundation for your incident response program. You will need a documented policy with an associated plan to lay the groundwork. You will need clearly defined roles and responsibilities, along with competent individuals who are trained and educated on the various facets of incident response. These are just a few of the basic elements you should look for in your assessment, which are covered in more detail as follows:

Incident Response Policy

Ensure an incident response policy has been developed and documented as part of the overall information security program. The policy should include the objectives and scope, as well as a section that assigns responsibility for identifying, documenting, and ensuring compliance with the relevant regulations and legal requirements. The policy should set clear direction and demonstrate executive management's support. The policy should contain an agreed-upon definition of the term "incident." It would also be beneficial to provide references to other documentation that supports the policy, such as procedures addressing incident triage and computer forensic handling. The policy should also reference the establishment of an incident response team that effectively and consistently responds to events impacting the organization, such as personnel actions, lawsuits, security incidents, and regulatory issues.

Computer Security Incident Response Team

Ensure a Computer Security Incident Response Team (CSIRT) is established as a service function responsible for receiving, reviewing, and responding to computer security incidents. The CSIRT is a group of employees who respond immediately to a variety of events, such as fraud, hacker intrusions, and confidentiality breaches. The CSIRT members devote their efforts to quickly re-establishing operations to its pre-event state. In addition, the CSIRT develops and deploys tools, procedures, and other mechanisms so that financial losses, business interruptions, and damage to your organization's reputation associated with such incidents are minimized. The CSIRT is also responsible for documenting all actions taken to restore the environment so that insurance, legal proceedings, and disciplinary actions can be fully supported. A CSIRT can either be formalized or an ad hoc team, and should have an executive sponsor with representation from departments such as Information Technology, Corporate Communications, Human Resources, Legal, Physical Security, and Business, Clinical, and Ancillary areas.

Incident Response Roles and Responsibilities

Confirm that incident response roles and responsibilities are defined and documented. One of the primary elements of an effectively managed CSIRT is the definition of roles and responsibilities. This should include assigning the level of authority for lead and supporting roles to make critical decisions, such as shutting down network connections, acquiring additional resources, and taking systems offline—or "wiping" them. Healthcare organizations often lack understanding of who should lead an incident response investigation, who should be involved, who has decision-making authority, and what roles should be played. By documenting and verifying that staff members understand their roles and responsibilities ahead of time, the organization can gain confidence that investigative issues are being addressed appropriately by the CSIRT when they occur. A good rule of thumb is to have every incident initially fall under attorney-client privilege whenever possible. The purpose of the attorney-client privilege is to protect from discovery in civil litigation those "confidential communications between an attorney and his client relating to a legal matter for which the client has sought professional advice."[4] When the privilege is asserted, it can prevent the disclosure of confidential communications. This is important because it allows your organization to investigate incidents and prepare for a potential lawsuit or regulatory inquiry without fear of having your communications revealed. If information regarding an incident is inappropriately divulged, this may compromise attorney-client privilege and become discoverable.

The CSIRT is authorized to take appropriate steps deemed necessary to contain, mitigate, or resolve a security incident. The team is responsible for investigating security incidents in a timely, cost-effective manner and reporting findings to management and other appropriate stakeholders as necessary.

Each of the following areas should have a primary and alternate member:

- Information technology.
- Help desk.
- Network.
- Servers.
- Compliance/legal/privacy office.
- Clinical and business applications.
- Internal audit.
- Physical security.

The following are general Incident Response Team Roles and Responsibilities:

Information technology:

- Designates a Recovery Coordinator who:
    - o Determines the nature and scope of the incident.
    - o Contacts members of the Incident Response Team.
    - o Determines which Incident Response Team members play an active role in the investigation.
    - o Escalates to management as appropriate.
    - o Contacts auxiliary departments as appropriate.
    - o Monitors progress of the investigation.
    - o Ensures evidence-gathering, chain of custody, and preservation are appropriate.
    - o Prepares a written summary of the incident and corrective action taken.

- o Provides proper training on incident handling.
- o Contacts qualified incident specialists for advice as needed.
- Help Desk
    - o Designated as the central point of contact for all incidents.
    - o Notifies Recovery Coordinator to activate Incident Response Team.
- Network
    - o Analyzes network traffic for signs of denial of service or other external attacks.
    - o Runs tracing tools such as sniffers, Transmission Control Protocol (TCP) port monitors, and event loggers.
    - o Looks for signs of network perimeter breaches.
    - o Contacts external Internet service provider for assistance in handling the incident.
    - o Takes action necessary to block traffic from suspected intruder.
- Servers
    - o Ensures all service packs and patches are current on mission-critical servers.
    - o Ensures backups are in place for all critical servers.
    - o Examines server logs for unusual activity.

Compliance/legal/privacy office:
- Coordinates activities with the Recovery Coordinator.
- Provides attorney-client privilege as necessary.
- Provides guidance on issues relating to legal, regulatory, and privacy issues throughout the investigation.
- Assists in developing appropriate communication to impacted parties.
- Assesses the need to change policies, procedures, and/or practices as a result of the incident.
- Advises on federal and state laws, regulatory requirements, and contractual arrangements.

Clinical and business applications:
- Monitors applications and services for signs of compromise or unauthorized access.
- Reviews audit logs of mission-critical servers for signs of suspicious activity.
- Contacts the Help Desk with any information relating to a suspected incident.
- Collects pertinent information regarding the incident at the request of the Recovery Coordinator.

Internal audit:
- Reviews systems to ensure compliance with information security policy and regulatory requirements.

- Performs appropriate audit test work to ensure mission-critical systems are current with service packs and patches.

- Reports any system control gaps to management for corrective action.

Physical security:

- Reviews facility and other physical security controls to ensure compliance with policy and regulatory requirements.

- Contacts the Help Desk with any information related to a suspected incident.

- Collects pertinent information regarding the incident at the request of the Recovery Coordinator.

Incident Response Plan

Ensure a plan is implemented, supported by technology, and based on the incident response policy. Incident escalation triggers need to be defined and based on asset prioritization, system or application type, and results of the incident analysis. The plan should specify the types of responses and techniques used, such as:

- Acquisition and analysis of data.

- Remediation.

- Referral to law enforcement.

- Escalation of incidents.

- Reporting of findings.

Incident identification and prioritization needs to be defined as well. This would include incident alerts from systems such as intrusion detection and firewalls and confirming there are appropriate routing procedures for evaluation and validation. Defined procedures that specify who needs to be notified when an incident occurs should be in place. Verify that procedures for forensic acquisition, analysis, and handling of data exist and include the platforms in your IT environment, such as Windows, Unix, Linux, or Macintoshes. Also, verify that procedures include the review and analysis of physical security logs to detect violations that correspond with the incidents. Ensure there are corrective action and remediation procedures that determine the tasks required for compromised systems. These can include patching, reconfiguring of settings, reloading data from backup media, and complete system restores. Verify that procedures include the development of an executive report of the investigation along with its findings, remediation steps, and recommendations. The report should be presented to senior management and be adequate for presentation in court if required. Agreements should be established with outside organizations, business partners, and associates using Service Level Agreement (SLA)-type language that addresses such issues as how incidents are handled, the notification and required response times, designated contacts, and communications with the public.

Breach notification procedures. Ensure the incident response plan specifically addresses breach notifications. Your organization should provide notification of a breach to patients who potentially have had their unencrypted personal information accessed or acquired by an unauthorized person. Patients should be notified in the most expedient manner possible and without unreasonable delay. Notification should be consistent with the needs of law enforcement or any measures necessary to determine the scope of the breach and restore the integrity of the compromised system. ARRA requires all notifications to be made "without unreasonable delay and in no case later than 60 calendar days after the discovery of a breach"[5] by the covered entity or Business Associate involved. The department or office responsible for controlling access to and security of the breached electronic equipment should compile a list of the names of those patients whose personal information was, or is reasonably believed to have been, accessed or acquired by an unauthorized person. This list should be compiled based on the laws of the state they reside in, since most states have specific notification laws. Depending on the circumstances, consideration should be given to notifying the major consumer credit reporting agencies about the breach and the patients affected. The breach notification should provide a brief description of the security breach, a contact for inquiries, and helpful references to individuals regarding identity theft and fraud. ARRA requires reporting of the breach to include the following:

(1) A brief description of what happened, including the date of the breach and the date of the discovery of the breach, if known.

(2) A description of the types of unsecured protected health information that were involved in the breach (such as full name, Social Security number, date of birth, home address, account number, or disability code).

(3) The steps individuals should take to protect themselves from potential harm resulting from the breach.

(4) A brief description of what the covered entity involved is doing to investigate the breach, to mitigate losses, and to protect against any further breaches.

(5) Contact procedures for individuals to ask questions or learn additional information, which shall include a toll-free telephone number, an e-mail address, Web site, or postal address.[5]

ARRA provides several methods of notice:

(1) INDIVIDUAL NOTICE – Notice required under this section to be provided to an individual, with respect to a breach, shall be provided promptly and in the following form:

(A) Written notification by first-class mail to the individual (or the next of kin of the individual if the individual is deceased) at the last known address of the individual or the next of kin, respectively, or, if specified as a preference by the individual, by electronic mail. The notification may be provided in one or more mailings as information is available.

(B) In the case in which there is insufficient, or out-of-date contact information (including a phone number, e-mail address, or any other form of appropriate communication) that precludes direct written (or, if specified by the individual under subparagraph (A), electronic) notification to the individual, a substitute form of notice shall be provided, including, in the case that there are 10 or more individuals for which there is insufficient or out-of-date contact information, a conspicuous posting for a period determined by the Secretary on the home page of the Web site of the covered entity involved or notice in major print or broadcast media, including major media in geographic areas where the individuals affected by the breach likely reside. Such a notice in media or Web posting will include a toll-free phone number where an individual can learn whether or not the individual's unsecured protected health information is possibly included in the breach.

(C) In any case deemed by the covered entity involved to require urgency because of possible imminent misuse of unsecured protected health information, the covered entity, in addition to notice provided under subparagraph (A) may provide information to individuals by telephone or other means, as appropriate.

(2) MEDIA NOTICE – Notice shall be provided to prominent media outlets serving a State or jurisdiction, following the discovery of a breach described in subsection (a), if the unsecured protected health information of more than 500 residents of such State or jurisdiction is, or is reasonably believed to have been, accessed, acquired, or disclosed during such breach.[5]

The content of the breach notification, and when appropriate, the content of both the Web site page and the press release should be reviewed and approved by management. Subsequent to the security breach notification, your organization can expect inquiries from notified patients, their relatives or spouse, and security vendors. All inquiries regarding the breach should be directed to your Public Affairs/Communications department in order to respond to any phone calls, e-mails, letters, or walk-in traffic.

Incident response training. Ensure CSIRT members are properly trained in incident response competencies by reviewing the results of your skills assessment and any gap areas identified. Often, healthcare organizations designate personnel to lead an incident response who have no previous investigative experience. Defining and developing training plans would improve CSIRT-member knowledge regarding proper principles and techniques. Enhancing the skills and knowledge of staff will provide improvements to the organization's incident response approach through better execution and decision making. Training course examples include tools for incident response, threat analysis, forensic techniques, chain-of-custody process, and legal standards.

Incident response metrics reporting. Ensure a process for collecting, maintaining, and reporting incident response metrics and trend analysis is implemented. Healthcare organizations typically lack an effective way to capture and track accurate incident metrics. Or when they do, it is usually a subset of all the incidents occurring within the organization. An Incident Response Tracking Database should be created and maintained to track all identified incidents. By centralizing all the incident response data collection and management, the resulting metrics and trending will provide a more accurate picture of your risk landscape. It also allows you to apply preventive and detective security controls and countermeasures more effectively. The security metrics should be designed so there is a relationship to the performance of the information security program and, if they were evaluated over a period of time, could determine whether the program was meeting your organization's objectives. Security metrics can be quantifiable, qualitative, tangible and intangible and developed based on a range of attributes. Metrics examples might include number of user sign-on changes for a specified period of time, number of internal and external security violations detected per week/month, and time between security alerts and remediation.

Incident response awareness training. Confirm there is an awareness program in place for management, IT staff, and the general user population. Users need to know how to identify an incident and where to report it. The training and awareness should address the varying needs and sensitivities of all users, with focused sessions for specific audiences. Management has a tendency to become anxious once informed about certain incidents. By developing and implementing an awareness-training program, the knowledge of every organizational member is increased, which allows each to more fully understand the importance of incident response, their individual responsibilities, and how to act accordingly.

Detection and Analysis

Although no two incidents are identically alike, the response process should be executed consistently. When the incident response program is activated, the CSIRT is deployed based on the suspected nature of the incident. The CSIRT's first task is to assess the situation and determine its nature and scope. Once a determination has been made, then the analysis begins. This is where the effectiveness of the preparation phase becomes critical. Your CSIRT should have the competency and expertise to perform under difficult circumstances and produce an outcome that resolves the incident. Policies, procedures, training, and teamwork all play a vital role and can affect the ultimate result if any of them are executed ineffectively.

Detection involves determining whether an incident has occurred, and, if one has occurred, then triaging the nature of the incident. The objective of the triage process is to gather information, assess the nature of the incident, and begin making decisions about how to respond to it. When the Response Coordinator is notified of a potential or confirmed incident, the following questions should be answered:

- What type of incident has occurred?
- What is the impact thus far?
- What is the projected impact?
- Who is involved?
- What is the scope?
- What can be done to contain the incident?
- What systems or applications have been affected?
- Are other systems or applications vulnerable?
- What actions have already been taken?
- What are the recommendations for proceeding?

Since incidents present a risk of legal action, all information and evidence gathered need to remain confidential to avoid accusations or rumors. The Response Coordinator should contact legal counsel before taking any action and determine if attorney-work privilege is necessary since it is unknown what will be uncovered. The Response

Coordinator should also contact physical security as necessary to provide access to secured locations and avoid setting off alarms or raising suspicions.

Evaluate simple mistakes to expose other related problems or vulnerabilities. Once the simple mistakes have been quantified or ruled out, it is much easier to determine the total scope of the incident. Examples of simple mistakes include errors in system configuration or an application program, hardware failures, and user or system administrator errors. Conduct a comprehensive Internet search to include blogs and forums to help find information pertaining to the incident.

Once the incident has been formally detected, review and analyze the data and evidence gathered. One of the first places to start reviewing evidence of the incident is in logs of the affected system(s). Determine if any unauthorized access or activity has occurred. Examine processes consuming excessive resources. Identify processes starting or running at unexpected times. Determine if there are any unusual processes that are not the result of normal, authorized activities. Review processes that prematurely terminate or multiple processes with similar names. Check previously inactive user accounts that suddenly begin to spawn processes and consume computer or network resources. Examine unexpected or previously disabled processes. Review any unusually large number of running processes. Correlate events between single and multiple sources.

Maintain a chain of custody on any log data collected. Document authorized or unauthorized access, the process names and startup times. Note the status of the process. Identify which user executed the process. Record the amount of system resources used by specific processes over time. Document the system and user processes and services executing at any given time. Determine the method by which each process is normally started and what authorization and privileges have been assigned to those processes.

If an incident is suspected to be occurring over a network, then capture network traffic through a packet sniffer. Configure the sniffer to record traffic that matches specified criteria to keep the volume of data manageable and to minimize the inadvertent capture of other information. Focus on network monitoring to detect inexplicable packets originating internally that are bound for the Internet.

Conduct an inventory on intellectual property (IP) and compare with the current inventory list. The inventory should categorize the different types of IP (proprietary knowledge, trade secrets, patents, copyrights, trademarks, etc.) and be accessible only to those with a need to know. Conduct an electronic and paper search to discover any misuse of IP. Document any misuse detected.

Gather and keep documentation used or referenced in the investigation, such as dated and signed notes, printouts, etc. Original handwritten notes should be copied and the original notes sealed as part of the chain of custody. Electronic data should be captured as soon as possible, and the process of making copies of the evidence should be witnessed. If any evidence is turned over to law enforcement, ensure every item is detailed and signed for as part of the chain of custody process.

Designate an evidence custodian to prove who has access to the evidence storage. If there is a key lock, each key should be stamped "do not duplicate." Ensure each person with access understands that he or she is required to control access to these items. Any person with access to the evidence may have to testify if the incident results in a court trial. Keep a log of all correspondence, phone calls, meetings, etc. that occur during the incident. Keep accurate and detailed notes to allow for quick retrieval of important facts as the need arises.

Once detected and analyzed, the incident should then be classified. Incident classification is identifying, understanding, and categorizing the incident. Effective incident classification helps route the response in an effective manner and ensure the proper personnel are involved.

Assign the incident an IMPACT of large, medium, or small based on the guidelines illustrated in Table 11-1.

Table 11-1: Incident Impact.

IMPACT	DESCRIPTION
Large	Incident prevents multiple users from performing tasks critical to normal operations. Incident may affect patient care or many users. Incident affects multiple users with VIP status.
Medium	Incident prevents or disrupts multiple users from performing tasks with little impact to normal operations. A single service is down or performance is severely degraded. Incident affects a single user with VIP status.
Small	A single service is degraded and users may be inconvenienced or a single user is affected.

Assign the incident an URGENCY of high, medium, or low based on the guidelines illustrated in Table 11-2.

Table 11-2: Incident Urgency.

URGENCY	DESCRIPTION
High	Incident has a direct negative effect on patient care delivery or patient safety, business operations, support or services.
Medium	Incident degrades or impairs patient care delivery or patient safety, business operations, support or services.
Low	Incident in which the impact is minimal or limited.

Apply incident determination from IMPACT and URGENCY tables against the following matrix to determine the PRIORITY LEVEL, as illustrated in Table 11-3.

Table 11-3: Incident Priority Level.

URGENCY	IMPACT		
	Large	Medium	Small
High	1	2	3
Medium	2	3	4
Low	3	4	5

The following Priority Levels from Table 11-4 determine the appropriate level of response:

1=Critical
2=Significant
3=Moderate
4=Negligible
5=None

Table 11-4: Incident Response.

PRIORITY	RESPONSE TIME*	DESCRIPTION
1	30 mins	Critical – Incident prevents multiple users from performing tasks critical to normal operations and may affect patient care in the same office or multiple offices. No work-around available.
2	30 mins	Significant – Incident prevents multiple or single users from performing tasks critical to normal operations. No work-around readily available.
3	4 hours	Moderate – Incident does not require immediate attention. Function is disrupted or impaired with little or no impact to the organization. A work-around is available.
4	4 hours	Negligible – Incident is non-critical in nature. Timing of the service is at the discretion of the user or availability of support resources.
5	8 hours	None – Incident is non-critical in nature. A single user is inconvenienced. The timing for providing the service is at the discretion of the provider.

* Response Time: The time that elapses between initial notification of the incident to the Help Desk and the time support personnel respond.

Containment, Eradication, and Recovery

After the detection and analysis phase, the incident evolves into something similar to a project, for which resources are added and removed as objectives are achieved or new problems arise. The goal of containment is to limit the scope and magnitude of an incident to keep it from worsening. It is important to secure the system or area. Do not alter the system in any way until a backup has been completed. Keep the area pristine and unaltered.

Determine the risk of continuing operations. Decide whether a system should be shut down entirely, disconnected from the network, or be allowed to continue to run in its normal operational status so that any activity on the system can be monitored. If a compromise is determined, then immediately disconnect the compromised system from the network until a forensic analysis is completed. If there are business reasons that preclude disconnection, then consider placing a firewall directly in front of the compromised system and establish an Access Control List (ACL) to preclude an attacker's access or filter incoming and outgoing connections to and from the compromised system at the network perimeter. Review logs and file signature databases from other systems on the same subnet and from systems that regularly connect to the affected system(s).

Focus network monitoring to detect inexplicable packets originating internally and bound for the Internet. Review network or Internet connections. Telnet and File Transfer Protocol (FTP) should be allowed only to systems that absolutely need to provide these services. Run as few services as possible on Web, Domain Name System (DNS) servers, and mail relay systems and ensure they are well protected.

Obtain a full disk-to-disk backup as soon as there are indications that a security-related incident has occurred on a system(s) using disk imaging. Use new media to avoid overwriting old information. Perform all digital evidence gathering and analysis on bit-by-bit duplicates of the originals. Be sure to thoroughly document all collection procedures to include when data were collected, what data were collected, how the data were collected, and by whom. Properly identify each step taken. To help maintain authenticity, be sure to keep the image creation time and MD5 hash creation time as close together as possible. If an error is made during the collection process, thoroughly document the error and go on. If in doubt, consult legal counsel on the proper evidence collection procedures for specific incidents.

Conduct a forensic investigation and analyze the evidence on the backup copy. Determine if there has been any compromise or unauthorized access to sensitive information. Establish whether a compromise occurred and the source or individual involved. Determine the timeframe of the compromise. Preserve all potential electronic evidence on a platform suitable for review and analysis by a court of law if needed. In the case of system compromise, change passwords on the compromised system and all systems with which it interfaces.

The goal of eradication is to mitigate the factor(s) that resulted in the incident. Determine cause and symptoms of the incident. Conduct a comprehensive review of the data and evidence gathered during the previous phases. If there is insufficient evidence to arrive at an exact understanding of how the incident occurred or exploited a weakness, then list all realistic possibilities based on available information. From what is possible, collectively develop scenarios to explain what has occurred.

Remove the cause of the incident. In the case of malware infestations, eradication requires removing the malware from all systems and media with antivirus software and other means necessary. Recognize the potential for reinfection, given that it may be difficult to disinfect all media to include backup media. In the case of network intrusions, determine whether the attacker has modified the compromised system in any way (i.e., alterations of system binaries and files, installation of attack programs, creation of "backdoors" into the compromised system).

Perform a vulnerability analysis by using a vulnerability scanning tool to determine whether configuration and software versions need to be updated. Confirm proper patches and security fixes have been applied. Ensure other platforms within the organization are not vulnerable to the factor(s) that allowed the compromise.

Improve your organization's defenses by implementing appropriate protection such as firewall and/or router filters, moving the system to a new name/IP address, or porting the machine's function to a more secure operating system. Verify the correct implementation of those protection procedures.

In the recovery phase, the task is to restore the environment to its normal business status. Restore the system by conducting a complete restoration from backups or reload the entire system. Ensure that no compromised code is being restored. If no backups were made prior to compromise, rebuild the system from CD-ROM or other trusted media and apply patches, or use a backup from a similar system that has not been compromised. Validate the system by verifying that the restore operation was successful and the system is back to its normal condition. Run the system through a test plan or its normal tasks while closely monitoring by a combination of techniques, such as network loggers and system log files.

Decide when to restore operations by briefing management and system owners on recovery tasks and provide recommendations as to when operations can be restored.

Once the system is back online, continue to monitor periodically. Prepare a report for management to include:

- The chronology of events.
- Actions taken during the incident.
- Estimates of damage/impact.
- Costs of the incident to include personnel time invested and time necessary to restore systems.
- Follow-on efforts needed.
- Policies or procedures that require updating.
- Efforts taken to minimize liabilities or negative exposure.

The following is a sample outline to be used when completing the incident report:

1. Executive Summary
   a. Include an overview of the incident.
   b. Include Impact, Urgency, and Priority Levels.
   c. Determine if compromise has been contained.
2. Background
3. Initial Analysis
4. Investigative Procedures
   a. Include forensic tools used during investigation.
5. Findings
   a. Number of accounts at risk, identify those stored and compromised.
   b. Type of account information at risk.
   c. Identify ALL systems analyzed. Include the following:
       i. Domain Name System (DNS) names.
       ii. Internet Protocol (IP) addresses.
       iii. Operating System (OS) version.
       iv. Function of system(s).
   d. Identify ALL compromised systems. Include the following:
       i. DNS names.
       ii. IP addresses.
       iii. OS version.
       iv. Function of system(s).
   e. Timeframe of compromise
   f. Any data exported by intruder
   g. Established how and source of compromise

6. Recommendations

7. Contact(s) and Incident Response Members Involved

The incident should not be closed until operations are restored to normal and problems are rectified. When all of the objectives are achieved and the incident is resolved, the life cycle process moves into the post-incident phase.

Post-Incident Activity

When the containment, eradication, and recovery phase is finished and operations are back to normal, it is time to analyze what happened and how your organization performed during the incident response. The goal in this phase is to learn from the incident by searching for lessons that will improve the response process in the future. Conduct a lessons learned meeting and summarize the incident from the incident report. During this meeting, the incident is analyzed to determine its root cause, and the effectiveness of the response is evaluated. Gather responses, disagreements, additions, and suggestions from all stakeholders. The following are sample questions to ask during the meeting:

- Was there sufficient preparation for the incident?
- Were there adequate resources available?
- Did detection occur promptly?
- What tools could have helped the process?
- Was the incident sufficiently contained?
- Was communication adequate?
- What difficulties were encountered?

It is important to conduct a root-cause analysis and identify any flaws or weaknesses that enabled the incident to affect your organization. The forensic analysis should allow you to sift through the electronic evidence to ascertain cause-and-effect relationships. Your organization should attempt to calculate the cost of your response, which would include any purchases and labor expenses. Create an action plan from the meeting by summarizing the outcome. Submit the plan to management with findings and a prioritized set of recommended changes, cost estimates, high-level project schedule, and the advantages/disadvantages of implementing the recommendations.

Finally, establish a process to annually review and test the incident response plan to ensure it remains viable and up-to-date. A current and complete incident response plan provides your organization with the confidence that the response strategy has been thoroughly mapped, that suitable measures will be taken in the event of an incident and that all personnel understand their response roles.

Risk Assessment

Threats that can ultimately impact your organization's information assets are constantly evolving. New systems and applications are continually being introduced into your IT environment with some potentially lacking proper security testing prior to implementation. Add to this the ever present and fallible nature of humans. All of this adds up to a dynamic environment that requires periodic and consistent revisiting to ensure threats and vulnerabilities are identified as early as possible so appropriate mitigation measures can be taken. As a result, periodic risk assessments, as discussed in Chapter 2, are an integral component of a successful and effective incident response program. The risk assessment should address such areas of risk as intellectual property, revenue impact from business interruptions, liability to business partners, and legal compliance with regulatory requirements and standards.

Incident Response Guidelines

By their random nature, incidents can be a challenge and more so in attempting to manage what is typically a disorganized and fluid situation. An incident response program can best position your organization to handle this type of challenge by incorporating several foundational guidelines:

Leadership. There is no special formula for leading a response to an incident. The basis for the leadership that is required can simply be the personality and character of an individual who leads and the relationship created with those who are led. Good leadership assesses the skills and capabilities of the individuals who will be involved in the response and adapts to the situation. It is imperative to create an incident response program that supports the overall life cycle from start to finish and provides the structure necessary to be effective. As a result, the program supports the CSIRT that works in unison and does not solely rely on one individual or leader.

Flexibility. Most incidents start out appearing to be one thing but end up as another, which makes these situations hard to plan for and predict. Therefore, it is important to take this uncertainty into account and allow your response to be flexible. This means that your CSIRT should apply the right tools for the right problem and be prepared to adapt and change given the situation. Successful management of disruptive incidents depends on a flexible incident response program that mobilizes and deactivates resources based on response needs.

Scalability. Your incident response program must be scalable to meet the needs of incidents, both large and small. Your approach should scale so resources can be summoned or released depending on the needs of an incident. This would include areas such as internal audit, legal, human resources, facilities, physical security, IT, and various clinical and business units.

Consistency. Personnel are added and removed as needed. However, because all personnel use consistent procedures and understand their roles and responsibilities, response and mitigation times are reduced. The goal is to consistently apply structure to disorder.

Structure. The structure must be able to expand or contract as the size or severity of the incident changes. Managing disruptive incidents requires quick decisions and, therefore, does not operate well under siloed bureaucracies following differing chains of command.

SUMMARY

The HITECH Act takes HIPAA enforcement from a reactive, complaint-driven system to a more proactive approach, driven by audits and enforcement activities that are funded by more stringent civil monetary penalties. As a result, a lack of compliance can become costly to your organization. However, failure to effectively respond and mitigate an incident can be costly to your organization as well. Losses may be suffered as a result of the failure itself or costs may be incurred when recovering from the incident, followed by more costs to secure systems and prevent further failure. Therefore, it is imperative for your organization to have a documented incident response policy and plan with defined roles and responsibilities and a well-trained team. These elements are marks of an effective incident response program, the implementation of which can result in preventing losses, preparing your organization for the next incident, and ultimately saving money in the process.

Discussion Questions

1. Why is an incident response policy important?
2. I doubt my manager has read the incident response policy document. Why should I?
3. As an employee, am I supposed to know all of the stuff contained in an incident response policy?
4. Why should my organization be concerned about incident response when we have not experienced any hacking or other events?
5. How do I know which patients to notify if a laptop is stolen?
6. Where can I get information about identity theft?

References

1. U.S. Securities and Exchange Commission. SEC approves new guidance for compliance with section 404 of Sarbanes-Oxley [online]. May 23, 2007. Accessed July 14, 2009. Available at: www.sec.gov/news/press/2007/2007-101.htm.

2. See page 112 of the Recovery Act: Available at http://frwebgate.access.gpo.gov/cgibin/getdoc.cgi?dbname=111_cong_bills&docid=f:h1enr.pdf. As of July 14, 2009.

3. Page 146 of American Recovery and Reinvestment Act located at http://frwebgate.access.gpo.gov/cgi-bin/getdoc.cgi?dbname=111_cong_public_laws&docid=f:publ005.pdf.

4. Scarfone K, Grance T, Masone K. Computer security incident handling guide: recommendations of the National Institute of Standards and Technology. NIST Special Publication 800-61;Rev 1. Accessed July 14, 2009. Available at: http://csrc.nist.gov/publications/nistpubs/800-61-rev1/SP800-61rev1.pdf.

5. Breach Notification Rule Accessed October 19, 2009. http://www.hhs.gov/ocr/privacy/hipaa/administrative/breachnotificationrule/index.html.

6. See page 147 of the Recovery Act: Available at http://frwebgate.access.gpo.gov/cgi-bin/getdoc.cgi?dbname=111_cong_public_laws&docid=f:publ005.pdf.

CHAPTER 12

Disaster Recovery and Business Continuity

Tom Walsh, CISSP

NEWER CONCEPTS IN CONTINUITY AND RECOVERY

In the past decade a deluge of new technology has integrated into the daily lives of business people, creating a greater dependency on that technology. As this book's focus is on privacy and security, an important question to ask at this point is whether business continuity and disaster recovery planning have kept pace with technology.

An example to consider occurred on July 29, 2008, while I was working at a hospital near Los Angeles; we experienced an earthquake of 5.4 magnitude, with an epicenter near Chino Hills (a community near Los Angeles). Within minutes, cell phones, as well as land lines, became nonfunctional, not because of damage from the earthquake, but due to an overload from the volume of simultaneously placed phone calls. Within this context, consider that most disaster recovery plans are based upon an organization's ability to quickly contact the right personnel to respond to an incident. How effective is the plan without a dial tone or cell phone connectivity?

In a related example, one of the lessons learned from those who stayed behind and worked in New Orleans area hospitals during Hurricane Katrina, is that even when land lines had failed and cell phones had no signal strength for voice communications, text messages were successfully transmitting. This is because text messaging uses smaller amounts of bandwidth. I tested this myself during the California earthquake.

Using e-mail, I sent a text message to my son's cell phone. My son, who was in Kansas, was able to receive my message when a call would not go through. Using text messaging via e-mail could be an alternative means for communication in a disaster. However, this information was not in the Hospital Incident Command System (HICS) plan, which relied solely on traditional telephone service being available to contact key employees. Since then, the plan has been updated to include information on how to send text messages using e-mail.

The hospital created a distribution list containing the cell phone numbers and carrier service used (needed for sending a text message via e-mail) of the key staff responsible for incident response. Now, the hospital's operator can create and send one text message, immediately reaching the cell phones of key managers and directors on the distribution list and saving time, which is critical in the first few moments of any incident or disaster. Figure 12-1 has a sample listing of the e-mail address structure for sending text messages via e-mail by some of the most common cell phone carriers.

Service Provider	Email Address for Text Message
Alltel Wireless	*number*@message.alltel.com
AT&T Wireless	*number*@txt.att.net
AT&T Mobility (formerly Cingular)	*number*@txt.att.net *number*@cingularme.com
Boost Mobile	*number*@myboostmobile.com
Cricket	*number*@sms.mycricket.com
Qwest	*number*@qwestmp.com
Sprint (PCS)	*number*@messaging.sprintpcs.com
Sprint (Nextel)	*number*@page.nextel.com
T-Mobile	*number*@tmomail.net
US Cellular	*number*@email.uscc.net
Verizon	*number*@vtext.com
Virgin Mobile (USA)	*number*@vmobl.com

Figure 12-1: **Sample E-Mail Addresses for Sending Text Messages. (From www. email-unlimited.com/stuff/send-email-to-phone.htm. Used by permission.)**

This chapter covers some newer concepts relating to business continuity and disaster recovery planning, such as the example about text messaging given earlier, and the need for cultural change away from the traditional planning.

COMPONENTS OF A SOUND DISASTER RECOVERY/BUSINESS CONTINUITY PLAN

Most organizations have either a business continuity plan (BCP)* or a disaster recovery plan (DRP), or hopefully both since each should be unique. While there are many similarities, it is worth noting the differences between a BCP and a DRP as outlined in Figure 12-2.

It has been shown that, during real-life disasters, companies with solid business continuity and/or disaster recovery plans survive a business disruption. The disaster that occurred on 9/11 in New York City, resulting from terrorist attacks, showed that

---

* Within the United States Federal government, the term, Continuity of Operations (COOP), is used for business continuity, since the government does not consider itself to be a "business." In this chapter, business continuity and continuity of operations will mean basically the same thing.

companies that do not have plans, or do not have decent plans, usually do not endure for long after a disaster strikes.

Business Continuity Planning	Disaster Recovery Planning
Addresses the operational procedures to allow the business to continue to perform its mission in a crisis situation	Addresses the technology and data needed to allow the business to continue to perform its mission in a crisis situation
The goal – Process recovery Ensuring ongoing business operations	The goal – Data recovery Recovering quickly from an outage
The plan's focus – People and processes Keeping vital business functions operating, even if only on a limited basis May include operational procedures in the absence of information technology	The plan's focus – Technology and data Systematically restoring mission critical information systems in the aftermath of a disastrous event affecting the data center or network operations center
The responsibility – Usually with business operations, facilities, or the safety engineer	The responsibility – Usually with the information technology (IT) or information services (IS) department
Strategy – Modeling the business	Strategy – Resiliency

Figure 12-2: The Differences Between Business Continuity and Disaster Recovery Plans.

How does an organization know if it has a solid plan? The simple answer is that any plan that helps the organization quickly recover and get back to business is solid. Aside from actually having to implement the plan, and perhaps learning the hard way that a plan is inadequate, how does an organization evaluate the soundness of its plans? Plans should have some the following characteristics:

- **Mission/business focus.** Maintaining high availability is no longer an option; it is a business necessity. Those responsible for writing either type of plan must have an in-depth understanding of business goals and priorities. While the purpose of a BCP (ensuring ongoing business operations) and a DRP (recovering quickly from an outage) vary slightly, both are in place ultimately to support the organization's mission and business operations. A common mistake is for the BCP and/or the DRP to be created without first conducting a Business Impact Analysis (BIA). Without first conducting a BIA, the plans determine the restoration priorities in a vacuum and possibly without an understanding of business workflows and dependencies which should drive the prioritization of response and recovery. Additionally, the BIA aids department managers in understanding their dependence on IT and how it impacts their ability to meet their department's mission.

- **Risk-based.** Before writing either a BCP or a DRP, a risk assessment or a hazard vulnerability assessment (HVA) should also be conducted. The HVA is used to identify threats (what could happen and the probability of things going wrong), current controls used to protect the business, and evaluate the potential impact on the business if the threat is realized. In the business world of diminishing resources, it makes sense that a sound plan be based upon reasonably anticipated threats, rather than trying to write a plan to address every conceivable threat. The challenge of any risk analysis is to quantify the impact of a business interruption.

- **Concise procedures.** "The bigger the binder, the better the plan, right?" Wrong. Being thorough does not mean attempting to address every possible threat or scenario. Consider this—in a crisis, will people take the time to sift through a plan in a huge binder to find what they need? Probably not. Other healthcare organizations have survived disasters with short, concise plans. On the other hand, if too little detail is provided, it may take longer for the organization to recover. Perhaps the best plan is based upon the "Goldilocks approach"— not too long, not too short, but just right.

- **Well-written.** The last thing you need in a crisis is a novel. In fact, checklist formats are often preferred over wordy paragraphs in these situations. An additional benefit is that the checklist serves as a log used to track completed tasks. Figure 12-3 is an example checklist.

✓	Task	Date & Time	Name	Status / Notes
Assessment				
	Quickly try to get a handle on the situation while waiting for additional help			
	Assess the scope of the incident or disaster:			
	Physical condition of the building / data center			
	Network connectivity – Internal / external			
	Telephone systems			
	Applications and/or systems affected			
	Estimate the overall impact of the incident			
Mobilization Procedures				
	Contact the members of the Incident Response Team (IRT) using the contact information in the Appendix			
	Call for additional help from IT staff and other key personnel using contact information in the Appendix			
	Have IRT members and IT staff report to the designated staging area			
	Require all other personnel responding to the incident to first check in (by phone or in person) with the Incident Commander to verify their role and assignments			
	Remind staff members not to discuss any details of the incident with their family or friends or with the news media			

Figure 12-3: Sample Checklist.

- **Easy to read.** Plans should be written in easy-to-read fonts and in a font size no smaller than 12-point. A good rule of thumb for gauging the readability of a plan is to try reading it in a completely dark room, using only a flashlight. Consider bolding text to make sure that important telephone numbers and contact information are easy to read.

- **Uses generic job titles rather than names.** People come and go and change roles. It is better to refer to job titles, such as the director of radiology, within the main body of the plan, rather than use the actual name of the current director. Actual names should only appear in the appendices section of the plan because this is the section of the plan that contains information that is frequently updated.

- **Defines the command structure and responsibilities.** Two common questions asked in a disaster situation: "Who is in charge? What can I do to help?"

  o **Incident command.** The plan should clearly address who is in charge and the process for succession of the role of incident commander. It can be unproductive and confusing in a crisis when two people are giving conflicting orders. Plans should be written to assume that the first person on the scene with the highest level of authority, or the most seniority by default, becomes the incident commander. This person retains the commander role until he or she is willingly replaced by someone else with more authority or seniority. A common mistake is that the plan is based upon the assumption that certain key individuals will always be available to take charge of the situation.

  o **Defined responsibilities.** Plans should outline roles and responsibilities of response team members in an easy-to-read, bulleted list. When writing the plan, it is important to make sure that the responsibilities are clearly delineated to avoid overlapping of duties.

- **Uses appendices.** Information that is subject to frequent changes should be listed in the appendices section rather than in the main body of the plan. Examples of information to keep in the appendices include names and contact information for senior management, the primary incident response team members and their alternates, departmental call lists, organizational charts, inventories, vendor contact and contract information, and other external organizations' contact information.

- **Specific instructions.** Specific instructions for evacuation, shutting down equipment, alternate workflows and processes, and stopping and resuming business activities need to be a part of the plan. Checklists and illustrations may be more helpful in this than verbose descriptions. Plans created in electronic format could include hypertext links to documents or files for more detailed instructions. Figure 12-4 provides ideas for creating and maintaining plans in electronic format.

- **Training requirements.** This information should be listed toward the back of the plan and should include training requirements for incident response team members, employees responsible for rescue or salvage operations, and general training requirements for all employees at an organizational level, such as familiarity with the code system within a hospital. Each department should also train its employees on downtime procedures and the location of the department's contingency plan.

- **Exercising and testing.** An untested plan is just a fantasy. Only when a plan is exercised and/or tested will some deficiencies in strategy and planning be discovered. A good plan has provisions for creating scenarios and ground rules to be followed for conducting periodic evaluation and testing.

- **Plan maintenance.** Phone numbers and other important contact information should be periodically reviewed and updated. Maintaining and controlling printed copies of the plans can be burdensome if the plan is primarily distributed in paper format. It is recommended that plans be maintained primarily in electronic format with very few paper copies (see Figure 12-4 on electronic plans for more information).

- **Senior management approval.** Plans, no matter how well-written, require review and support from senior management. Even when senior management was involved in the development of the original plan, it is still a good idea to get their input and approval again. Over the years, business priorities may have changed and the business assumptions upon which the foundation of the original plan was created may have eroded. Senior management should also at least have an opportunity to review any results from exercising or testing the plan. Management does not like surprises, and therefore, needs to know if the current plans are inadequate. Senior management's approval could be in the form of a dated memo or their signature at the very beginning of the plan.

Traditional disaster recovery procedures required printed copies of the plan to be assigned and tracked. Often directors and managers working in information technology were told to keep a copy of the plan with them. Many kept a copy of the plan in the vehicle in which they would normally drive to work. While it sounds like a good idea, often it wasn't feasible or practical. The person responsible for the administration and maintenance of the plan would keep an inventory of who had a copy of the plan. Updating the plan would require the staff to bring their binder to the administrator so that old pages could be replaced with updated pages.

Reasons for leveraging technology and storing plans *securely** on a USB drive include:

- **Effortless to transport.** Carrying a USB drive is preferred to carrying a three-inch binder filled with paper

- **Easier to read.** Plans can be more easily read on a computer or laptop screen. The size of documents can be expanded making it easier to read smaller print fonts. In the event that there is a loss of power, no problem. Almost all organizations have laptops readily available. The average laptop can run four to six hours without electricity, depending on the battery pack installed. Additionally, monitors and laptop screens are backlit, making an electronic plan easier to read in the dark.

- **Faster for finding information.** Having a plan in electronic format allows for key word searches within the document, as well as hypertext links that can be used to find additional information such as power on or shut down procedures for a server, or linking to a spreadsheet storing inventory, and system configuration information.

- **Trouble-free updating.** When the plan needs updating, no more hunting down copies of the plans to remove old pages and insert new ones. Instead, everyone carrying a copy of the plan plugs their USB device into their computer workstation and downloads the latest version of the plan from a network drive folder.

It is still a good idea to have at least one or two paper copies of the plan. One copy should be securely stored off-site, preferably at the alternate site used for disaster recovery.

* If the plan is kept in some form of portable electronic media, consider either password protecting the files or using encryption.

Figure 12-4: Electronic Plans.

Figure 12-5 provides a checklist for assessing either a BCP or a DRP.

Evaluation Criteria	Status
Was a business impact analysis (BIA) conducted and signed off by key stakeholders prior to developing business continuity and disaster recovery strategies and plans?	
Does the plan specify the meaning of "disaster," include a flow chart, or define the triggers for declaring a disaster and activating the plan (including who has the authority to activate the plan)?	
Does the plan include emergency evacuation procedures?	
Are essential departments and business functions that cannot be interrupted identified in the plan?	
Does the plan heavily depend on telephone and cell phone communication systems working?	
Do response team members know where to report for duty following the activation of the plan?	
Are there provisions in the plan for addressing the situation when family members accompany an incident response team member when they report for duty?	
Is there a checklist of emergency preparedness items (equipment, tools, and supplies) that incident response team members are expected to have when responding to a disaster or an incident?	
Are there at least one or two copies of the plan in paper format, with at least one copy at the alternate recovery site?	
Does the plan address how communication with employees, patients, physicians, and business partners will be maintained?	
Are there instructions, directions, and/or maps for moving and restarting operations at an alternate facility?	
Does the plan prioritize the order for restoring information systems?	
Does the plan describe critical system dependencies such as interfaces or network connectivity?	
Does the plan describe the location and instructions for obtaining access to media and vital records kept in an off-site storage facility?	
Are lists of equipment, tools, or supplies necessary for salvaging electronic equipment in the plan?	
Are there provisions in the plan to empower employees to make emergency purchases of needed equipment and supplies?	
Have contracts with vendors been written that specify expected service level agreements for emergencies such as quick shipments and preauthorized purchase agreements?	
Does the plan provide instructions for hiring temporary workers and/or redeployment of staff?	
Are there samples of paper documents or forms, which are used in the absence of information systems, included with the plan?	
Is the public spokesperson for the organization identified in the plan?	
Are there prewritten scripts for communications with the public and news media?	
Has the plan been exercised or tested within the last year?	
Does the plan require a post disaster debrief meeting to evaluate the plan's effectiveness?	
Has the contact list of employees and vendors been validated for accuracy?	
Is there a link between change control process and the disaster recovery plan?	
Has the plan been reviewed by an impartial third-party?	

Figure 12-5: Checklist for Assessing Plans.

Plan Structure

Figure 12-6 provides a suggested outline for a BCP. Figure 12-7 provides a suggested outline for a DRP. The plans have many similarities. Another resource for developing the structure of a plan can be found in the National Institute of Standards and Technology (NIST) Special Publication 800-34 Contingency Planning Guide for Information Technology Systems.

Document Change History and Plan Approval

Overview

- Goals and objectives
- Scope
- Assumptions and exceptions

Activation

- Declaration
- Evacuation (if needed)
- Notification

Response

- Responsibilities
- Mobilization procedures
  - Response teams
  - Public Relations
- Assessment and control
- Security and safety
- Escalation procedures

Recovery

- Restoring critical business processes
- Business resumption procedures
- Emergency procedures

Restoration (Back to Normal Operations)

- Terminating emergency procedures
- Plan deactivation

Training

- Audience and content

Exercises and Tests

- Developing scenarios
- Coordinating and scheduling
- Reporting

Plan Responsibility and Maintenance

- Distribution
- Version Control

Glossary of Terms and Abbreviations

Figure 12-6: Suggested Outline for a Business Continuity Plan.

Document Change History and Plan Approval

Overview

- Goals and objectives
- Scope
- Assumptions and exceptions

Activation

- Declaration
- Evacuation (if needed) and equipment shutdown procedures
- Notification

Response

- Responsibilities
  - Incident commander
  - Incident response teams

Assessment and Control

- Safety and security
- Damage assessment
- Salvage

Recovery

- Activation of alternate recovery site (if needed)
- Resource management and logistics
- Procedures for restoring critical information systems

Emergency Mode Operations

- Emergency procedures for information technology department

Restoration to Normal Operations

- Systems cut-over
- Plan deactivation

Training

- Audience and content

Exercises and Tests

- Developing scenarios
- Coordinating and scheduling
- Reporting

Plan Responsibility and Maintenance

- Distribution
- Version Control

Glossary of Terms and Abbreviations

Figure 12-7: Suggested Outline for a Disaster Recovery Plan.

RECOVERY OBJECTIVES—CAN YOUR CURRENT PLAN SUPPORT THE MISSION?

Because shorter recovery times are critical in a digital age, it is essential that the appropriate solution be selected for data and system resiliency. Generally speaking, it is easier to design resiliency into a system rather than go back and acquire a recovery solution.

There are two terms used regarding recovery objectives:

Recovery Time Objective (RTO) is the maximum tolerable downtime or interruption in access to an information system that a department could handle before the impact would be unacceptable to either patient care or business operations. Depending on the criticality of the mission of the department and existing workarounds or manual processes, RTOs can range from minutes to days. Figure 12-8 illustrates sample RTOs for some hospital departments.

Intensive Care Unit	30 min
Surgery	1 hr
Pharmacy	1 hr
Medical/Surgical Units	1 hr
Cardiology	2 hrs
Health Information Management	2 hrs
Emergency Department	4 hrs
Dietary Services	4 hrs
Radiology	4 hrs
Admitting (Patient Access)	8 hrs
Respiratory Care	12 hrs
Lab	1 day
Environmental Services	1 day
Finance	2 days
Billing & Patient Accounting	2 days
Human Resources	2 days
Facilities Maintenance	3 days
Marketing	1 week

Figure 12-8: Sample RTOs for Some Hospital Departments.

Recovery Point Objective (RPO) is the potential loss of information due to the frequency of the backups. For example, if backups are created daily, the RPO equals 24 hours. If data are restored from a backup, there is a potential loss of 24 hours' worth of transactions or work. Yet, while this may be an unacceptable loss, daily backups are still the norm.

The BIA will also identify gaps between current restoration capabilities and what was identified by the various departments as needed to support patient care and business objectives. For example, if there is no redundancy or failover of a system and the current recovery strategy would be to drop ship new hardware and rebuild the system, then the recovery time objective (RTO) for that particular system would be a minimum of two days. If in the BIA, several departments identified the system as critical, requiring a recovery time of fewer than four hours, then there is a gap of 44 hours (two days for recovery or 48 hours – 4 hours (RTO) = 44 hours). Likewise, if daily backups are created, then even if the system could be restored in fewer than two days, there is still the added potential loss of 24 hours worth of data or transactions between the time the system was last backed up and when it crashed. Senior leadership should validate the priorities and recovery objectives stated by each department and decide how gaps in restoration capabilities will be addressed—either by improving system availability or by reducing the expectations of departments.

Resource Challenges

Financial funding and management backing are two of the primary challenges most often identified by business continuity planning professionals, especially as organizations struggle with economic hard times. Because business continuity and disaster recovery are perceived as "just-in-case" measures that take away from an organization's bottom line, it can be difficult to justify the allocation of resources. The costs for full redundancy for all systems is impractical. However, as previously noted, gaps may exist between current capability and expectations. These gaps could help justify improved data backup and recovery strategies for the most critical systems.

Support also means providing adequate staff and training. Participation in exercises and tests is frequently viewed as counterproductive and take staff away from their normal job duties. With most hospitals facing nursing storages, many have had to layoff staff to meet budget restrictions; it is difficult to gather management's support for allowing staff time to participate in drills. Even when drills are conducted, they are usually scaled back, limited in scope, and only conducted out of necessity to meet regulatory requirements.

The EHR-accessibility dilemma. How long can clinicians and physicians go without access to patient information? How would the quality of treatment be affected if clinicians and physicians could not get access to previous lab results or vital signs? The answers drive the recovery objectives for an EHR. In some cases, even 30 minutes of downtime can be unacceptable, especially as healthcare organizations become more digital. In some cases, using paper as the backup for system interruptions may no longer be a viable option.

Clinical departments that depend upon the EHR will have to develop alternative ways of providing care and obtaining information when the EHR system is unavailable. These workaround procedures should be spelled out in departmental contingency plans and/or downtime procedures.

For hospitals, the business continuity plan would also need to address clinical workflows and ancillary systems that interface with the primary clinical information system containing physician orders and clinical documentation. This information is as equally important to patient care and can include the history and physical (H&P), laboratory results, reports from diagnostic imaging procedures done in radiology, and medications from pharmacy.

Because of their criticality, EHR systems need to either be replicated or have frequent backups. Replication often involves having multiple systems or redundant systems, which can be expensive and often difficult to justify. Please see this chapter's section on backup trends for more information.

Another consideration for access to patient information is the need to balance access to that information in an emergency situation with privacy requirements. However, patient health and safety take precedence over privacy. In October 2008, the Office for Civil Rights in HHS issued a clarification of when certain provisions of the HIPAA Privacy Rule can be suspended during a national or public health emergency.

Workable downtime strategies. The BCP is the organizationwide umbrella plan and the DRP is the plan utilized in some type of internal disaster to information systems. But for planned or minor downtimes, departments must implement their contingency plan or downtime procedures as part of the business continuity strategy.

Departmental contingency plans, also known as downtime procedures, are temporary workaround procedures to provide continuous patient care and maintain the flow of information for business operations. These plans are implemented during scheduled system downtimes or unplanned interruptions in service. Departmental contingency plans:

- Identify which applications and information systems are used by the department to function.

- Determine the criticality of those applications and information systems.

- Describe manual* or workaround procedures implemented to offset the temporary loss of access to information systems.

- Outline escalation procedures for prolonged downtimes.

- Define how data created and captured on paper can be entered into the information systems once they have been restored to prevent data synchronization errors.

- Contain test procedures for validating the integrity of data once an information system is restored.

The plan should outline an approach based upon the information systems identified in the BIA. Employees should receive some education on the department's contingency plans and downtime procedures as part of their orientation to the department and periodically as reminders of what to do when there is an interruption in information systems. Education will improve the time required for the workforce to locate and implement the plans.

Often when the department does have downtime procedures, they usually only address the primary clinical information system (provider organizations) or claims processing (payor organizations). Departments may not realize the number of information technology applications or systems they use. For the contingency plan to be complete, it must address all of the applications and systems used by the department. To facilitate the writing of departmental contingency plans, the individual(s) responsible for disaster recovery should provide a template.

---

*   As technology dependency grows and baby boomers retire from the workforce, organizations are losing the ability to fall back to some type of manual system.

Because the goal is to quickly recover the business, time is important. The time required for restoring systems must be factored into the gap analysis between the recovery objectives of the business and the current capability. Operational steps that must be considered to fully account for the RTO include the time for:

- Retrieving backup media which includes requesting and transporting the media from off-site and/or storage.
  - o It could take several hours to retrieve the backup media from a commercial off-site storage facility.
- Obtaining a different computer system platform to be used for restoration.
- Loading an operating system and application software.
- Loading the series of backups in the proper sequential order, such as last full backup and then each incremental or differential backup.
  - o It may take anywhere from a few hours for a simple system to a couple of weeks for a large, complex system such as a picture archiving and communications system (PACS); the backup technologies used are also a factor.
  - o It takes far longer to restore data from a backup tape than from data that has been backed up on a storage area network (SAN).
- Testing the system.
- Validating the integrity of the data.

Sometimes an organization may not need to have all the data restored in order to get back to an acceptable level of operational readiness. For example, for a PACS system, initially the most recent year's worth of images may be sufficient for the short term.

Recovery strategies should be built around resiliency and speed. Resiliency implies that interruptions are only temporary setbacks and the organization can and will recover. While having good plans are important, anything that an organization can do to prevent a business interruption is definitely more desirable.

Backup trends. System recovery depends on restoring applications and data from *backups*—a retrievable, exact copy of information and data on some type of media. *Media* are the materials or devices that are used to store information or data in any format including magnetic tapes, hard drives, removable hard disk drives (RHDD), CD ROMs, DVDs, magneto optical disks, USB-memory devices, and in some rare cases, floppy diskettes and microfiche. Storage media have a cost usually directly related to their storage capacity. The frequency for making backups is determined by the criticality of the information and the difficulty in recreating the data. *Restoration* refers to the process of retrieving the data off the backup media and loading it back into a computer system. For a variety of reasons, backups will sometimes fail. Therefore, backups need to be regularly tested to verify that the processes work and that the data can be restored. When media is physically transported, there needs to be accountability and security. Wherever feasible, backup media should also be encrypted. Figure 12-9 highlights how some healthcare organizations found out the hard way what happens when backup media is not properly secured.

Listed here are examples of incidents regarding lost or stolen backup media that were in the news. These "real-life stories" are always good for convincing management when security improvements are needed.

Organization	Date(s) of Incident	Type of Incident	Patients Affected
Providence Health & Services (Seattle)	September 2005 - March 2006	Unencrypted backup tapes, optical disks, and laptops were lost or stolen	386,000
The University of Miami	March 17, 2008	A case of six computer back-up tapes was stolen from a vehicle	2.1 million
The University of Utah Hospitals & Clinics	June 2, 2008	Theft of backup tapes containing billing data	2.2 million

To protect media when they are sent off-site for storage, healthcare organizations should consider implementing the following controls:

1) Verify that all backup media are transferred in secured, locked containers.
2) Use barcode scanning, a log sheet, or a signed manifest for tracking media movements and for maintaining accountability.
3) Use a reputable courier for transporting media.
4) Verify that couriers know how to report incidents.
5) Encrypt the backup media, if feasible.
6) Periodically, review the security controls at the off-site storage facility.
7) Conduct periodic inventories of backup media.
8) Destroy backup media following best practices after they are no longer needed for business or legal reasons.

Figure 12-9: Lessons Learned from Unsecured Backup Media.

Most organizations back up their applications and systems daily, which means that up to 24 hours worth of information previously entered and stored on some systems could be lost if a system crashed and was restored from backup. Given the volume of business and the number of possible lost transactions, this could potentially be devastating and unacceptable. Backup technology improves the availability of data, reduces the RPO, and reduces the amount of data or transactions that may have been lost as a result of a system being restored from backup media. Therefore, the careful evaluation of backup technologies ensures the selection of the ones that are best suited for meeting the expectations of the various departments. Some of the common backup technologies in use today include the following:

Magnetic tape. Used for data storage since the early years of computing, magnetic tape is a cost-effective media. Tapes are contained within some type of cartridge or cassette used in either separate tape drives or as part of an automated tape library or storage management system that does not require much operator intervention. While the tape media may be cost-effective, an automated tape library or storage management system is an expensive investment.

Disk-to-disk or disk mirroring. Although it costs more than magnetic tape, this method of backup is preferred for its speed and flexibility. Data from the primary storage disk are duplicated on another target disk through a network connection. Data can be written instantaneously or periodically to the target disk, which is highly desirable for applications or systems that have an RPO and RTO of zero or near zero. The downside is that disk mirroring can introduce some latency and reduce the production system's performance. Organizations with alternate recovery sites often use two storage area networks (SAN), one at the primary data center and its backup SAN located at the recovery site as disk mirroring.

Online backup solutions or remote copy. This backup solution uses a backup target disk that is maintained by another company and connected to the primary disk through the Internet. Periodic snapshots or updates are transmitted using file compression to reduce bandwidth. A *snapshot* is a copy of memory, which may include the contents of memory and hardware registers, taken periodically to restore the system in the event of failure. The advantages of this system is that data are stored securely off-site but available at anytime, anywhere for disaster recovery. Upfront, there are no capital costs for the remote copy storage management solution, but there are monthly expenses based on the amount of data being backed up. A high-speed network connection is required as bandwidth is always a concern when doing data replication over any distance.

Most organizations are using a hybrid approach to enterprise backups for systems residing in their data centers, using a combination of software, hardware such as mirrored systems, SANs, and tape storage systems for automatically creating backups. Regardless of the technology used, the key is to have at least one set of backups securely stored off-site, away from the primary data center.

The system administrators of departmental systems, such as the laboratory information system (LIS), PACS*, or pharmacy drug dispensing cart systems, have the responsibility for the creation and implementation of a data backup plan especially if the system is hosted in their own departments and not being automatically handled using an enterprise backup solution.

Typically, backups are scheduled to run automatically at night when the backups are least likely to impact patient care and business operations. However, the demand for memory storage is growing exponentially causing backup and recovery problems. Daily backups used to take only a few hours, but may now take longer than 24 hours to do a full backup. In some cases, systems have grown so large that a full recovery may be impractical. Explanations for the memory and storage growth include:

- **Users are saving everything.** Most organizations recommend that users store their work on network file servers and not the internal hard drives of computer workstations. A lack of well-defined retention policies and enforcement can be a contributing factor.

- **Images.** To provide better continuity of care, the trend is toward integrating images from several different sources into a single PACS repository system. Newer PACS with three-dimensional capability are using two to six times the file size over 2-Dimensional images.

---

* PACS are normally supported by the Radiology department, the Biomed (Clinical Engineering) department, or a vendor. These systems can be challenging to back up.

Data Backup Plans

Each application and information system should have a formal data backup plan. Documented in the plan are:

- Backup frequency (daily, weekly, monthly, quarterly, yearly, etc.)

  Note: *Reducing the potential loss of data requires more frequent data replication or backup.*

- Backup type (incremental, differential, or full)
- Storage technology or media type (SAN, tapes, optical disks, etc.)
- Media labeling (date created, system, data classification or sensitivity)
- Storage (on-site, off-site) and transportation procedures
- Rotation procedures (primarily for tape media)
- Media retention (one year, six years, seven years, 10 years, forever, etc.)
- Encryption requirements
- Responsibilities for ensuring backups are created (system administrator, data custodian, night shift operator, etc.)
- Testing procedures to validate data recovery and integrity

Testing Backups

Backups need to be periodically tested to verify that the backup process is working properly and prevent the possibility of unrecoverable data caused by corrupted media. This is especially true with magnetic tapes which get rotated and reused. Over time there is an increased possibility of failure because tapes have a lifespan and should be discontinued per the manufacturer's specifications. Unfortunately, some organizations will continue to reuse a tape until the system generates an error while trying to store data on the tape. Others have learned their lesson the hard way after trying to retrieve data from corrupted backup media.

Testing the backups can be challenging. The testing process usually requires a different computing platform (hardware, operating system, software application, or all three) for restoring data from backups; otherwise the restoration process could overwrite the existing data on the system. In some cases, systems have test or training environments where data restoration tests could take place. If there is only a production environment, then a second computing platform may be required. The availability of spare equipment to use for testing can also be an issue.

Periodically, system administrators may recover specific files or data from a backup. If and when this occurs, the system administrator should document the recovery as a test of the backup media and a partial test of the DRP. The rationale is that, if some data or files can be successfully retrieved, then the backup media must be good and the assumption is made that the rest of the data could also be successfully restored if needed.

Regulatory Requirements for Data Backups

Figure 12-10 outlines the HIPAA Security Rule implementation specifications as they pertain to data backup. In light of the e-Discovery Rule, organizations are required to create retention and destruction policies. These policies need to be considered when creating a data backup plan. Retention of backups could also be an issue for healthcare organizations which must comply with the Sarbanes-Oxley Act (SOX). If an organization accepts credit cards for payment (co-payments, gift shop, cafeteria, patient bills, etc.) and stores cardholder data in electronic format, then they also have to comply with the Payment Card Industry (PCI) Data Security Standards which have specific requirements for protecting backup media.

There are three implementation specifications that deal with backups.

§164.308(a)(7)(ii)(A) Data backup plan (Required)
Establish and implement procedures to create and maintain retrievable exact copies of electronic protected health information.

§164.310(d)(2)(iii) Accountability (Addressable)
Maintain a record of the movements of hardware and electronic media and any person responsible therefore.

§164.310(d)(2)(iv) Data backup and storage (Addressable)
Create a retrievable, exact copy of electronic protected health information, when needed, before movement of equipment.

The following questions pertain to data backups and come from the Centers for Medicare and Medicaid Services (CMS) white papers

- Does the backup plan include storage of backups in a safe, secure place?

- Is a process implemented for maintaining a record of the movements of, and person(s) responsible for, hardware and electronic media containing EPHI?

- Have all types of hardware and electronic media that must be tracked been identified, such as hard drives, magnetic tapes or disks, optical disks or digital memory cards?

- Is a process implemented for creating a retrievable, exact copy of EPHI, when needed, before movement of equipment?

- Does the process identify situations when creating a retrievable, exact copy of EPHI is required and situations when not required before movement of equipment?

- Does the process identify who is responsible for creating a retrievable, exact copy of EPHI before movement of equipment?

Figure 12-10: HIPAA Security Rule and Data Backups.

WHAT ARE THE REAL COSTS ASSOCIATED WITH A DISASTER?

Healthcare organizations may react to dips in the economy by cutting costs. Since IT is an overhead department and disaster recovery planning is viewed as overhead to IT, estimating the real potential impact and costs if a disaster were to occur, may be the information security professional's only hope for justifying resources. The Business Impact Analysis (BIA) is probably the best place to start for estimating costs associated with a disaster. During the BIA, each revenue-generating department estimates their average daily charges and/or potential revenue billed for their services. It is important to note that if the organization has solid business continuity and departmental contingency plans that the revenue may not be totally lost. Instead it may be that the charges were tracked manually on paper forms and will get updated into the patient billing system at a later time. However, even using a manual/paper method for tracking charges will probably result in some loss of transactions or billing charges. For example, if a system's daily backup was completed at 1 a.m. and the system later crashes that same day at 3 p.m., when the system is restored from the backup, the last data entry or transaction will have been around 1 a.m. All of the transactions that occurred between 1 a.m. and 3 p.m. (a 14-hour span) may be lost.

Measureable Costs

Estimating the real costs associated with or trying to maintain the continuity of business operations depends on many variables including the type and magnitude of the business interruption or disaster. Listed below are some areas where costs may be incurred.

- **Lost revenue from missed charges, delays in billing and collections.** The lack of incoming revenue could severely impact the business operations. The BIA should include the average daily revenue generated by each department to help quantify potential financial losses. Realistically, this does not mean that a business interruption would result in all of this revenue being lost. Hopefully, within the departmental contingency plans, departments will address how charges would be captured and reentered into the systems once they are restored.

  Some outpatient services and some elective procedures would probably be postponed due to the risks of providing services without sufficient information. In some extreme cases, patients may choose to schedule their appointments with another healthcare provider rather than wait. This could possibly result in a decrease in revenue from a decrease in patient visits.

- **Emergency purchases.** During a crisis, it may be difficult to take the time to shop around to find the best bargain. If the disaster is regional such as an earthquake, other businesses may be competing for limited resources. In this situation, organizations should plan and budget to pay premium prices for equipment, tools, and supplies which include overnight shipping expenses.

- **Recovery at an alternate site.** Costs for recovery vary greatly and are primarily based upon the RTO which drives the disaster recovery strategy, and the number of information systems that must be recovered after a disaster. Figure 12-11 briefly explains each of the strategies and their advantages and disadvantages.

  There are monthly expenses related to either the cost of ownership of an alternate location or contracts with companies providing disaster recovery services. Costs will vary based on location, the type of data center available for recovery (hot, warm, or cold site), and upon the number of information systems to be recovered.

Recovery Strategy		Description	RTO	Advantages	Disadvantages
Alternate facility owned by the organization	Hot site[1]	Requires duplication or failover capability of critical applications, systems, and the network infrastructure supporting them	<2 hours	• Shortest recovery time • Easy to test backups and recovery plans	• Most expensive
	Warm site[2]	Requires duplication of most critical systems and basic network infrastructure; has the physical and environmental controls in place	<1 day	• Moderately priced • Basic infrastructure with some equipment	• Not as easy to test plans • May not be enough floor space to recover all information systems
	Cold site[3]	Physical space that is reserved and converted into data center only after a disaster is declared	>5 days	• Least expensive • Space that is readily available	• Longest recovery time • No equipment is available; it must be ordered and installed • No way to test plans
Remote Hosting Services[4]		The organization's systems are hosted in remote data center	<2 hours	• Third party assumes risk and is responsible for appropriate physical and environmental controls and some redundancy • The facility may not be affected by the same disaster facing the organization	• Can be as expensive as owning an alternate location (hosting facility) • Ease of use (hosting facility); IT staff must travel to the facility to work on systems • Organization does not own or control the application (ASP or SaaS)
		An application and associated hardware is owned and hosted by a service provider (Application Service Provider – ASP or Software as a Service – SaaS)			
Business recovery centers and service bureaus[5]		Businesses that specialize in providing hot or warm sites and in some cases, workspace for operational staff	>2 days	• Cheaper than ownership of an alternate data center; monthly contract costs are viewed as insurance • Generally located far enough away that the facility is not affected by the same disaster facing the healthcare organization	• Costs go up when a disaster is declared • Facility may not always be available; first come, first served[6] • The equipment at these facilities is owned by the recovery service • Clients are only allowed short-term use of facility; prices go up based upon length of use • Employees may not be willing to leave their family during a regional disaster to travel to a recovery site

Figure 12-11: Recovery Strategy Comparisons.

Recovery Strategy	Description	RTO	Advantages	Disadvantages
Mobile site	A specialized tractor trailer–a data center on wheels that is delivered to the facility, normally within 72 hours after declaring a disaster	>3 days	• Most vendors have specified response times averaging 72 hours • Can be parked adjacent to existing facility	• Roads may not be passable making it difficult to deliver the trailer • Trailer may not contain exact duplicates of equipment
Quick ship	A contract with vendors and suppliers for guaranteeing a drop shipment of critical equipment and supplies as needed	>4 days	• Inexpensive until the services are needed	• May not be practical during a regional disaster or in meeting an RTO of less than four days
Advance reciprocal arrangement[7]	An agreement between two businesses that in the event of a disaster, one company is allowed to use the other business' data center as a recovery site	>5 days	• Inexpensive • Only better than no strategy at all	• Seldom works well and difficult to find a willing partner with enough floor space in their data center • Assumes that the other site has not been impacted by the same disaster • Not easy to test plans
No recovery strategy	The decision not to have a strategy is not recommended; it is however, still a strategy	>2 weeks	• Inexpensive until a disaster strikes	• If a disaster does strike, chances are that the organization will never completely recover • Violates HIPAA Security Rule

Footnotes

1. Equipment at the alternate site is owned and usually older equipment is placed there after it is replaced by newer hardware.

2. Most healthcare organizations have some type of alternate location that functions as a warm site.

3. The use of a warm site or cold site would also require quick ship agreements with vendors and suppliers which may not be practical during a regional disaster or in meeting an RTO of less than four days.

4. This strategy relies on the ability to access applications and systems via a private network or the Internet.

5. Leasing a commercial hot site (IBM, SunGard, EMC, HP, etc.) is costly and that is why many healthcare organizations have abandoned this strategy.

6. Vendors have been known to overextend their resources which cause problems during large-scale regional disasters.

7. This strategy seldom works well especially when dealing with regional disasters that affect both businesses.

Figure 12-11: Recovery Strategy Comparisons. (cont.)

Workforce expenses. Smaller healthcare organizations may not have the luxury of having employees cross-trained. While no one employee is indispensable, the absence of one or two key employees may cause confusion and a disruption of workflow. Key employees and contractors should have been identified in the BIA. To supplement the workforce, the organization may have to hire temporary workers, specialists, or consultants. Employees may be required to work overtime. Hourly employees would have to be paid a premium (time and a half) for their overtime.

Workers may be displaced and forced to work at a different location, causing some inconvenience. Depending how far away the alternate work site is from their original job site, employees or the organization may have to incur the costs of additional travel (gasoline, bus fare, train fare, etc.).

Insurance. Annual expenses may include *business interruption insurance*—insurance coverage that provides protection (subject to the policy provisions) for the loss of earnings and the expenses resulting from covered damages resulting in an interruption of normal business operations.

Penalties or late fees for payments due, missed discounts for early payments. In a disaster, payments due to other businesses could be delayed. Many businesses would likely be cooperative if the situation was explained to them along with some reasonable estimate as to when they could expect payment. A few may show some compassion and forgo penalty fees associated with late payments. However, most businesses function for one purpose only—to make money. It is better to plan that businesses would enforce penalty fees. Late payments may impact an organization's credit ratings, resulting in higher interest rates for future loans.

Depending on when the disaster occurs in the financial cycle or fiscal year, filings and payment of federal and state taxes could be delayed if the organization requests an extension.

Legal—Malpractice claims or lawsuits. United States is a litigious nation. A disaster may result in health and safety issues for patients and the workforce.

Patient care could possibly be compromised in the absence of the electronic health record, images, test results, dictated reports, or other information needed to make important patient care decisions. It is worth noting that patients have been treated for years without the help of computers. Therefore, in most cases, caregivers would continue to treat patients even in the absence of information technology, especially in critical care areas or in situations where the treatment is obvious, such as a broken finger, and/or where the patient is very familiar with his or her own medical history.

If workforce members were hurt on the job as a result of the disaster, workman's compensation claims may be filed. Worse, if a patient died or an employee was killed on the job as a result of the disaster, a wrongful death suit may be filed, especially if the organization could be proven to have been negligent for inadequate disaster planning.

Regulatory compliance. The likelihood of the federal government fining a healthcare organization for noncompliance with HIPAA standards pertaining to business continuity and disaster recovery planning is low. While the risk is low, executives and officers are still potentially culpable for not allocating the necessary resources to ensure the continuity of business.

Intangible Costs
Other indirect costs that may be associated with business interruptions or disasters and could be difficult to estimate or measure include:

Productivity loss and workforce morale. Long-term interruptions of information from computer systems may lead to frustration from physicians and clinicians due to the inability to access patient information. The alternate work location may be smaller and lacking some of the equipment, tools, and supplies they need to perform their jobs efficiently. The challenges of working around system outages while being expected to maintain daily operations can weaken employee morale.

Damaged reputation. Long-term disruptions in services could prove to be embarrassing. Maintaining a good reputation is generally a priority for most organizations. When there is a regional disaster such as a tornado, patients are more understanding of the challenges of operating a hospital and running a business under those conditions. However, when there is an internal disruption, such as a water pipe breaking and flooding the data center, patients may be less tolerant. Patients do not want to hear excuses such as, "Our computers are down today."

SUMMARY

A sound business continuity and disaster recovery plan can ensure resiliency, especially when plans are created based upon needs and expectations of the business. As healthcare organizations move away from paper-based systems patient medical records move toward electronic systems. Any gaps between recovery objectives as determined by the executive management for supporting the organization's mission and the recovery capabilities of critical information systems must be addressed. Workable downtime strategies include establishing departmental contingency plans and downtime procedures. Backup trends are moving away from daily backups toward more frequent snapshots to minimize lost transactions during any system interruptions. While having good plans are important, anything that an organization can do to prevent a business interruption is definitely more desirable. The real costs associated with a disaster can serve as justification for such improvements to prevent interruptions.

Discussion Questions

Some selected questions from the CMS white papers on the HIPAA Security Rule, "Sample questions for covered entities to consider"[*]:

1. What is the ePHI that must be backed up?
2. Does the backup plan include storage of backups in a safe, secure place?
3. Is the organization's frequency of backups appropriate for its environment?
4. Does the disaster recovery plan address issues specific to the covered entity's operating environment?
5. Does the plan address what data is to be restored?
6. Is a copy of the disaster recovery plan readily accessible at more than one location?
7. Does the organization's plan balance the need to protect the data with the organization's need to access the data?
8. Does the emergency mode operation plan include possible manual procedures for security protection that can be implemented as needed?
9. Are the processes for restoring data from backups, disaster recovery, and emergency mode operation documented?
10. Do those responsible for performing contingency planning tasks understand their responsibilities?

---

[*] HIPAA Security Series #2, *Security Standards: Administrative Safeguards,* created by CMS.

11. Have those responsible actually performed a test of the procedures?
12. Have the results of each test been documented and any problems with the test reviewed and corrected?

CHAPTER 13

Developing an Effective Compliance Strategy

Sharon Finney

ARE WE COMPLIANT?

This is the question most often asked by hospital management and the board. This is the question that most information security officers find difficult to answer.

Compliance programs are by no means a new concept to healthcare organizations. This aspect has been a part of the daily life of running any healthcare organization for years. The problem is that most compliance programs today deal with clinical protocols, the medical record, coding practices, and HIPAA privacy among other areas. This means that, whereas in the past information security, because of its technical nature, was relegated to those "techie" people, this structure is now rapidly changing. Organizations are learning that the technology is only one part of an effective information security program and that, due to changes in the way regulations are being enforced, compliance, internal audit, legal, and risk management play equally important roles. In fact, the knowledge and skill of these diverse groups are required to develop and implement an effective compliance strategy.

Healthcare organizations tried to deal with compliance to the HIPAA Security Rule in the same way they dealt with the HIPAA Privacy Rule. Compliance with the HIPAA Privacy Rule was predominately related to workflow and how confidential information was handled in the workflow process. This allowed compliance to handle the requirements of this rule through adequate policies, procedures, and education programs. However, this would not be the case with the HIPAA Security Rule, and most organizations quickly realized that this was not an effective strategy. Because of the technical nature of this rule, the entire process was moved to the IT group. Subsequently, the IT group did what they do very well. They looked for technology solutions to technological problems. As a result, they implemented technologies to secure e-mail, lock down workstations, activate screen savers, and a host of other technical solutions.

This is the technical interpretation of the HIPAA Security Rule. At the same time, IT wrote numerous policies and procedures based on technical best practices and technical standards, while compliance also wrote policies and procedures to satisfy compliance requirements of the rule, such as risk assessment and risk management. These policies and procedures should have been developed together to achieve a unified information security compliance methodology.

Because the compliance, risk, and technology functions did not converge during the initial implementation phase, most healthcare organizations struggle with information security compliance. Information security compliance should always begin with the risk assessment process. However, at the time the HIPAA Security Rule became effective, information technology departments did not possess adequate risk assessment knowledge and skill. The risk assessment knowledge and skill resided in risk management, legal, internal audit, and/or compliance. Unfortunately the IT group did not speak "risk language," and the compliance/risk groups did not speak "techie." With information security compliance relegated to IT, risk assessments were performed, but most were technology-focused and did not take into consideration other aspects of compliance. As a result, these technology solutions were only applied to solve the technical security problems; they were not applied to solve compliance, risk, audit, or legal issues. In other words, we started in the middle with both compliance and IT working backwards toward the beginning and the end. The problem we face today is that the policies and procedures we have in place are not supported by how the technology has been implemented and how it is managed. Organizations did not document what they do but what they should do. This has created an environment of non-compliance, not only with applicable standards but also organizational policies and procedures. To realize the ultimate benefit of an effective information security compliance program, information technology; compliance; risk management; legal; and internal audit functions must converge.

Please note that in this chapter, references to data in terms of ePHI or card holder data do not exist, except when referring to the scope of specific regulatory requirements. Information (data) is referred to as information assets. This is deliberate, as the time has passed for healthcare organizations to quibble over whether a system or database or network stores, processes, or transmits ePHI or credit card data. Maintaining and managing the information assets related to patients and business is performed on every computing device in the organization every day, period, end of story.

You cannot develop an effective information security compliance strategy without doing some legwork. It is imperative to get the right group to the table to make initial decisions on purpose, goals, scope, and responsibilities.

In this chapter, we will cover the fundamentals of developing an effective compliance strategy. I would love to say that you will find in this material some revolutionary idea that will make developing and implementing an information security compliance strategy easy, but alas no. If you are looking for glamour and glitz you will find little of that here. This is hard work. Implementing technology is easy. Ensuring that the organization is using the capabilities of that technology to establish compliance is not. It requires a well-planned strategy, deliberate execution of the plan, diligent monitoring of outcomes, and consistent corrective action. As shown in Figure 13-1, the compliance process is a never ending story that revolves around a sound strategy.

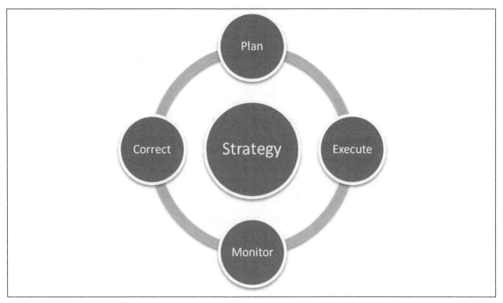

Figure 13-1: Compliance Process.

WHO'S INVITED TO THE PARTY?

Information security is truly a cross-functional discipline. It spans compliance, information technology, internal audit, legal and risk management (Figure 13-2). Of course not all organizations are fortunate enough to have individual departments to cover all these areas, and, in fact, some of the functions may be outsourced, such as legal services.

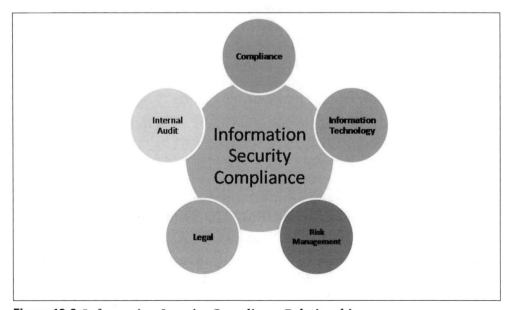

Figure 13-2: Information Security Compliance Relationships.

Regardless of who performs these functions and where they sit on the organizational chart, these are the subject matter that experts needed to define and scope an information security compliance program. It is highly recommended that this group be formalized as a committee or council within the organizational structure. A compliance program is a journey, not a destination, so continued management governance is imperative to keep the program in alignment with the business and the ever-changing regulatory quagmire.

THE SEVEN ELEMENTS

The HHS OIG developed a series of compliance program guidance publications for multiple healthcare and healthcare-related organizations. Each of these guidance publications referenced seven common elements of a comprehensive compliance program, as depicted in Figure 13-3. The following was adapted from the HHS OIG: Publication of the OIG Compliance Program for Hospitals, *Federal Register* 63 (35):8987, February 23, 1998.

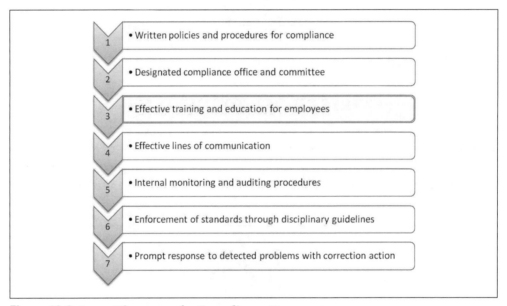

1 • Written policies and procedures for compliance

2 • Designated compliance office and committee

3 • Effective training and education for employees

4 • Effective lines of communication

5 • Internal monitoring and auditing procedures

6 • Enforcement of standards through disciplinary guidelines

7 • Prompt response to detected problems with correction action

Figure 13-3: Seven Elements of a Compliance Program.

Since most healthcare organizations are already using these seven elements as the guiding principles of other compliance efforts, leverage this: It is more efficient and cost-effective to integrate into an existing compliance program than to maintain multiple efforts.

WHAT IS AN INFORMATION SECURITY COMPLIANCE PROGRAM?

In order to develop a strategy, the organization must define and agree upon the purpose of the Information Security Compliance Program (ISCP). "A management plan composed of policies and procedures to accomplish uniformity, consistency, and conformity in securing information assets that fulfills organizational and regulatory requirements."

Whew! That was easy. Now we need to define the goals of our ISCP. The following is a sample set of goals:

1. Ensure the confidentiality, availability, and integrity of information assets.
2. Ensure compliance with federal and state regulations and organizational information security policies and procedures.
3. Provide and monitor correct action recommendations for continued compliance improvement.

Establishing a Scope and Avoiding 'Scope Creep'

It's going to get a little harder now. Let's talk about the scope of the program. No organization begins at the end, but you must begin with the end in mind. As a result, it is important to return to the information security compliance relationships shown in Figure 13-2, and consider each element based on the organizational structure, ability of the organization to provide resources, and whether the necessary knowledge base and skills exist within the organization. Figure 13-4 shows some of the decisions that will help define scope.

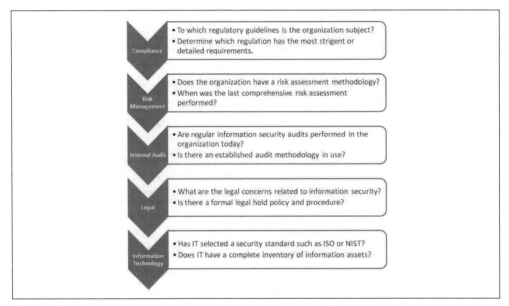

Figure 13-4: Scoping Your Information Security Compliance Program.

The second item that will help you avoid becoming overwhelmed is the comprehensive risk assessment. This will focus compliance efforts based on overall risk to the organization. Almost every standard that healthcare organizations are subjected to requires regular risk assessment. It is imperative to integrate information security compliance with the risk assessment process. This allows an organization to avoid working on the right things at the wrong time. An organization cannot do everything at once. There is only so much time, resource, and money to allocate in a period of time. Using the risk assessment will help the organization focus efforts on compliance tasks that balance regulatory compliance risk, technical security risk, and risk of compromise.

Regulatory Requirements and the Compliance Matrix

Every organization is a bit unique and so we will move from the general to more specific requirements. We will first define the federal regulations that impact healthcare organizations and then move on to industry specifics, such as Joint Commission and finally other regulations that may or may not impact a healthcare organization depending on its business model.

There is a great deal of crossover in the various industry and regulatory requirements. Developing a compliance matrix that cross references the requirements and control objectives from each regulation will help minimize duplication of effort and allow the organization to respond to the question "Are we compliant?"

HIPAA. Information security professionals have a love-hate relationship with HIPAA. As a first step in requiring healthcare organizations to address information security issues, HIPAA now provides a starting point for developing the compliance matrix. However, in and of itself HIPAA does not provide the necessary level of detailed control objectives. It is necessary to reference other available standards and regulatory requirements from organizations such as NIST.

In 2008, CMS began active enforcement of the HIPAA Security Rule. They realize, and HHS has confirmed, that voluntary enforcement does not work. Even if an organization escapes the fines that CMS may impose for non-compliance, the organization still incurs heavy costs in time and possible project delays due to reassigning resources to the audit response. It is much more efficient and cost-effective to plan for compliance.

FISMA. The Federal Information Security Management Act enacted in 2002, was meant to strongly encourage federal government agencies and federal contractors to implement appropriate security measures. The difference between HIPAA and FISMA is that FISMA actually defines the processes to be implemented and details control objectives within each process. These processes are based on a series of Federal Information Processing Standards (FIPS) documents, the NIST SP-800 series, and other legislation such as HIPAA. Think HIPAA on steroids for the federal government.

Many healthcare organizations assume that, because they are not federal agencies, this regulation does not apply. This assumption is erroneous. The two primary agencies that heavily regulate and audit healthcare organizations, CMS and OIG, are federal agencies. Although technically healthcare organizations are not "covered entities" under this act it is reasonable to assume that many of the control objectives may be applied during an audit. In any event, FISMA should be understood and considered as a part of the overall compliance strategy.

FISMA is based on a set of processes that follow a combination of FIPS, NIST SP-800 series, and other pertinent legislation related to federal agency information processing, storage, and systems. Table 13-1 spells out how the FISMA compliance process is defined.

As you can see from this list, FISMA is well-aligned with other standards of its type. The FIPS documents and NIST special publications provide much needed compliance and technical implementation guidance. Using HIPAA, FISMA, FIPS, and NIST together helps to build a comprehensive information security compliance program that has substance and is credentialed with the very organizations that are charged with ensuring healthcare organization regulatory compliance.

FRCP. The Federal Rules of Civil Procedure (FRCP) and more specifically, Rules 26–37 covering discovery are drawing information security, compliance, and legal ever closer. Litigation is generally handled by compliance and legal. However, changes to the FRCP to include electronic discovery have made information security and IT integral parts of discovery response and preservation. Judges are not looking kindly on organizations that do not have in place proper policies and procedures to preserve and produce evidence as requested.

Table 13-1: FISMA Compliance Process.

1. Determine system boundaries.

2. Determine system types and perform FIPS-199 categorization.

3. Document the system.

4. Perform risk assessment.

5. Select and implement security controls.

6. Certify the system.

7. Accredit the system.

8. Monitor continuously.

The primary focus of information security efforts, to date, has been to ensure confidentiality of information assets. The recent changes to legal discovery requirements bring the elements of information availability and integrity to the forefront of the compliance strategy. The inability to respond could be a costly mistake.

The Joint Commission. Healthcare organizations are very familiar with maintaining compliance with Joint Commission requirements. In recent years The Joint Commission has become increasingly cognizant of the role that information assets play in standards of care and patient safety. Although the primary focus of The Joint Commission is on the patient care process, they are delving more and more into the security specifics of systems used as a part of the patient care process.

The Joint Commission accreditation and certification standards have included an information management section for years. As healthcare organizations move to more dependence on electronic information to improve patient safety and operational efficiency, we will see the Information Management (IM) standards of implementation mature and an increased focus in this area during the accreditation and certification process.

In today's healthcare organization, the confidentiality, integrity, and availability of information are critical to providing a safe care environment. Therefore, the goals of The Joint Commission requirements must be considered when developing an information security compliance strategy.

Other regulatory requirements. In recent years, healthcare organizations have evolved not only into centers of care but financial institutions. Organizations today use credit reports; process credit/debit cards; debit bank accounts, establish payment plans, and maintain a wealth of financial information on every patient. The good news is that organizations have been responsive to the increasing financial burden of healthcare on the patient. The bad news is that healthcare organizations are now subject to many of the regulatory requirements imposed upon the financial industry.

Payment Card Industry Data Security Standard. The Payment Card Industry Council was founded by some of the largest financial institutions in the world. Its function is to promote the security of card holder data by establishing a data security standard. This standard applies to any organization, that processes payment cards, including healthcare organizations. The requirements for compliance vary depending on how many transactions the organization processes and how those transactions are processed. Many financial institutions are requiring customers that process a large quantity of transactions to provide attestation of compliance with this standard.

The Payment Card Industry Data Security Standard (PCI DSS) is predominantly a technical standard. It is focused on the protection of cardholder data and is based on twelve well-defined requirements. In the most recent 1.2 version of the standard, each of the 12 requirements is broken down into specific control objectives, as depicted in Table 13-2. This standard is a technical auditor's dream. It is specific, technologically detailed, and control objectives are measurable.

Table 13-2: The 12 Requirements of PCI DSS.

Requirement 1: Install and maintain firewall configuration to protect cardholder data
Requirement 2: Do not use vendor-supplied defaults for system passwords and other security parameters
Requirement 3: Protect stored cardholder data
Requirement 4: Encrypt transmission of cardholder data across open, public networks
Requirement 5: Use and regularly update anti-virus software
Requirement 6: Develop and maintain secure systems and applications
Requirement 7: Restrict access to cardholder data based on business need-to-know
Requirement 8: Assign a unique ID to each person with computer access
Requirement 9: Restrict physical access to cardholder data
Requirement 10: Track and control all access to network resources and cardholder data
Requirement 11: Regularly test security systems and processes
Requirement 12: Maintain a policy that addresses information security

As healthcare organizations continue to be innovative to meet the financial demands of providing healthcare services, compliance with financial industry standards like PCI DSS will be increasingly important.

FACTA. In October 2007, the FTC published the final rules to implement sections 114 and 315 of the Fair and Accurate Credit Report Act of 2003. You will hear these sections commonly referred to as the "Red Flag" rules. The final rule requires financial institutions or creditors that maintain consumer account information where there is a foreseeable risk of "identity theft" to implement an identity-theft protection program. The rule further defines 26 events that may trigger a red flag.

Healthcare organizations are consumer information gold mines. The likelihood of such a wealth of information being exploited for identity theft purposes is a risk that must be addressed.

State disclosure law. As of 2008, 38 states have passed laws requiring organizations to notify consumers in the event that their personal information is compromised. Most states have followed the basic premises set forth in California's SB 1386. However, some states have begun to strengthen this legislation with more stringent requirements and additional penalties for non-compliance during an event.

SUMMARY

The days of voluntary information security compliance have passed. Non-compliance has real measurable costs that can be realized in actual dollars, disruption of business processes, and risk to patients and the organization's reputation. As the custodians for massive amounts of personal information, healthcare organizations have both a legal and ethical responsibility to implement an information security program and ensure that program is maintained and continually improved through compliance.

For information security compliance to become a business enabler and not a barrier, information security processes that support compliance need to become imbedded in the workflow. Healthcare organizations have used this methodology for medical records, EMTALA, and other compliance initiatives. This leads to the true benefit of an effective compliance program, continual improvement. Effective compliance programs not only look for areas of non-compliance but create an environment wherein input from the workforce is used to create additional efficiencies. W Edwards Deming, considered the father of modern quality systems, once said, "It is not enough to do your best, you must know what to do, and then do your best".

Let's summarize the steps (Figure 13-5).

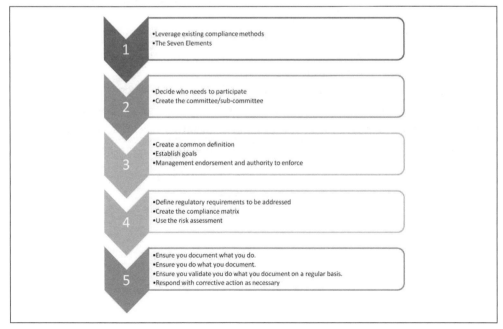

Figure 13-5: Steps to an Effective Compliance Strategy.

This does not happen all at once. There is no silver bullet. Developing and maintaining an effective information security compliance program requires the organization to dedicate time, money, and resource. The good news is that healthcare organizations already have established compliance methodologies. So don't write a new novel just because this particular area happens to include technology. Simply write a new chapter to extend the existing program methodology to include IT and information security. This will be the most efficient and effective way of maintaining a standardized approach and credentialing the program through appropriate separation of duties.

Discussion Questions

1. What level of importance does your organization place on maintaining compliance?
2. Has the organization historically dedicated time, money, and resources to compliance efforts? If so, what groups have been involved in those efforts?
3. Do the compliance, information technology, finance, risk, legal, and internal audit groups currently have a collaborative relationship? If so, is this formalized in a council or committee?
4. What group or groups are currently responsible for information security within your organization?
5. To which legal and regulatory requirements related to information security is your organization subject?
6. Does the organization perform regular risk assessments? If so, are the results of the risk assessments communicated to leadership?
7. As a member of leadership for your organization, are you familiar with the information security policies that are currently in force?
8. Do you recall any internal communication in the last twelve months specifically related to information security? If so, what was the subject of that communication? Do you remember any of the details?
9. Does the organization have an established employee training and education mechanism that includes some type of information security training? If so, discuss three elements from that training module.
10. As a member of leadership, do you receive regular reports or updates on the frequency, severity, and response to security incidents within your organization? If yes, discuss the components of those reports. If no, discuss what you feel that leadership needs to know related to security incidents in the organization.

CHAPTER 14

Managing Security with Outsourcing Partners

Terrell W. Herzig, MSHI, CISSP

OUTSOURCING IT AND POTENTIAL RISK

The healthcare delivery industry is nearing a decade-long refinement of its relationship between healthcare delivery and the use of IT. Viable software applications, combined with an exploding volume of complex medical information, have put many healthcare organizations on the path to next generation clinical systems that physicians and nurses will routinely use. Much is expected from these substantial investments, with their potential to be fully realized. Meanwhile, IT department staff and budgets are doubling and, in extreme cases, tripling due to the substantial software, hardware, communications, security, and business continuity and disaster-recovery investments required to maintain operations.

Although obtaining business value from IT must be a shared responsibility of all senior management within the healthcare organization, the CIO must be prepared to lead efforts and address questions that top executives, boards, and government sponsors will inevitably ask: How do we address the organizational and technical management challenges, as well as the clinical and business applications' infrastructure? Many healthcare organizations struggle to understand whether they are equipped to be an integrated healthcare delivery organization or one postured to only achieve a higher standard of automation.

Healthcare is unique in its need to support widespread and diverse user bases in mission critical and life critical situations, with a diverse platform of IT and medical devices that must comply with an increasing explosion of healthcare-specific regulations and standards. Despite this criticality and because this infrastructure is inherently invisible when the technology works well, CIOs often find it difficult to make the case to make and expand infrastructural improvements. This challenge is heightened during economic recessions and downturns, especially when coupled with the expectation of constrained reimbursements. This situation almost always triggers reactive spending controls.

Many healthcare organizations suffer from the inability to staff and retain sufficient skill sets to make such IT infrastructures viable. Many organizations will examine or turn to the use of healthcare-targeted system integration/implementation specialist firms, consulting practices, and select outsourcing and remote-hosting services. In some extremes, healthcare providers have outsourced their entire IT operations and many other activities that management perceives as non-core processes.

Some healthcare organizations have leveraged their IT investments to transform their clinical care delivery and improve quality, both in the inpatient and ambulatory models. These organizations have come to embrace enterprise-wide business intelligence. Business intelligence crosses both business/financial and clinical perspectives, leveraging both internal and available external data.

Healthcare consumers, having seen how technology has helped them in the retail, banking, and entertainment industries, are becoming increasingly dissatisfied with aspects of their healthcare delivery organizations. Inconvenient scheduling, lack of care coordination, dated patient-provider communications methods, and limited inpatient access to the online environment are considered to be barriers to building brand loyalty.

The healthcare delivery organization needs to plan how to meet the IT demands of their patients. The current working population is working longer hours, while also managing the care of their children and elderly parents. Healthcare organizations, especially acute-care hospitals, often define their key "customer" not as the patient but as the referring physician. Healthcare delivery organizations need to transform from inward-facing and physician-focused to outward-facing organizations that leverage IT to partner with patients and non-clinical family caregivers to build brand loyalty.

To accomplish this mission, healthcare delivery organizations must embrace healthcare data standards and information exchanges to improve coordination across the boundaries of disparate healthcare delivery organizations. For example, the use of technologies such as telemedicine can form a continuous engagement with the patient through their use of home monitoring.

To leverage technology, many healthcare organizations will find it necessary to engage various outsourcing services for the very reasons previously defined. However, healthcare delivery organizations should engage such services with caution and not blindly outsource their IT resources in an effort to save money.

This chapter examines some of the core areas of outsourcing IT and the possible risks the organization may face with outsourced operations. For the organization that is considering moving toward the outsourcing market, here are suggestions of what to look for when entering into contractual relationships with external outsourcing entities.

Outsourcing System Integration and Application Development

With the emergence of new delivery methods, such as third-generation computer-based patient record systems (CPR) and advanced integration, tools have the potential to not only improve the administrative and financial processes of healthcare systems, but to also deliver safer, more consistent, and more cost-effective patient care. This fact is recognized in ARRA, signed into law in February 2009. A section of this act, called HITECH, sets mandates for the adoption of EHRs, PHRs, and the creation of standards and processes to develop health information exchanges.

To accomplish these goals, healthcare organizations must leverage their IT operations in response to specific needs, which include the following:

- CPR-system implementation and optimization.

- Performance measurement.

- Improved business intelligence capabilities.

- Development of HIEs.

- Improved revenue cycle management.

- Addressing IT complexity through standardization.

For many healthcare delivery organizations, fulfilling these needs will involve enlisting external experts that, if selected and used appropriately, could provide assistance with fundamental operations, such as application development, procurement implementation, integration, and clinical process improvements.

CPR systems can significantly aid clinicians in the delivery of patient care. These systems enable major improvements in the quality and consistency of care and can move the healthcare organization closer to the practice of evidence-based medicine. They can also help the organization adhere to government regulations, conduct better data reporting, and become more efficient with business operations.

The healthcare delivery organization must refocus its attention from implementation to impact. The installation of a CPR system is not a one-time IT project but a clinical transformation that involves culture, governance, and clinical workflow. As a result, external consulting companies may be employed to supplement internal skills in the areas of change management, process redesign, clinician engagement, and training.

The United States has recognized the importance of establishing programs to share patient information among multiple healthcare organizations. These programs are called health information exchanges (HIE), regional health information organizations (RHIO), and electronic health records (EHR). The primary purpose of such programs is information sharing, although they can facilitate information analysis and patient health management.

The benefits of exchanging patient information include improving the quality of healthcare and the reduction of medical errors and are accomplished by making information available to the correct healthcare giver at the right time, improving the convenience of care, and reducing waste (including redundant testing) and fraud. Patients become empowered to better manage their own health. Reporting of information to public health agencies is improved.

HIE programs face important challenges, including the development of viable financial models; development of the content for shared records; establishing the best way to engage vendors; identification of patients; and acceptable approaches to privacy, security, and consent.

Government and private healthcare payors are recognizing a wide variation in outcomes among healthcare organizations. As a result, payment methodologies designed to encourage conformance with evidence-based quality metrics are being developed. To measure and improve performance, organizations must become more efficient at data collection. Business intelligence systems can play an important part in organization process and outcome measurement, as these healthcare organizations have a huge volume of data for which business intelligence systems could assist in managing and improving business. With the advent of CPR applications and performance-based measurement methodologies, a need to invest in integrated clinical and financial business intelligence tools now exists. However, packaged solutions are unlikely to meet the full range of needs of larger healthcare organizations. Therefore, healthcare delivery organizations may need to develop or customize data warehouses, extraction, transformational, and loading processes, or analysis and reporting services. Often, organizations lack sufficient IT skills to select the appropriate technology platforms, design appropriate data models and processes, and then deploy and optimize the solution.

Healthcare organizations are under constant cost pressures from those who pay for medical services. This pressure requires a greater need for attention to cost-accounting systems and an understanding of how much it costs to deliver care and receive payment for that care. In response, healthcare delivery organizations are becoming aware of advances in activity-based accounting used heavily by the manufacturing and retail sectors. Software vendors and IT service providers are beginning to offer healthcare specific activity-based accounting solutions.

As the healthcare IT environment is becoming increasingly complex, healthcare organizations are confronting more complexity in areas such as IT service management and delivery, application development, project management, and IT operations management. Organizations are now turning to guidance from process frameworks, such as the Information Technology Infrastructure Library (ITIL), Control Objectives and Information Related Technology (CobiT), and Capability Maturity Model Integration (CMMI).

ITIL is most frequently the framework choice for internal operation processes because it is specific and prescriptive and can be extended to accommodate a particular domain. ITIL, a publicly available set of guidelines for the best practice of IT services management, is a process framework for integrated IT service support and delivery processes used to manage IT operations' environments. Many organizations have turned to outsourcing, managed services, and remote hosting to shift some responsibility to external agencies.

Recommendations. Healthcare organizations considering the use of external service providers should:

- Ensure the contract covers:
  - Staff retention (lock down key members of the project team for a defined period of time).
  - An exit clause that can be used should the provider be acquired by another company/vendor.

- Ensure the location of all resources is explicitly stated in the contract. If an offshore service is engaged, ensure data ownership and privacy issues are adequately addressed in the contract. Use of offshore and blended delivery models is commonplace.

- Select partners with a demonstrated expertise in interfacing and integrating the organization's applications.

- Research and educate yourself on the advantages and disadvantages of new delivery models and make an informed choice.

- Use the presence or absence of provider certifications as a way to compare and contrast consultancies.

- Ensure the service promotes the same commitment to quality and service standards held by your organization.

- Work to reduce the defection of your key staff members because of the increasing scarcity of skilled healthcare IT staff.

- Ensure the company under consideration has deep clinical IT experience, strong expertise in the specific vendor system, and a strong, satisfied client base.

- Evaluate whether the vendor has a vested interest in a particular vendor, application, or service methodology.

Business Process Outsourcing

So what exactly is business process outsourcing? Gartner defines business process outsourcing as the "delegation of one or more IT-intensive business processes to an external provider that, in turn, owns, administrates, and manages the selected processes based on defined and measurable performance metrics."[1] Examples of common business processes that are typically outsourced include logistics, procurement, human resources, finance and accounting, and other administrative or customer-facing business functions. Healthcare delivery organizations are beginning to outsource clinical business operations, such as laboratory, radiology, and retinal imaging. Market drivers for healthcare business process outsourcing include:

- The need for healthcare delivery organizations to concentrate on what they do best, which is continuing to focus on improving clinical delivery. As a result, it is often clear that help is needed from external organizations to make clinical, administrative, and financial back-office processes more efficient. Organizations that cannot perform these processes as well as their peers look to outsourcers to provide these functions. An additional driver is the difficulty healthcare organizations in many regions have in recruiting and retaining skilled resources.

- The need to reduce costs. Many healthcare organizations believe that outsourcing business processes will reduce their costs. These organizations are particularly looking to take advantage of the cost savings associated with moving services delivery to proven offshore locations where labor is less expensive. Although such relationships can reduce costs in healthcare, they must be carefully managed to ensure that the anticipated cost savings are actually achieved.

- The opportunity to shift risks for service delivery to external organizations. Some business process outsourcing deals are for fixed-price delivery. Under these agreements, the outsourcer assumes some of the risks by holding to a fixed price (a per-transaction price). The healthcare provider benefits by having a predictable price for the service.

- The opportunity to consolidate back-office infrastructure. Multi-hospital care delivery organizations are seeking to cut costs. A major source of inefficiency is that typically each hospital has its own back-office infrastructure, resulting in the duplication of work, variability of data and processes, and difficulty sharing best practices. As a result, organizations are increasingly interested in ways to perform back-office functions in shared operations. Such ventures are not easy to establish, and many turn to external experts to establish and run these centers.

Recommendations. Healthcare organizations considering business process outsourcing should:

- Determine if it is more appropriate to reach your goals via internal change with external consulting than a complete outsourcing of business operations.

- Examine the amount of time it takes to reach value with the provider. This particular market sector is changing quickly.

- Make sure the organization has a business plan that includes potential growth, since telemedicine is quickly maturing. Some larger organizations with expertise may find they can gain additional business opportunities.

- Keep in mind cultural/language issues if offshoring these functions.

- Remember the legal issues pertaining to privacy and information security.

- Avoid providers that continue to pursue lowest-cost locations.

- Scrutinize their track records when evaluating potential providers, especially in offerings related to the more technical capabilities, such as telemedicine and teleradiology services.

IT Outsourcing

According to Gartner in 2008, worldwide IT outsourcing in healthcare has grown more than 11percent since 2006 and is forecasted to have an annual growth rate of more than 9 percent through 2011.[1] With new delivery methods emerging, IT outsourcing has the potential to improve administrative and financial processes of healthcare delivery organizations. Depending on the size and location of the healthcare organization, external help may be needed in the following areas:

- The potential to shift decision making from the IT departments to the business units.

- Faster turnaround in realizing value from IT services.

- Cost reductions.

- Shortages of skilled staff.

- Skill set shortages.

- Desire for increased quality of service.
- Desire to move internal staff to higher value work.
- Assistance with the restructuring of internal IT.
- Need to share resources among disparate healthcare organizations.
- Access to newer technologies.
- Improved disaster recovery services.
- Legacy system transitions.

Increasingly, departments other than IT within healthcare delivery organizations are making decisions to outsource services and technology. This shift is driving the adoption of SaaS and remote application hosting, in which clients receive specific software solutions that do not require extensive customization. Organizations participating in these practices must be aware of the privacy and security risks that come with these outsourcing models. Later in the chapter, contractual issues surrounding outsourcing campaigns are examined. Of special interest are the privacy and security of the organization's data in prospect of offshore outsourcing.

Healthcare delivery organizations are also exploring new hosting models, such as the previously mentioned SaaS, remote application maintenance, and application hosting. These hosting models offer reduced time to value, reduced implementation times, and, frequently, reduced training times. They also may help reduce the cost and complexity of support issues with the provision of remote maintenance opportunities. Many application vendors are shifting to outsourcing their own support venues and then contracting back to the organization with guarantees of faster support and turnaround. However, strict attention must be paid to the contract details as well as the possible risk exposure to the organization. In many cases, the vendor may want extensive open connectivity to their outsourced support centers. By engaging in remote support activities without the proper security and privacy safeguards, the organization's networks could be open to global threats.

Many healthcare organizations believe that outsourcing all or part of their IT functions will reduce IT costs. Although cost savings, cost containment, or predictability of cost should be parts of an outsourcing agreement, the largest failures of outsource projects can be traced back to the fact that cost savings were the prime or sole motivation for the project.

Often healthcare providers are struggling to attract and retain qualified IT professionals because healthcare has traditionally paid its IT staff less than other industries (such as financial services), and IT professionals are concentrated in urban areas, whereas hospitals are typically geographically dispersed.[1]

As IT continues its explosive evolution, especially in the healthcare market, internal IT skills are often lagging and may be insufficient to implement new, major initiatives. Healthcare organizations will often reduce training budgets to reduce costs, further perpetuating the loss of skill.

Many hospitals have underinvested in project management, implementation, and support capabilities. This lack of investment has left internal staff with little training in and abilities for emerging standards for quality service delivery. The result is that the use of standards such as CMMI, Total Quality Management (TQM), and ITIL is rare among healthcare providers.

As organizations analyze their IT needs, they are increasingly deciding to use external organizations for lower-value work, such as help desk support and call center operations. This will often free up resources for more-strategic IT management responsibilities.

Healthcare delivery organizations that understand they must improve IT services will often use external IT providers to gain centralization, while attempting to avoid political turf battles. In European countries, healthcare operations have already moved to enterprise-wide centralized IT services. In the United States, the trend seems to be decentralized departmental based services. Such decentralized operations can lead to replication of services that result in increased costs, reduced efficiency, incompatible technologies/solutions, and, of course, privacy and security concerns.

The search for economies of scale will often not only collapse independent IT departments into internal enterprise-wide centralized IT support but has implications beyond the walls of the healthcare organization. The drives for economies could present themselves in two forms: multi-organizational centralization and shared services. The key difference between a shared-resource model vs. centralization is ownership. Shared services can be outsourced to independent firms and can provide services cross-enterprise to independently controlled healthcare organizations.

New technologies that assist with IT management continue to mature and emerge in the marketplace. Many healthcare organizations cannot afford to purchase these new technologies or do not have the internal resources to manage them. IT outsources will deliver these new technologies and automations within the context of outsourcing contracts.

Healthcare organizations rely on IT systems to manage the administrative, financial, and clinical applications critical to their operations. However, few organizations have developed the robust infrastructures required for disaster recovery and operational availability. As healthcare facilities continue to build reliance on IT systems for patient treatment and real-time clinical operations, system continuity and disaster recovery issues are becoming important patient safety issues. Healthcare providers are increasingly considering professional external support to deliver the required levels of recovery capability. While external support can assist an organization, the level and type of support must receive careful planning and consideration.

Recommendations. Healthcare providers considering IT outsourcing should:

• Ensure the use of outsourcing as part of an overall outsourcing strategy and not as a quick fix in an attempt to reduce costs.

• Ensure the commitment of senior management to an outsourcing strategy. This means not only to a commitment with the service provider, but also to the internal organization and the changes that will be needed to make the deal a successful venture. Internal changes could include the creation of new roles, redeployment of staff, and the acceptance of new business processes. These changes should predate the move to outsourcing. If the organization is not appropriately focused on outsourcing, it could fail to yield the desired result. Organizations hoping to maximize costs from such investments will not be thrilled with the costs it will encounter to bring the outsourced functions back into the organization.

- Decide whether the organization is to embrace full or partial outsourcing. Outsourcing can range from the entire IT operation to just printer maintenance. Often, by starting small, the size and scope can increase as the outsourcing relationship evolves. Relationship mistakes at this level are less costly and more easily fixed than they are in the massive move. Full outsourcing carries significant risks and ties the organization to an external provider. An important fact to remember is that the IT infrastructure consists of multiple components, such as desktop support, Web site hosting, and network maintenance, and each component is relatively discrete. This component element could give the healthcare delivery organization an opportunity to evaluate the capabilities of providers without making substantial commitments. Be aware, however, that the larger the organization and the more integrated its IT, the more interdependencies exist. Fracturing off components perceived to have lower value to the organization can impact and hinder the overall delivery of services.

- Invest in advanced competencies to successfully manage multiple outsourcing providers if using outsourcing as a pillar of a business strategy. Even with well-defined strategies and best-in-class sourcing management, contracts will be troubled without the appropriate people to manage outsourcing dynamics, communication issues, and terms and conditions.

- When evaluating and selecting potential providers, choose a provider with a demonstrated and proven understanding of healthcare in the local environment, which includes legislation, regulations, reporting requirements, clinical and administrative workflows, and the specific healthcare applications in use within the organization. [1]

Reducing Risks When Building Outsourcing Contracts

Healthcare organizations that decide to enter into outsourcing contracts must be aware of changes within the language of its typical contractual offerings. If the organization is utilizing national providers, it must consider the legal ramifications for operations related to the states in which the work is being performed. Often organizations focus only on the scope of work and fail to address the local legal and regulatory requirements.

Healthcare organizations entering into outsourcing agreements must be prepared for the inevitable subcontract outsourcing service providers may elect to pursue. Although the outsourcing contract is entered into with a firm based onshore, that firm may choose to move some work components to offshore providers. Healthcare organizations that enter into the outsourcing relationship must be certain of legal protections for complications that could arise from provider-initiated offshoring.

Healthcare organizations that directly establish global outsourcing agreements may mistakenly believe the terms and conditions of their domestic contracts are the same as those of their in-country providers. This misconception can lead to contractual risks for liability, regulatory compliance, legal enforceability, service performance, and privacy/security breaches.

Structuring outsourcing contracts will require preparation, research, time, and judiciousness to ensure that the contract appropriately mitigates as much risk as possible. Outsourcing contracts structured with onshore providers will not work as templates for offshore outsourcing without significant modification.

Global contracting issues are generally easier to address for countries in which global providers have dealt with many foreign organizations, and therefore, officials understand and appreciate customer concerns about risks and risk mitigation. The greatest risks for global outsourcing come from emerging countries that are recent entrants into the outsourcing market.

Recommendations. Areas of offshore contracts that may need modification include:

- Proprietary rights.
- Security and confidentiality.
- Legal compliance.
- Fees and payment terms.
- Personnel.
- Term length and conditions.
- Use of subcontractors.
- Service transition and definition.
- Assets and third parties.
- Warranties.
- Insurance.
- Limitations of liability and indemnification.[2]

When contracting with global outsourcing providers, healthcare organizations should be aware of the attitude toward intellectual property rights. The healthcare organization must understand the outsource provider's cultural attitude toward intellectual property and the means they have to enforce their rights. In some countries, data and intellectual property rights are lax and little is done by the foreign governments to monitor and enforce property rights. When contractually discussing intellectual property rights, healthcare organizations must stipulate what defines "work" and how it is produced to develop a clear understanding of what defines intellectual property and when it is breached.

When healthcare organizations are making decisions to globally outsource services, data security requirements are often overlooked or given minimal attention. Before signing a contract, a healthcare organization must compare its internal security and privacy practices with the practices of the outsourcing provider. If the outsourcing provider is not offering the same protections, the contract should remain unsigned until the risk is mitigated.[2]

Outsourcing providers should mirror the healthcare organization's data security requirements, confidentiality, and legal obligations. Privacy laws differ by country and geographical location.

The outsourcing provider's subcontractors and third parties must also be held to the same security and privacy provisions. If subcontractors are to be used, a healthcare organization can contractually include the right to examine any subcontractor's business, processes, and security standards to ensure they are acceptable. The contract should stipulate that, if deficiencies are found or if the contractor is in an undesirable location, the organization has the right to reject the contracting firm or any specific individuals.

Determine and agree on auditing standards and procedures. Auditing is especially important if the provider's staff largely operates in a foreign location. Identify all locations that the provider will use to conduct business and make sure the contract acknowledges the healthcare organization's audit rights and concerns. If the contract does not include the appropriate auditing standards and procedures, the organization may have audit rights only within the provider's flagship operations center and not in the higher risk locations.

Regarding outsourcing, concerns arise related to how the service provider controls its environment, the standards and processes used, and the audit methodologies applied. Outsourcing does not negate the need to comply with laws and regulations, nor can regulatory compliance be outsourced. Controls can be contractually enforced, but accountability always resides with the service recipient.

The contract must stipulate what potential audits may occur and identify audits for healthcare and financial sectors, as well as any possible governmental regulatory audits. To ensure access to the provider's facility and records, the contract should stipulate who will be performing the audits, including internal auditors, outside auditing professionals, or regulatory examiners.

Before entering into global contracts, outsourcing providers and recipients must determine which country's legal system will govern and provide jurisdiction if disputes arise. Dispute resolution procedures and arbitration locations must be stipulated. The legal compatibility between countries must be considered. Finally, legal guidance must be sought from lawyers with international law experience.

While fees and payment terms may seem straightforward, problems can arise if these terms are not dealt with in contract language. When working in global economies, the currency to be used for payments must be decided. Typically, the recipient pays the outsource provider in local (recipient) currency. However, the stability of the outsource provider's country should be considered. An economic analysis should be performed to determine if paying the outsource provider in its local currency is cost effective. The contract should specify how exchange rates will be addressed.

Global outsourcing can trigger unforeseen tax consequences because work is shifted from in-country to foreign providers. Healthcare organizations often seek offshore contracts as a way to reduce costs. However, hidden costs could erode the anticipated savings.

Frequently healthcare providers utilizing global service providers do not consider issues such as business hours, time zones, and holiday schedules. If the service provider is to provide important support roles, it is critical to contractually define expectations relating to these issues. Failure to do so can impact operations and cause unforeseen business problems.

If healthcare organizations utilize offshore contracts for supplies, then it is necessary to address Customs regulations and shipping times within the contract. If healthcare organizations are outsourcing services that stipulate the use of particular computer equipment, hardware, and software, then the laws governing the export or import of such systems must be examined. It may be illegal to ship certain products to certain countries.

Outsource service providers often warrant items within a deal, such as the ability to perform services by having certain skills, resources, or expertise. A loophole may appear, however, if the outsource provider warrants certain legal compliance without clarifications.

Finally, decide what constitutes a "failure to perform." Limitations of liability place a financial cap for damages on the service provider and recipient if a breaching party fails to perform obligations under the agreement. However, the definition of "failure" is often vague. Local foreign laws may exist with respect to what liability can be limited.

SUMMARY

Outsourcing options continue to rapidly evolve. Therefore, healthcare organizations must regularly review their service requirements and develop overall strategies if they wish to embark on successful outsourcing partnerships.

Healthcare organizations must maintain the appropriate level of ownership for governance and secure service delivery. The organizations must have accurate and usable service-level definitions and agreements to shape integration and service requirements. In the absence of such agreements, providers are left to their own devices as to how to map business and technology processes.

If healthcare organizations develop their strategic IT business processes, they may see opportunities to become the outsourcing providers this chapter has discussed. With the market lagging in skill sets, it is possible that some healthcare organizations may find opportunities to offer outsourcing products within their own internal skill mix.

Discussion Questions

1. What issues should be examined first when considering outsourcing system integration and development tasks?
2. Discuss the market drivers for business process outsourcing.
3. Discuss the benefits of outsourcing IT services, and contrast those benefits against the risks to the flow of information across a healthcare facility.
4. Compare the risks between a domestic outsourcing contract and a similar contract with a foreign company.

References

1. Edwards J, Lovelock JD. Care Delivery Organization Business Process Outsourcing: Market Drivers and Key Players. Gartner Industry Research. [G00155729]. April 18, 2008. New York, NY.
2. Edwards J, Lovelock JD. Care Delivery Organization IT Outsourcing: Market Drivers and Key Players. Gartner Industry Research ID Number G00154191. January 22, 2008. New York, NY.

CHAPTER 15

Physical Security

Terrell W. Herzig, MSHI, CISSP

PROTECTING THE FACILITY IN THE PHYSICAL ENVIRONMENT

In no other industry does the need for physical security and controls conflict with the nature of doing business than in healthcare. Healthcare facilities must be open and accessible to their patients on a 24-hour-a-day basis, making achieving security far more difficult. To prove my point, ask anyone where he or she would take shelter during a natural disaster, and most will respond with the local hospital.

Further, hospitals contain massive amounts of information technology, imaging systems, and life-support equipment. They also daily process thousands of payment and financial transactions. They maintain some of the most sensitive information available within their medical records and digital systems.

In the early days of computers, the information resources within healthcare facilities were housed in mainframes that resided in a central data processing facility, usually located near the business office. Much of the security was focused on the physical security protections of these areas. Controls concentrated on physical restriction from personnel by using locks and alarms, and environmental controls to ensure equipment was protected from heat and moisture.

Distributed systems and movement of IT into patient care areas have changed the dynamics surrounding the security of information resources. Physical security is as much a concern today as it was 20 years ago. Mobile computing devices, such as laptops, personal digital assistants (PDAs), and sophisticated biomedical diagnostic equipment have given the healthcare facility the ability to carry information outside the limiting physical environment.

Ever-changing world threats from natural disasters and terrorism have demanded faster response times for first responders. The same healthcare facilities, on which the public will depend in moments of need, have themselves become critical infrastructure facilities in danger from terrorist attacks.

One challenge for information security professionals is to understand the physical challenges associated with protecting the facility in the physical environment. Physical security has long been documented with specific technologies, such as closed-circuit cameras (CCT) and alarm systems. These systems are often maintained by different groups working within different environments. Traditional security staff focus on personnel and access controls, while IT security professionals tend to focus on the logical controls. This dichotomy often results in the lack of coordination and a competition over budget resources.

In areas where physical security and information security work together, both will begin to realize their goals are the same: protecting the valuable resources of the organization.

THE POSSIBLE CONVERGENCE OF INFORMATION AND PHYSICAL SECURITY

Traditionally, physical security and information security have been seen as discrete disciplines. Each has its own management hierarchy—physical security located in facilities management and information security located within IT. However, many organizations, especially in healthcare, have recognized a common intersection between the two, with mutual technologies now existing for physical and information security. Probably the most prevalent of these technologies is the common access card, which can be used to enter a parking deck, a building, or a computer system through access control technology.

Dividing access control into logical access control, which is the use of mechanisms related to information to provide access control; and physical access control, which is the use of physical mechanisms to provide access control, is well-established. However, physical control has more than one meaning: It is also used to mean control of access to any physical resource (typically buildings and parking structures). The intersection of physical and information security is much broader.

This is not a recommendation to converge these two under one management structure. Two very different cultures are involved, and each requires distinctly different management styles. However, cost savings and an increase in security can be accomplished by recognizing that the two can work together.

THE ABCs OF PHYSICAL SECURITY

The goal of a physical security program is to provide a safe environment for patients and clinical staff. The measures employed to accomplish this goal include locks, cameras, card access systems, fire suppression, backup power, and additional disaster recovery technologies. In today's distributed environment, personal computers and laptops are also considered critical resources, and physical security must go beyond the computer room to address these resources.

Physical security is often the most visible means of security because the controls used in physical security are visible to insiders as well as outsiders. People can see locks, cable locking equipment, CCTV cameras, alarms, and security guards. These types of controls act as a deterrent and a visual cue as to the state of the facility's security posture.

If a would-be intruder's first impression is that this facility has several physical security measures in place, he may determine that there is too much work needed to circumvent the controls to gain access to the facility. With physical access, an intruder can bypass or disable logical controls. Due to this inherent danger, physical security is a very basic component of an organization's security plan.

Like other security goals, the objective of physical security is to ensure the systems and their resources are readily available to all who need them. The integrity of the systems must be ensured, and the confidentiality of the data must be protected. It is, therefore, a combination of all security controls, including physical controls, that provides a level of assurance that confidentiality, integrity, and availability will be maintained.

A physical attack can be launched against any element of an IT system, from the physical equipment to its storage systems to the personnel who run and maintain the systems. If the attack is successful, it can compromise the integrity and confidentiality of the resource or make it unavailable to authorized users. This would be catastrophic in a healthcare setting.

Threats can interrupt the normal operations of IT systems. IT outages can have a tremendous impact on patient care and revenue. Whether intentional or accidental, damaged equipment can cause corruption of data and can increase the cost of doing business because replacement equipment must be purchased. In many cases, replacement equipment for healthcare systems is not available within the local community and may require extensive shipping, setup, and recovery times.

When planning or auditing physical security, an in-depth risk assessment should be conducted. This risk analysis should focus on existing threats and determine where countermeasures would be most cost-effective. This does not mean, however, that potential threats should be ignored.

Electrical Power

Computers depend on electrical power to operate. So do ventilators and life-saving equipment. Therefore, most hospitals and healthcare organizations are prepared with backup power and filtering. Healthcare facilities should have both emergency generators and full-time uninterruptable power systems (UPS), as well as dedicated filtered power. However, generators take time to initiate once a power failure has been detected. While waiting for the generators to provide power, non-UPS will reset, reboot, or shutdown. With few minor variations, UPS-run equipment full-time from batteries, converting the DC battery source current to AC. The batteries are recharged continuously from the AC power source. In the event of a power failure, the batteries will continue to supply the required current for a short time, depending on the current drain on the system. UPS should always be tested for run-time tolerances and battery condition. Once the generator is fully ready, the current is supplied to the UPS from the generator, restoring the charging function until the primary power source is returned to service.

UPS are not limited to supporting IT functions. UPS are required for continuous life-support functions (i.e., operating room and surgical environments) and physical components such as access card readers and door lock systems.

Large UPS come integrated with power filtering and conditioning circuits. This technology works to ensure that the quality of the electricity being supplied to the protected device is as stable and clean (free from sags, spikes, brownouts, etc.) as possible.

Aside from a total loss of power, power degradation could occur anywhere with the power transmission operation. Possible power degradations include the following:

Brownouts. A reduction of voltage from the power utility, often in response to power demands exceeding the supplier's capacity.

Sags and dips. A very short period of low voltage. Most voltage sags occur within the facility and are often the result of starting a large motor or other power-hungry device. Sags and dips can originate from the utility company as the result of a circuit fault.

Surge. A sudden rise in voltage. A strong power surge can damage or destroy unprotected computers and processor systems. A surge can also stress other electrical components, such as light bulbs and electrical motors.

Transient events. These occurrences are usually caused by line noise or a disturbance superimposed on the supply circuit and cause fluctuations in electrical power.

Interference. When electrical currents flow through a wire or some other form of conductor, a corresponding proportional electromagnetic field develops around the conductor. As the current increases, the electromagnetic field increases in strength. Since we receive our power from a utility company in the form of AC current, a continuous rising and falling electromagnetic field proportionate in size to the current flowing through the wire surrounds most conductors. This magnetic field and its relative motion is now sufficient to generate (or induce) an electric current in a nearby conductor. This changing field can cause interference.

Interference (sometimes referred to as *noise*) is a random disturbance that can interfere with the operations of electronic devices. Two types of common interference include electromagnetic interference (EMI) and radio frequency interference (RFI). *EMI* is defined as the interference within a circuit, for example, the disturbance on a computer monitor when a nearby electric motor starts. *RFI* is the reception of radio signals. It is similar to EMI but at a higher frequency (cycles per second). Small electrical discharges can generate RFI and can be created by electrical systems and devices.

Static controls. Static discharge and sensitive computer hardware do not do well together. Have you ever walked across a carpeted floor or rug, reached out to touch a doorknob, and received a shock from the build-up of static electricity? The amount of voltage involved in a static shock is impressive: walk across that carpet floor and touch a grounded object and that voltage can be 10,000 to 12,000 volts.

Several variables come into play when trying to determine how much static voltage is created. Two of the most important include the materials involved and the level of humidity present in the air. Computer-based integrated circuits can be damaged or destroyed by static voltages as low as 400 volts.

To reduce the risk of static damage, consider installing carpets with anti-static features, such as special filaments, that reduce static electricity. Monitor the humidity levels in the computer room, and install controls to regulate the humidity levels. Finally, anti-static sprays and special anti-static mats should be used around computer equipment.

Best Practices for Electrical Power

Healthcare facilities depend on clean, stable electrical power. To help ensure this goal, consider the following:

- Maintain alternate power supplies, including a balanced combination of UPS and generator services, in the event of an outage in the primary source.

- Secure dedicated feeder circuits and dedicated circuits from more than one power grid or utility substation.

- Install and maintain appropriate access controls to breaker panels and supply boxes.

- Install Emergency Power Off (EPO) switches that are easily accessible in the computer room areas.

- Install and maintain monitoring equipment that can detect and record frequencies of the electrical power, voltage, and amplitude changes. Consider some of the newer systems that can also report on load and line current over time.

- Evaluate and test to ensure enough backup power to conduct orderly shutdowns of computer equipment.

- Stage startup and shutdown of equipment to avoid inrush current problems.

- Examine cable runs, use of radio and RF equipment, and the spacing of fluorescent lights to minimize the possibilities of interference.

Water Damage

Information systems are easily damaged by water leaks, condensation, and other water sources. Common water problems are broken pipes, fire suppression systems, and the improper installation of air conditioning systems, condensers, and evaporative coolers. Facilities should be routinely checked for signs of mold and mildew. Mold and mildew are not only good indicators of water and moisture problems, but also create health problems. Left untreated, mold and mildew can grow and potentially make the workspace uninhabitable—a disaster in a healthcare environment.

A most effective approach to reduce the risk of water damage is to be aware of the location of the computer room in relation to water sources. Make sure the computer room is not located under areas that use large supplies of water. For example, make sure that bathrooms, wash areas, showers, kitchens, water mains, and drain waste stands are not located over the computer operations area.

Another consideration is the location of the computer facility within the building. Is the computer room located in the basement? What happens if flood waters enter the building? What about a fire in the building? Ultimately, water runs down. The last place to locate the computer facility is in the basement of a building. This is especially true in healthcare environments for which the availability of computer resources is absolutely essential to patient care.

The debate continues about where in a building is the best location for computer rooms. Many people will disagree, but I recommend the center of the building. The logic is simple: It is not in the basement, so a substantial volume of water, usually not occurring outside of a basement, would be required to affect operation of the equipment.

Some argue that the basement acts as protective bunker. While I agree, I think the risk of water damage from flood or fire outweighs the protective gain of the bunker effect.

When examining plumbing within the computer room, it is important to remember to examine under raised floors for pipes and valves. Install water sensors under the raised floor. I can personally vouch for their effectiveness. We recently had a supply pipe main break in a stairwell. Water sprayed from the pipe with great force, and it easily seeped under the stairwell door, through the sheet rock of a hallway and under (you guessed it) the raised floor of the computer room. The sensors responded instantly. This event occurred at 2 a.m. on a weekend. The operations team was alerted and immediately located the problem. Within minutes, the main was shut down, and potential damage was averted. Never underestimate the effectiveness of well-placed sensors and shutoff valves.

Finally, as part of your disaster-preparedness contracts, consider establishing contracts with recovery service providers. In the event of a fire or a limited flood, having a contract in place with a recovery service can mean the difference between a well-managed downtime event and disaster declaration. Recovery services specialize in rapid response and clean-up of fires and water floods to help minimize damages and the possible development of mold and mildew. Along these same lines, it may be necessary to have access to rental companies that can supply large fans, commercial dehumidifiers, disinfectants, and sanitizers.

Heating, Ventilation, and Air Conditioning

Heating, ventilation, and air conditioning (HVAC) equipment represent multiple challenges for the healthcare facility. Not only are air quality and quantity important in patient care areas, they impact IT areas as well, including their placement in relation to computer rooms. For example, is the HVAC system adequately designed to prevent unauthorized access to the facility via the HVAC components?

Modern HVAC components rely on network connectivity for reporting, monitoring, and making adjustments. Cases are documented in which hackers have gained control of HVAC systems and remotely controlled the temperatures of offices or entire buildings. Therefore, the use and control of HVAC from remote locations should be a primary concern.

In March 1995, terrorists released sarin, a nerve gas, at several points in the Tokyo subway system, killing 12 individuals and injuring more than 5,500. As healthcare facilities are considered critical national infrastructures, the risk of harmful agents being introduced into the facility from HVAC intake points is a valid concern.

The HVAC controls for the computer center should be separate from the other HVAC controls in the building. This setup allows for more adequate zoning and control of the areas that contain sensitive processing equipment. If possible, consider using a totally separate air conditioning system for the computer center.

Fire Controls

Fire controls should be in place for prevention, detection, and suppression. Fire prevention controls are those controls that would help avoid problems before they occur. The goal of fire detection is to recognize a fire while it is small and containable.

The last level of fire control is suppression, how to contain and extinguish the fire in the event of an emergency.

Containment will utilize a combination of controls and barriers, including fire safety-rated barriers (floors, ceilings, and walls), vents, dampers, and controls within the HVAC system to keep the smoke and fire from spreading. Suppression utilizes fixed or portable extinguishing systems, such as water or chemical based solutions.

All systems combine to make what is referred to as a "fire protection" system. The system overall effectively minimizes the risk of damage due to fire and the safety of staff and patients. Life safety issues include alarms, communication systems, evacuation plans, exit routes, and refuge areas. Healthcare facilities are not only concerned with the safety of their workforce but have the safety of their patients in mind as well.

In computer areas, combustible materials, such as paper sources, tapes, toners, and other materials that can be both flammable and toxic, must be well-managed. Combustible materials should be stored in areas that provide adequate protection to allow staff to escape the facility. The oxide materials on tapes can generate toxic smoke clouds that could overcome staff members as they attempt escape from the facility. Consider fire-resistant containers and cabinets in which to store these materials.

Hand-held fire extinguishers come in a variety of ratings, each predetermined to be effective with certain types of fires. Computer rooms should keep a supply of "ABC" hand-held extinguishers within easy reach of the equipment. "ABC" extinguishers are appropriate because they are designed to work on combustible solids (Class A), combustible liquids (Class B), and electricity (Class C).

Some facilities utilize water-based, automatic overhead sprinklers. When activated, they spray water from sprinkler heads. One problem associated with the use of water for fire suppression in a computer room is that a computer fire often involves electricity. Since unpure water is a conductor of electricity, it can compound a problem instead of helping it. When possible, electrical equipment should be shut off before activating water-based extinguisher systems. The electrical kill switch can be used to immediately cut all power to the equipment room.

Water-based extinguisher systems may come in two types, a pre-action or "dry pipe" installation or the more popular "wet pipe" system. In the conventional wet pipe system, the water is held back by a sprinkler head and immediately released when a sensor unit activates. The wet pipe system can prematurely release water if the sensor malfunctions or the sprinkler head breaks. Care must be taken when working around wet pipe systems to avoid the potential for accidental breaks. In a dry pipe system, the water is held back remotely by a valve that is actuated by a sensing system.

PERIMETER AND GROUNDS SECURITY

Perimeter security controls are intended to provide the first layer of defense in a multi-layered approach. Physical security barriers are used to impede or control the flow of personnel through entry and exit points. They are designed to reduce the number of entry and exit points, delay intruders for possible interception, and protect personnel from hostile actions. While it may not be readily noticeable, two types of protective barriers exist. The first barriers are referred to as natural barriers and consist of natural protective barriers such as thickets, heavy bushes, bodies of water, and other terrain that is difficult to cross. Natural barriers are often employed around perimeter areas and adjacent to wide open spaces for easy monitoring. Landscaping can be used as a natural barrier to enhance security. When configured with lighting systems, it can also serve to enhance personal safety.

The second common type of barrier is the physical barrier. Structural barriers involve such manmade barriers as fences, gates, bollards, and facility walls. Gates, ranging from simple swing arms to elaborate rolling gates, serve as moveable barriers. Gates also serve as capture or entrapment devices and can range from limiting access of vehicles to restraining entry and exit of pedestrian traffic.

Bollards are a type of vehicle barrier. Just about everyone has seen them in action, but few may have realized what they are called. The bollard is a heavy duty post that provides traffic control and the protection of property premises. These barriers prevent intentional or accidental ramming of property from vehicles. Well-designed facilities will employ bollards around service entrances, guest drop off and pickups, and especially around emergency department areas. Once again, these physical structures are often fitted with lighting to help increase personal safety.

Lighting

Effective lighting has been demonstrated to reduce the likelihood of criminal activities. If bad behavior can be readily observed, then that serves as a deterrent. While many security analysts fail to consider lighting during the planning stages of a physical security program, it is essential to an integrated physical security system. Good, effective lighting is achieved by having bright levels of illumination.

Several common types of protective lighting systems exist:

- Standby lighting is similar to the continuous lighting systems found within the facility. The difference is they are not continuously lit but are automated or manually activated when suspicious activity is suspected.

- Emergency lighting is limited to use during times of power outage and operates from battery sources for the duration of the downtime.

- Trip lighting is activated by some trigger event, such as an intruder crossing a sensor.

- Continuous lighting is the most common protective lighting system and consists of a series of fixed floods or other bright light source.

Surveillance Devices

Good physical security systems should include multiple surveillance systems, arranged internally and externally of the facility. Devices include video surveillance, motion detectors, and infrared or audio detectors.

The most common surveillance control is the closed circuit television system, or CCTV. The CCTV system consists of video cameras connected by wired or wireless technologies to transmit video images back to a central monitoring facility. CCTV technology has advanced significantly over the past several years. Today's CCTV systems can transmit high-definition color images in very low light, resulting in more detail. With the advent of wired and wireless network technologies, CCTV cameras no longer require expensive, long cable runs to central monitoring stations. With Ethernet network technology, CCTV cameras can transmit their images across IP-based networks and can be accessed by security staff with Web browsers. These cameras can also be programmed to record only when motion is detected without having to deploy separate hardware motion sensors.

Entry Points—Doors and Windows

In healthcare facilities, doors need to open and close quickly. It is important that the doors provide tight physical security when closed but unlock and open quickly during patient transport or emergencies. Special patient care areas, such as psychology wards, observation rooms, and emergency departments, need solid door systems that can be closed to safely restrict access to particular populations. Regulations also stipulate the use of physical controls, such as doors and walls, to have special fire and security ratings.

When it comes to selecting the correct door for a particular task, regulatory bodies and building codes have defined the appropriate technological requirements. These requirements consist of many factors, including the acceptable door type; such as hollow or solid core doors, the type of door frame, lock sets, hinge type and placement, and fire-resistance ratings.

A typical door is a hollow core door. The top, bottom, and sides are structural members covered with thin sheets of veneer. Hollow core doors are not adequate for many corporate structures, especially healthcare facilities. They are easily broken, cut, or kicked in and are not fire-resistant.

Solid-core doors are composed of a structural inner part that is integral to the support frames of the top, bottom, and sides. The inner core can be constructed from various materials like metal, foam, or press-wood. Fire resistant solid-core doors contain composite, block, or gypsum materials that are structurally more fire-retardant. Solid-core doors require better constructed walls for support. A solid-core door mounted in a drywall wall can be circumvented by kicking in the drywall and bypassing the door completely.

Doors are installed in door frames. The door frame is the weakest element of a door assembly. Because it is the weakest element, intruders wishing to gain access will attack the door frame first. For this reason, hinges and strike plates should be firmly secured. Hinges should not be accessible from unsecure areas, and hinge pins should be welded or pinned in place.

Emergency exits must be equipped with panic bars. Panic bars are door-locking devices that are activated by touch to unlock the door and provide quick exit. Panic bars are designed to allow rapid exit from inside, while keeping intruders locked out from the outside.

A special system that utilizes two locking doors within a length of hallway, whereby the first door must close and lock prior to the unlocking of the second door, is called a *mantrap*. In a mantrap, an individual must produce adequate identification to gain access through the second door. This arrangement reduces the flow of traffic through an area by allowing one individual through the two-door system at a time. If an individual cannot authenticate through the second door, he is trapped between the two doors.

Windows

The most common form of residential window is standard plate glass, which is easy to cut and easy to break. As a result, the plate glass window provides little security. The next product up from plate glass is tempered glass. Tempered glass is more break-resistant than plate glass. Once the tempered glass is punctured, it will break into small fragments. As a result, tempered glass is less prone to injure bystanders. However, this feature also means that the tempered glass window must be pre-formed to the correct opening size as the glass cannot be cut.

In addition, windows can be made from acrylics and polymers. While very resistant to breaking, acrylics are flammable and produce toxic smoke and fumes in fires. Therefore, they are not appropriate for use in healthcare organizations. Acrylic windows also scratch easily and can be cut or sawed.

Glass-clad polycarbonate windows combine the best qualities of glass and plastic. Windows made from this material are resistant to abrasions, chemicals, and fires and are usually anti-ballistic. However, such windows are extremely expensive and usually only found in areas with high-security needs.

Laminated glass is made by bonding a plastic inner layer between two outer layers of glass under high heat and pressure. When the glass is broken, it does not separate significantly from the inner layer. Increasing the number of layers can strengthen the resistance to impact. Laminated glass is more expensive than plate or tempered glass and cannot be cut. Thus it has to be ordered to size. Windshields in automobiles are made from laminated glass.

Wired glass is made by embedding wire mesh within two layers of glass. The glass will tend to cling to the wire, preventing the glass from shattering when it is broken.

Locks

The lock is the most used and accepted physical security device. Locking mechanisms are designed to keep the un-honest person out, but for the unauthorized determined individual, the lock is simply a temporary deterrent. Locks can be bypassed, and most keys can be duplicated. Circumventing a lock can take time, but all locks are subject to force. Special tools and techniques may be needed to gain entry. Because of these vulnerabilities, door locks should be used as one layer in a multi-layer security solution.

High-security locks use special keyways, tumblers, and other features to deter picking, drilling, and other means of attack. The type of lock to use depends on what item needs protecting and the amount of accessibility required. Locks currently available in the market include the following:

Key locks. A key lock requires a key to open the lock. An expert can usually pick key locks in a matter of minutes.

Combination locks. Combination locks use a sequence of numbers in a specific order to open the lock. The lock contains wheels and a dial face. The more wheels present, the better the protection of the lock.

Electronic combination locks. Electronic combination locks use a push button number interface that activates a solenoid device to operate the lock.

Deadbolt locks. The deadbolt lock utilizes a bolt inserted into the frame of the door for additional security. The bolt slides into the door frame casing to provide a stronger resistance to force.

Smart locks. Smart locks are designed for limited access and usually consist of a programmed plastic card that is inserted into the locking device. A magnetic strip on the card allows the lock to read the identity of the individual and interrogate a central computer system to determine access eligibility.

Effective control must be maintained to ensure that locks, keys, and combinations are used appropriately. All facilities should have a lock-and-key control system. Key control consists of documenting who has access to keys and should include sign-outs, inventory, and destruction procedures. The key control program must be capable of dealing with lost keys and lock replacements.[1]

Master keying. A master key system is usually used in large facilities. This system contains a "master key" and a system of submaster keys. The master key can open any lock in the facility, although each lock has its own unique (submaster) key. The lock is designed to work with two different keys. The submaster key opens its specific lock, and the master key opens many locks in the system.

When locks are master keyed, a plan must be developed to establish the scope of keys. All master and submaster keys must be identified and documented. The documentation must identify the doors, the users, and the quantity of each key.

DATA CENTER AND COMPUTER ROOM SECURITY

In healthcare facilities, the data center and computer room contain the most sensitive patient information that is accessed throughout the organization. This site is usually the central site for all patient data storage and processing. As a result, this area of the health system must meet the most stringent physical safeguards.

Having a number of technicians, systems analysts, network engineers, programmers, and managers needing access to a facility is not uncommon. Many people will have need to access only certain areas within the room or floor. For this reason, many data centers employ a sophisticated card access system to control access to computing resources.

Smart cards contain microchips that provide the card with processing, storage, and encryption technology. Use credentials can be stored on the card in an encrypted form. When presented to an electronic lock with a reader, the data are read from the card, and the individual's access is confirmed on a secure central computer at a different secure location.

If traffic volume is high, an RF proximity smart card may be used. This smart card allows the lock to communicate with the individual's access card via encrypted radio communications as the individual approaches and is in range of the lock. If the individual is authenticated, the door unlocks to allow him access.

By using this locking mechanism, access can be granted according to a use-based, defined role, or individual need. By stationing card readers and locking entry ways around special areas, access can be limited. A user's access can be quickly terminated. Most healthcare facilities that employ this technology integrate the account management as they do other medical application systems.

Once access is gained to the data center, inventory control becomes a sensitive issue. Only authorized individuals should be given approval to bring equipment in and out of the facility. Inventory devices are often integrated within staging areas to monitor the movement of computer systems. Inventory devices utilize Radio Frequency ID or RFID systems. RFID systems use electronic tags affixed to equipment to send serial numbers and inventory numbers to wireless receivers, strategically located at exit points. Devices, capable of reading the ID numbers on the tagged equipment, quickly interrogate an inventory database for approval to remove the equipment before the user reaches the door. If the tagged equipment has not been "cleared" to exit the facility, automatic door locks quickly stop the unauthorized exit.

Additional physical protection of computer equipment can be employed by using mechanisms to lock and retain the computer equipment. The most common form of this physical security are equipment racks that can be fastened to the floor. The racks can be enclosed with lockable panels that prevent unauthorized access to rack components.

Buildings planned for housing sensitive documents and computing equipment should be made with walls that extend from the floor to the ceiling plate. It is not uncommon in some construction practices to install a drop ceiling and build the wall only to the drop ceiling. This exposes enough room for individuals to remove the ceiling tiles and climb over the wall.

Best Practices for Data Center Security

Access control

- Given the sensitivity of healthcare information, consider using electronic badges or smart cards to authenticate access. Using these systems allows for logging the travel habits of computer room users.

- Door alarms should be used and tested frequently. The door alarm can be configured to inform security every time the door is opened or if it is left open for a period of time.

- Access control lists should be posted on the outside of the door indicating who is allowed unescorted access to the facility.

- Visitors should be required to sign in and document the reason for their visit. No visitors should be allowed in the computer room without escort. On the visitation log, notate the visitor's escort.

- Access control policies should document who has access and at what times.

- Key control procedures and audits must be followed.

- Secondary access doors must be securely locked from the inside. Deploy monitoring technologies such as CCTV and alarm systems to verify their security posture.

- Audit lock combinations, keys, and/or access lists.

- Routinely audit access logs.

- Deploy CCTV cameras throughout the data center to monitor access and equipment status.

- Deploy CCTV monitoring external doors to the facility and all visitor areas.

Site location

- Locate the data center within the building as close to the center of the structure as possible and away from visitor and public traffic.
- Locate the data center away from windows.
- Examine and verify proper placement of wiring, sensors, thermostats, humidity detectors, fire sensors, water, and waste pipes.
- Clearly mark all exits, emergency power shutdown controls, emergency extinguisher systems, and cutoff valves (include both water and gas).

Walls

- Walls of the data or computer center should not form an external wall of the building.
- Floors, walls, and ceilings should not adjoin areas over which the security administrator does not have control.
- Walls should extend slab to slab.
- Shatter-resistant glass should be used in doors or other appropriate areas.

Doors

- Should be solid core and fire safety-rated.
- Should not open out.
- Should have fixed hinges within the door frame and no less than three hinges each.
- Should have door frames permanently mounted to the adjoining wall studs.
- Should have emergency locking procedures tested.

HVAC

- HVAC should be on a separate system from the rest of the building. If the HVAC system is remotely monitored, a risk assessment of the monitoring systems should be conducted to identify possible threats and risks.
- Ducts and vents should be designed to mitigate possible use by an intruder.
- The data center should contain its own dedicated set of temperature and humidity controls.
- A positive pressure air system should be installed.

Power

- Backup generators and UPS should be installed and maintained. Plan to have a minimum amount of by-stand time to adequately shut down systems in the event of an outage, which is tested monthly.
- Electrical systems should be separate from other parts of the building.

- Electrical and telecom closets must be secured and access-restricted.
- Cables and wiring should be properly secured and inspected routinely.
- Emergency lighting must be installed and working correctly.
- Emergency power off switches should be located at all exit locations.
- The emergency power off switch should be encased in a clear protective covering.

Fire

- Routinely examine extinguishing systems for leaks or damage.
- Locate emergency extinguishers near equipment racks.
- Install and confirm fire sensors and detection equipment.
- Document emergency plans and test the plans.
- Install water sensors under raised floors.
- Inspect under raised floors for damage to cables.

Awareness and Training

To have a high-quality security program, proper training is necessary. Educate personnel on techniques used against the physical controls to gain unauthorized access. Discuss and review social engineering practices that can be used to attempt access to the facility.

Consult with police and have them present to help train personnel on appropriate physical safeguards and practices. The objective of a security program is to acquaint the workforce with the reasons for security controls and to ensure their cooperation.

An ongoing continuous awareness program will reinforce the importance of security to each workforce member and the importance of their specific responsibilities.

Drills and Testing

To keep personnel aware of their responsibilities, develop a testing plan. Ask security personnel to conduct a test of the plan. Practice emergency evacuation drills or simulated emergencies. These exercises will help prepare and train employees in the event of a real emergency.

PHYSICAL SECURITY CONSIDERATIONS FOR NEW CONSTRUCTION AND REMODELING

Physical security for new buildings and construction should begin early in the design phase. The plan should be reviewed throughout the life cycle of the construction process. With new construction, many concerns need to be addressed.

Location

The location of the facility must be reviewed prior to construction. The location of a facility dictates many controls that may be needed. For example, if the facility is to be located in an area with a high crime rate, the perimeter and parking areas will need additional security controls. These controls could include additional lighting, emergency call boxes, perimeter fencing, cameras, and guard patrols. Additional considerations may be necessary in areas with high public exposure.

One highly public area is a hospital's emergency department. Most emergency departments have closed-circuit cameras and guard stations. If the facility is located in a high-crime area, it may need to increase the presence of security personnel, change the entrance and exit design to accommodate a more secure access plan, and add physical barriers for crowd control purposes.

Location also means identifying risks related to natural disasters. What is the occurrence rate of natural phenomena, such as earthquakes, tornados, hurricanes, floods, and landslides for this location? When planning a new facility, building codes and regulatory requirements will often assist with the actual design choices for the physical construction. For example, earthquake- and hurricane-prone locations have many building code requirements for building reinforcement. Physical security needs may be easily overlooked. Plan for the physical security needs of the facility in the event each of these natural disasters were to occur.

Physical security must be in place to handle the mode of operation the facility may find itself in after a disaster. Ask yourself the questions: Can I control access to the facility if doors, windows and walls are compromised? Can I provide safety for the occupants of the facility in the event of disaster in which multiple physical access controls are defeated or not available?

Evaluate and assess the potential impact to the facility from different areas around and throughout the hospital. What controls will be needed if the hospital finds itself in the midst of a flood or under materials from a land slide? Does the facility have sufficient physical controls to allow it to operate while awaiting help from distant rescue efforts? Does the facility have positive air-flow systems (the air flows out, not in) to enable operation in environmental disasters, such as hazardous chemical spills? A properly designed physical security plan should protect access to mechanical and utility areas, data and phone circuits, and air handlers and HVAC systems.

Isolate lobbies, mailrooms, loading docks, and storage areas, as these areas provide easy and convenient entry to buildings. In the event of a threat, these areas should be easy to control by isolating their access. Building access from similar public areas should be limited by security controls and/or security staff. Any side entry doors that circumvent established security checkpoints should be strictly controlled. How often has a laptop or other piece of expensive equipment been stolen because someone propped open a security door to take a smoke break?

Equipment Location and Technology Convergence

Successful selection and installation of security equipment are paramount to the effectiveness of controls. Closed circuit systems can be expensive if they use the old coaxial cable runs, popular with earlier cameras. Camera selection and location should be well-planned, both indoor and outdoor. Is there a need in a particular area for Pan/Tilt/Zoom (PTZ) cameras? PTZ cameras can be installed strategically in wide spaces to minimize the number of cameras needed, while providing coverage with overlaps. PTZ systems move on special mounts and zoom across wide areas to magnify and monitor activities. The selection of camera systems should also take into consideration the temperature range of the area in which the camera is to be placed.

Indoor camera selection should focus on the need to have the camera in plain sight or as a covert camera, hidden from public view. Most likely, the cameras selected will be a mixture, depending on the area of the facility being monitored. Lobbies and other public areas best utilize cameras placed in plain sight, while staff areas use covert cameras.

Video equipment, alarm systems, access authorization systems, gates, and door locks generate data that need collecting and processing to provide adequate information. Controlling data streams, their integrity, and their security are paramount. Video and card key systems are often installed with "dark" network and cabling infrastructures to prevent tampering with the data from other network or IT systems.

In new facilities, examine infrastructure needs carefully as they substantially impact the budget for physical security. With technologies such as IP-based cameras, door controls, access authentication, and alarm monitoring, it is possible to use network resources with a minimum of secondary infrastructures. With IP-based systems, the same cabling architecture that is used for the data communication network can serve as a carrier for physical security systems. TCP/IP-based security products utilize Ethernet networks to move video and other communication data. These networks can use VLAN technology to restrict access to the data. Quality of service controls within the network environment aid in providing consistent response rates. TCP/IP-based security cameras record image data to servers, much like information from any other network device. Hard-drive storage of security images, surveillance, and event logs allow for faster retrieval than videotape-based systems. While video recorder costs have dropped over the years, having security data in an electronic format offers search and retrieval capabilities not available with videotape. Many healthcare organizations may find that they can further reduce new construction costs by utilizing integrated wiring to provide services over one cable media format, as opposed to running multiple cable configurations for dedicated functions such as data, voice, nurse call, CCTV, and other applications.

While physical security systems that utilize digital technology offer new capabilities, they can also present issues if not installed correctly and operated efficiently. IP-based monitoring systems may not perform well if sufficient care is not taken to ensure the information from the facility's patient systems and security systems are properly integrated. Careful network analysis must be performed to verify operation at acceptable frame rates, while not interfering with the facility's other network needs. Storage of video on site will require appropriately designed network storage systems to maintain the volume of data generated.

When planning to implement physical security in digital technology, consider the human factors. I have witnessed security staff trying to send huge video files via e-mail. People are usually the weak link in any IT system, and it is no different in physical security systems. Viruses and malware will often find their way to sensitive IT-based recorders and monitoring equipment.

Considerations for Leased or Rented Property

Leased and rental properties are common for healthcare operations. Facilities are often leased without adequately considering the physical safeguards of the facility. Lease and rental contracts should not be signed until an adequate site survey is performed to determine the controls in place, the risk exposure, and the responsible party for remediating identified threats.

Leased or rented facilities provide additional challenges not usually faced in new constructions. Replacing existing infrastructure can cost considerably more than new construction. Old materials may need to be removed, new routes may have to be constructed, and all regulatory codes must be followed. It is not uncommon to find cabling thrown through ceilings that may not be up to building code standards. Once the old cabling is replaced with new technology, other structural components may need updating to code. These revisions translate into unexpected expenditures. If the intent is to lease a facility short term, the cost of the renovations may not be worth the benefit.

Hospitals also present challenges to retrofitting a facility. Certain areas of the facility may require special care if retrofitting systems. For example, remodeling and retrofitting operating rooms and sterile environments present problems for security. Do the existing doors and windows meet security and regulatory requirements? Again, a thorough pre-assessment should be conducted which can provide management with cost assessments before the final contract is negotiated.

How will physical locks and key sharing be arranged? Depending on the size of the leased property and the previous use of the property, door locks and key management systems will need to be modified. These modifications may require replacing locks and master key systems. How are these modifications addressed in the lease contract? Who will be responsible for the costs?

Physical Security Considerations for Desktop Workstations and Portable Devices

While the bulk of this chapter has examined physical security of the facility, it is equally important to consider the physical security requirements for portable devices, workstations, and biomedical equipment. Often IT departments fail to consider such devices as candidates for theft. Depending on the size and location of the healthcare facility, easy access to the facility may make it a potential target for the theft of personal computers and portable devices. Workstations come in smaller sizes and are easier to carry. With the disappearance of bulky cathode-ray tubes and the proliferation of LCD monitors, an individual could carry a functional personal computer with one arm.

To prevent the theft of computer systems, it is critical for users to be vigilant in their security practices. Computer equipment should always be locked away. Even if an office space is to be left unintended for only a brief time, one should lock the door.

In public areas, it may be necessary to lock portable devices in filing cabinets or desk drawers. Workstations and portable devices that must remain in publicly accessible areas should be locked to a permanent fixture with a cable lock device or housed in special cabinets that can be physically secured when not in use. Never assume a portable device is immune from theft due to familiar surroundings. The following are some considerations for securing both workstations and portable devices:

- Encrypt it—if the device contains sensitive information. If it can't be encrypted, be sure the device is physically secured to a fixed location. This includes portable biomedical equipment. While the equipment may be portable, it should be locked in a room or secured to permanent infrastructure when not in use.

- Password-protect the device.

- Keep the portable device with you at all times. If traveling, be careful NOT to leave the device unattended in public locations, especially restaurants and other public locations.

- Do *not* leave the portable device in your hotel room unattended.

- If traveling in an automobile, do not leave the portable device in a visible location. If at all possible, carry the device with you or lock it in the trunk of the vehicle.

- Consider using bags or carry cases that do not call attention to the fact you are carrying a portable device.

- Purchase locking devices that allow you to secure the portable device to fixtures such as furniture. A variety of locking devices is available, and some come with an alarm system to help detect tampering.

- Back-up your data. In the event the device is lost or stolen, it should not contain the sole source of your data.

- Consider purchasing products that allow you to track the device and remotely wipe the data.

- Label the device with anti-theft labels that leave identifiers on the device if the labels are removed.

SUMMARY

Controlling access to information resources involves more than technical and logical controls; it includes limiting the physical access to the resources. As healthcare organizations continue to rely and expand their information infrastructure, the threats to these systems also become more sophisticated. The physical security environment is quickly becoming more complex and more difficult to protect for several reasons:

- More individuals are working outside the traditional care space.

- More people are carrying powerful mobile communication devices. Such devices come equipped with large memories and are capable of carrying a lot of sensitive information. These devices commonly lack many of the standard security implementations to which normal devices are subject.

- The utilization of laptops instead of desktops continues to grow quickly.

- USB mass storage technology makes data theft difficult to detect or deter.

- Social engineering is becoming more prevalent. Attacks are becoming more diverse and multi-disciplined.

- Identity theft is at the forefront of healthcare organizations. In healthcare operations, financial gain may come from identity theft or medical fraud. The problem has gained a lot of attention because of the large amounts of sensitive, private information available to large groups of individuals. This problem crosses into the physical security area in the protection and disposal of media (including paper sources). Consider the value of a single record of identity information made available on the black market. Reports have indicated individual identity information and credit card data usually sell for about $50 per record. Extrapolating this data to the amount stored on a common backup tape could make one lost tape worth more than $1 million dollars. Healthcare organizations are ripe with this kind of information and must ensure that this information is physically secure.

Discussion Questions

1. Discuss the components of a physical security plan.
2. What areas need to be considered when planning for the power needs of an IT department?
3. In what ways would HVAC and Fire Controls need to be integrated?
4. What should be included in a perimeter security assessment?
5. What issues are most important when discussing data center and computer room security?

Reference

1. Krause M, Tipton H. *Information Security Management Handbook*. Auerbach Publications. New York, NY; 2003.

CHAPTER 16

Effective Security Programs Enable Clinical and Business Improvements

Mary Anne S. Canant, MBA, CISA, CISSP

THE NEED FOR IMPROVEMENT

In the wake of high-profile information security breaches and the realization of their financial and reputational impact, organizations now devote considerable attention to data loss prevention. Breaches often make headlines and their costs are measured in forensic-hours and fees for notification and credit protection. At what cost, however, do healthcare systems and hospitals operate with inefficient or ineffective processes driven by poor data governance models? What performance improvements could be achieved using data that are accurate, timely, reliable, relevant, complete, and protected? How might patient-physician relationships be improved if patients were confident in the state of their privacy? How might processes be improved and clinical and business objectives be advanced if data governance programs were effective?

The primary drivers for effective data security and governance are the need to deliver quality outcomes (both clinical and business), comply with regulations, and increase business agility. Effective governance involves people, processes, and technology. Of these, technology is typically the least problematic. People and processes are the biggest challenges. To resolve data security and quality problems and achieve significant gains in efficiencies and effectiveness, organizations must focus on processes and the people responsible for their implementation.

Because lapses in security and quality can be injurious to brand, stakeholder value, and operational performance, the chief information security officer (CISO) faces a new test of leadership.[1] This chapter defines the need for CISOs to align security projects and communications with clinical and business objectives. It encourages the development of a knowledge environment—one that fosters continuous improvement and enables high-performance clinical and business processes. It describes the qualities and behaviors of successful information security officers and the essential disciplines needed to build alliances.

Align Security Programs with Clinical and Business Objectives

Ken Morris, CISO, Adecco, advises other security officers to ensure that each security project maps to their organization's strategic objectives. "You have to be ruthless when it comes to making tough decisions about the kind of information security investments you are willing to authorize and support. Ensuring that your security investments support your business strategy is a critical litmus test for any CISO. Every discrete security project must align with corporate strategy in order to make the cut. Otherwise, the project is not going to drive your business forward."[2]

The CISO should understand how information security risks impact operational performance, brand protection, and shareholder value. This understanding will help keep projects focused on appropriate risk and in alignment with clinical, operational, and financial objectives. In the following passage, Michael R. Waldrum, MD, COO, UAB Health System, links quality information to clinical objectives.

"In order to make good healthcare decisions and take care of patients better you have to have the right information at the point of care in order to provide the highest quality of care you can."[3] Clinicians recognize the value of quality data. It enables the delivery of safe, effective patient care. Healthcare system and hospital administrators recognize the value of quality data. It enables sound business decisions.

The security function is evolving. From its relatively sluggish start in the healthcare industry, it is maturing rapidly in response to changes in the scope and complexity of technology and the publics' growing demand for confidentiality and affordable, quality outcomes.

As the need for security increases, its impact on the bottom line gains visibility. The impact is explained by Paul Connelly, CISO for Hospital Corporation of America (HCA). "In the healthcare industry, our business leaders know that every dollar spent on security is a dollar not spent on caring for patients or improving the ability to attract patients and doctors. So as a CISO, whether we're able to deliver concrete, measurable value to these leaders can rise or fall entirely on whether we're able to explain security's contribution to bottom-line business results. We have to be able to do this in a manner that links security with the business vision, communicates the real costs of security, and demonstrates a flexible, comprehensively structured approach that's based on leading industry benchmarks and solid risk-management practices. The steps for making the strategy actionable help avoid the common pitfalls that result in strategies being nicely printed and put into binders that sit on shelves gathering dust. Letting that happen can doom a security program and CISO to being on the outside looking in, in terms of integration as a critical component of business operations. This can be the difference between success and failure."[4]

The ability to align security programs with the vision, mission, and objectives of the organization requires that security officers acquire a more comprehensive perspective and broader knowledge of the organization.

Create a Knowledge Environment

"A knowledge environment is the collection of social practices and technological and physical arrangements intended to facilitate collaborative knowledge building, decision-making, inference, or discovery. The purpose of a knowledge environment is to facilitate consistent knowledge outcomes revealed as learning, communication, goals, decisions, etc."[5]

The CISO's job is to support and protect the organization, and knowledge is the security officer's most powerful tool. The job requires that the security officer maintain knowledge of the:

- Healthcare industry.
- Challenges facing the industry and those specific to the organization.
- Competition.
- Local, regional, and national markets and their impact.
- Clinical, business, operational, financial, and reputational risks and their implications.
- Financials, lines of service, patient mix, payor mix, and staffing challenges.
- Business and operational objectives, strategies, and performance plans.

This knowledge should be the basis for developing security policy and training and awareness programs, prioritizing data governance and security activities, and formulating business cases for change, improvements, and innovations.

Design rules and standards for specific audiences recognize that their willingness to read and follow this guidance will be limited if its benefit and applicability is not apparent. Why should end-users sift through standards that are relevant only to IT operations or development? It's an inefficient use of time.

Realize that policy alone does not affect behavioral change and is ineffective in reducing risk. Policies must be coupled with education, enforcement, and reinforcement. A policy that details the organization's position on security is meaningless without continual user education and awareness.

Design ongoing security awareness and training programs so that employees and contractors understand and know how to fulfill their roles and responsibilities in maintaining secure data and systems. Making individuals more aware that data can be lost, stolen, or manipulated, however, does not necessarily translate into making data safer. Individuals must recognize that security failures and attacks have a real potential to negatively affect clinical and business goals. Individuals should understand how risk will benefit them personally and professionally.

Create a culture of awareness. Start by helping information owners conceptualize and assess the risk potential for their use of information and IT services. This promotes consciousness and shifts responsibility to those with greater understanding of the business objectives.

Work toward an environment in which information owners, not the IT or security teams, have ultimate responsibility for the security of those assets. Risk is most effectively managed when it is the responsibility of line of business (LOB) managers. Help management design risk assessments as repeatable processes so that the organization's overall security posture improves with each pass. Recognize that improvements become more effective when the results of the assessments are shared. Transparency fosters stability. Encourage transparency among clinical, business, and support units. It provides learning opportunities and helps interdependent areas coordinate threat responses.

For a security program to be effective, managers at all levels need to enforce it and demonstrate compliance. This level of support requires that managers have an understanding of security, compliance, continuity, and privacy—and their impact on risk and risk management. This level of support requires that CISOs earn the trust and cooperation of many stakeholders. Security professionals cannot effect change throughout an organization without reaching out to the organization. Creating and maintaining a risk-aware culture requires considerable communication skills. To establish and maintain credibility with management across the enterprise, CISOs should strengthen their soft skills and job qualifications.

Strengthen Job Qualifications and Soft Skills

Effective leadership requires a clear vision, the ability to communicate its relevance, and the managerial discipline to deliver its full value.[1] The ability to deliver value requires that security officers polish or acquire new skill sets. CISOs must ensure that clinical and business leaders understand that data governance and security are foundational requirements for innovation and improvements. Otherwise, leaders may view security projects as expenses and impairments to their productivity.

Gary Eppinger, CISO, Rockwell Automation, comments on the CISO's new skill requirements. "The most effective CISOs today aren't just experts in technology; they're experts in how technology must be positioned and implemented to support the business. That represents a quantum shift in the balance and breadth of skills that a CISO must be able to bring to the organization, because now rather than being just a 'technology guru,' a CISO must also be at home with the skills necessary for leadership, business management, executive communications, fiscal planning, and risk management."[7]

Security officers can improve their effectiveness and transform security's role using the disciplines listed in Table 16-1 and demonstrating personal qualifications outlined in Table 16-2.

In addition to technical skills and prior experience, a successful information security executive possesses the personal qualifications described in Table 16-2.

The CISO requires visibility and accountability to ensure that the organization can determine whether security practices are conducted effectively. The CISO requires authority to gain support of senior and LOB management. The CISO requires strong alliances that foster collaboration. Gartner consultant, Jay Heiser, advises security officers to form relationships. "Seek out influential individuals on the board of directors, among senior executive management, and in every LOB. Use them as agents of influence to drive necessary risk-related cultural change across the enterprise."[10]

Build Trust and Alliances

"Misplaced trust is ruinous," advises Daniel E. Greer, "both in business and in life. Trust makes it possible to proceed where proof is lacking. As an end, trust is worth the

Table 16-1: Strategic Disciplines Required for Security Transformation.[8] (Adapted from PwC Atlas, p.55.)

Discipline	Action
Assess	Understand where you are and where you want to be.
Analyze	Conduct analyses that will give you actionable insight.t
Strategize	Build a strategic implementation roadmap.
Align	Maintain strategy as a dynamic, continuous process.
Communicate	Improve consensus-building, messaging, and reporting.

Table 16-2: Personal Qualifications.[9] (Adapted from PwC Atlas, p.55.)

Qualifications	Demonstrable Behaviors
Excellent communication skills	Act as a liaison between many different groups with different world views, objectives and needs. Persuade management to adopt new and possibly unpopular courses of action.
Good relationship management skills	Work with and through a lot of people. Act in an advisory role to convince and persuade others.
Ability to manage many important projects simultaneously	Be an excellent project manager. Delegate work and manage people outside an information security group.
Ability to resolve conflicts between security and business objectives	See the pros and cons of differing courses of action. Choose and negotiate compromises.
Ability to see the big picture	Synthesize information from different sources. Maintain broad views and respond to the organization's business needs.
Basic familiarity with information security technology	Know the best technology to apply in response to the organization's needs. Maintain familiarity with methods used, processes employed, and business reasons cited to justify security measures.
Real world hands-on experience	Avoid using the organization as the proving ground for untested theories or ideas. Bring prior experience to bear on the problems the organization faces.
Commitment to staying on top of the technology	Stay abreast of recent developments in the information security field. Apply knowledge to avoid unnecessarily costly, burdensome, and antiquated solutions.
Honesty and high-integrity character	Maintain a clean criminal and credit record. Be an exemplary employee and a paragon of virtue and honesty.
Familiarity with information security management	Master the elements of an information security organizational infrastructure. Know and use generally accepted information security management tools.
Tolerance for ambiguity and uncertainty	Be able to make defensible decisions when important or critical information is unavailable. Recognize the complexities and interdependencies of information security problems.

Table 16-2: Personal Qualifications.[9] (Adapted from PwC Atlas, p.55.) (cont.)

Qualifications	Demonstrable Behaviors
Demonstrated good judgment	Maintain a good track record of decision-making in varied situations even when management pressure and quick responses are important factors. Recognize that judgments could profoundly affect the future of the organization.
Ability to work independently	Be able to work independently without direct supervision or encouragement. Be creative, proactive, and inspired by a vision of how things could be.
A certain amount of polish	Inspire respect and admiration. Maintain a professional appearance and demeanor.

price. Without trust, information is largely useless."[11] Once perceived as untrusting and intent on stifling connectivity and innovation, security professionals are increasingly identified as advisors of how clinical, business, and technological objectives can be achieved while maintaining compliance with policy and regulations. The mission of the security function has been reformulated as a business enabler.

To ensure that security initiatives align fully with business objectives, a CISO should establish strong working relationships with senior executives, LOBs, and other key stakeholders. In its report on information security and business innovation, RSA promotes building relationships and winning influence. "It's one thing to have great innovation-enabling security strategies in mind, but converting your plans into action requires building relationships and having organizational influence. To really become part of your company's business innovation process, to be there at the table for new initiatives and add significant value, you have to win over a lot of people."[12]

In its analysis of The Global State of Security® 2008,* survey (a worldwide security survey conducted by PricewaterhouseCoopers, CIO Magazine, and CSO Magazine), PwC states that "healthcare systems and hospitals that manage information security effectively within their clinical and business units can increase value, reduce risk, and improve operational efficiency." The survey shows, however, that 40 percent of health provider respondents reported "that their organization does not actively engage both business and IT decision makers in addressing information security issues."[13]

The CISO needs to drive the organization's perception of the security program. The goal is to help constituents internalize and accept the CISO's message. This requires good communication and crystal-clear reporting.

PwC suggests that CISOs customize communications to each constituent's concerns and explicitly align security with a role in supporting their objectives. "Are you addressing senior corporate executives at the C-suite level, business-unit leadership, or IT managers and administrators? Are you reaching out through e-mail, hand delivering a comprehensive report or conducting weekly planning meetings? Are you communicating in action and behavior, as well as through written and electronic

---

* Survey respondents included over 7,000 CEOs, CFOs, CIOs, CSOs, vice presidents, and directors of IT and information security with 252 respondents (3.5 percent of survey) in the healthcare provider sector.

means? Are you training, coaching, and mentoring your security staff to extend, support, and explain the communications objectives you have defined?"[14]

Take the time to develop good skills in listening, conversing, and exchanging information with other business and IT leaders. Take an interest in their points of view and build rapport at a personal level. Carefully target risk awareness communications to each constituent's interests and concerns. Table 16-3 provides examples.

Table 16-3: CISO's Approach to Communications.[15] (Adapted from PwC Atlas, p.55.)

Constituent	Constituent's Concerns	CISO's Approach
CEO	Earnings; profitability; stakeholder value; enterprise risk	Consider internal and external pressures and how quality data can improve decisions.
CFO	Assets, liabilities, income, and expenses; bad debt; Medicare pay for performance programs; Medicaid reductions; financial penalties and sanctions	Present security objectives in the language and context of financial issues. Consider security's current and future impact to the organization's assets, liabilities, income and expenses. Consider how the security addresses the overall risk management strategy.
CIO	Maintaining alignment with clinical and business objectives; business continuity, portfolio management; capacity; attracting and retaining skilled staff; service levels	Consider how security supports technology innovation and promotes sound project and portfolio management.
COO	Quality metrics; performance improvements; core business improvements; operational efficiencies; delivering value and service	Consider how security will impact quality improvements, service strategies, operational availability, business process integrity, and continuous operational improvement.
Medical staff	Patient care; preventable events	Consider how security impacts data integrity and system availability; how security is integrated with service levels.
Nursing staff	Patient care, preventable events; work environment	Consider how security and technology can increase performance.
Researchers	Funding; access to clinical data; recruiting research subjects; IT support; data management training for staff	Consider how security impacts access to data and the ability to recruit clinical subjects. Consider how more reliable technologies can attract funding sources.
LOB management	Core business improvements; meeting business objectives and budgets	Consider how business objectives are impacted by data errors, data loss, and IT failures.
Patients	Quality care; access; affordable prices; confidentiality	Consider new ways to increase patient awareness of identity theft and medical identity theft.

Elizabeth King, VP Information Management Services for Starbucks, provides CISOs advice on thinking like a CFO. "CISO's fiscal and fiduciary responsibilities require fundamental skills; among them is proficiency in translating the implications of security into financial terms with the appropriate level of transparency and clarity. Present your business case in a way that others on the executive management team will understand. Think like a CFO, your ability to deliver results may depend on your ability to communicate what security costs and what it delivers."[16]

Security officers should communicate and build alliances with all stakeholders to ensure that the security program is aligned with their clinical and business objectives and that it effectively addresses risk.

Full Circle: The Impact of an Effective Security Program

Healthcare systems and hospitals that manage information security effectively within their clinical and business units can increase value, reduce risk, and improve operational efficiency. Using security to enable the exchange of medical information within and across organizations helps maintain a competitive posture. Aligning security projects with business goals can ensure that those projects deliver real-world business value. Successful projects increase credibility.

Vendors label their IT and information security solutions as "business enablers." In healthcare systems and hospitals, administrators, medical, nursing, and support staff, and IT and security professionals earn that label when each assumes responsibility for their role in the organization's security program.

Discussion Questions

1. As CISO, you are responsible for developing and presenting an annual, enterprise-wide, information security program to a senior executive committee. Describe how you plan to gain support for the program in advance of your presentation.

2. Management hired a technical heavyweight to build an information security program after your organization suffered two high-profile security breaches. The new CISO recruited highly technical data security analysts and implemented strong technical controls. Executive management lost confidence in the CISO and her program, however, as data breaches continued. You have served with distinction in several clinical and operational areas of the healthcare system and management has asked you to serve as the interim security officer. You have always wanted greater involvement in data center operations although you have limited technical experience. How do you gain the trust of the security team and begin transitioning to a more balanced security program?

3. You worked as a security officer in the highly-regulated, compliance-driven nuclear power industry. Now, you have joined a very progressive healthcare system whose management recognizes that not all risk is bad. The management team expects you to manage information security risks judiciously, to mitigate it when possible, and to prepare the organization to respond effectively and efficiently when necessary. What steps will you take to transition from a compliance-driven security program to a risk-based program that supports clinical and business objectives?

4. Your organization's new executive management team wants to reduce costs and has expressed interest in outsourcing a number of IT functions—including information security. As an astute manager, you want to prepare two compelling arguments—one that supports in-house coverage and another that supports an outsourcing program. In each case you want to retain the superb security team you built over the past five years. Describe your plans.

References

1. PricewaterhouseCoopers, How to Align Security With Your Strategic Business Objectives, *Security ATLAS™ Guidebook*, http://www.pwc.com/extweb/service.nsf/docid/dbb0bdc50e3ac5c785256f3b0080 36fd/$file/security_atlas_guidebook.pdf, accessed July 18, 2009.

2. K Morris, quoted in PricewaterhouseCoopers, *Security ATLAS™ Guidebook*, 3.

3. MR Waldrum, quoted by Sun MicroSystems,
    http://www.sun.com/customers/software/uab.xml. accessed July 18,2009.

4. P Connelly, quoted in PricewaterhouseCoopers, *Security ATLAS™ Guidebook*, 45.

5. Knowledge Environment, Wikipedia, http://en.wikipedia.org/wiki/Knowledge_environment, accessed July 19, 2009.

6. PricewaterhouseCoopers, *Security ATLAS™ Guidebook*, 1.

7. G Eppinger, quoted in PricewaterhouseCoopers, *Security ATLAS™ Guidebook*, 57.

8. PricewaterhouseCoopers, *Security ATLAS™ Guidebook*, 11.

9. CC Wood. *Information Security Roles and Responsibilities Made Easy*, Version 2, April 2005, Appendix B, ISBN 1-881585-12-3.

10. J Heiser, Tutorial on How to Move Beyond Security Awareness to Create a Risk-Conscious Culture, G00156433, Gartner Research, Stamford CT, April 11, 2008.

11. D E Geer, Why Information Security Matters, Cutter Consortium Business IT Strategies Vol.7, No.3, 2004.

12. RSA, The Time is Now: Making Information Security Strategic to Business Innovation, https://rsa-email.rsa.com/servlet/website/ResponseForm?klHEu.263-8b.25VT.40hkt, accessed July 19, 2009, 14.

13. PricewaterhouseCoopers, *connectedthinking, The Global State of Information Security® 2008, http://www.pwc.com/en_GX/gx/information-security-survey/pdf/global_info_survey_health_provider.pdf, accessed July 19, 2009.

14. PricewaterhouseCoopers, *Security ATLAS™ Guidebook*, 55.

15. PricewaterhouseCoopers, *Security ATLAS™ Guidebook*, 55.

16. E King, quoted in PricewaterhouseCoopers, *Security ATLAS™ Guidebook*, 18.

CHAPTER 17

The Foundations of Information Assurance

Mary Anne S. Canant, MBA, CISA, CISSP

BROADENING THE PERSPECTIVE OF GOVERNANCE

Governing bodies are under intense scrutiny as trust erodes in capital markets, the nation's regulatory system, and an increasing number of organizations and their leaders. A board of directors is obligated to act in the interest of stakeholders. In this, they must exercise a set of responsibilities and practices that provides strategic direction and ensures that executive leadership achieves the organization's objectives, manages risk appropriately, and uses resources responsibly.[1] In their Policy Governance Model, John Carver and Miriam Carver note that if a board's effectiveness noticeably diminishes, stakeholders take new interest in its composition, conduct, and decision-making capabilities.[2]

Under current economic conditions, stakeholders are demanding stronger governance with closer board oversight, greater transparency in business practices, and increased accountability for risk management and asset protection. Demand extends beyond increased accountability for the protection of assets represented on a financial balance sheet. Information and the knowledge derived from it are among an organization's most valuable assets. As with other critical resources, information requires a level of protection achieved only through effective management and assured only through effective board oversight.

New regulations, laws, and industry standards hold an organization's directors and officers accountable for protecting personally identifiable information, credit card information, individual health information, and consumer privacy. For healthcare providers, the consequences of ineffective controls over information can be costly. Consequences can include compromised patient care, reduced public trust, reputational damage to the organization and its leaders, brand erosion, identity theft, medical identity theft, financial penalties and costs, and undermining of the organization's mission.

Demand for stronger governance extends beyond requirements for transparency in financial reporting. Healthcare providers have increasing requirements for non-financial data reporting—including clinical quality measures, adverse events, and inappropriate disclosure of personally identifiable information and credit card information. Other requests for non-financial data include media requests, hospital association/health system data surveys, and Web site content (operational indicators, quality measures, clinical program information, etc.).[3]

Stakeholders are asking for transparency. They want not-for-profits to justify their tax-exempt status and to articulate the benefits provided to the community, the performance level they are achieving, and the fairness of their pricing—especially in caring for the indigent, uninsured, and underinsured.[4]

The growth of healthcare consumerism is generating increased demand for access to provider price and quality data that can help consumers make healthcare purchase decisions.[5] Clinicians now share accountability for quality performance information along with board members and executive management who are accountable for the accuracy, relevancy, and reliability of all reportable information.

Why has non-financial information lacked attention for so long? One reason is that current accounting standards do not represent this type of information. Non-financial information has no "book value" and is neither understood nor controlled as are other, more tangible, corporate assets. Doug Laney, Director of Global Services Marketing for BMC Software, writes of information's three-dimensional problem—extreme velocity, volume, and variety. He identifies these characteristics as impairments to inventorying and cataloging information assets. In the following passage, Laney identifies the need for valuation. "For long term assurance, determining and deploying an enterprise information architecture that controls, coordinates, and monitors data from capture to consumption can mitigate information-related risks significantly. As or more important, a well-defined information architecture enables information to be leveraged with more confidence and consistency in driving improved business process effectiveness, and, ultimately, information's bottom line value."[6]

Healthcare futurist Joe Flower promotes an accelerated use of data technologies. He sees them as requisites for meeting the demands for healthcare reform and healthcare providers' survival. He recognizes that more technologies will be needed to support evidence-based medicine, digitized processes, data transparency, and automation to drive productivity and quality measurements and monitoring. He expects that reform and survival will be driven by data with every data system tracking its actions in ways that can be monitored and queried. This also means every manual effort will be examined with a "lean manufacturing" style for potential automation with reduction in transaction costs and error.[7] The future of healthcare requires that providers digitize, automate, and streamline. "Expect a much higher component of data technologies tying it all together," notes Flower, "which means an expanded need for tech geeks skilled in healthcare information technology."[8]

The need for healthcare systems and hospitals to improve the content, quality, integrity, and availability of information they provide to decision makers has never been greater.[3] The need for assurance of the confidentiality, integrity, authentication, availability, and non-repudiation of information and information systems has also never been greater.

This chapter expresses the need for healthcare system and hospital leaders to broaden their perspective of governance to include the effective management of information-related risks. It describes an information assurance process and proposes a method of implementation based on an informed directorate. This would comprise layered responsibility for assurance activities with feedback loops designed for dynamic regulation of risk control and acceptance decisions.

A WELL-INFORMED DIRECTORATE

The Institute of Internal Auditors (IIA) recognizes a broader view of governance in its statement on information assurance. "While there is a continuing need for attestation of the validity of financial statements, there is an increasing demand for assurance that information is secure and supporting technologies function properly and are adequately and efficiently protected from harm and disruption."[9]

An organization's health relies on sound decisions—those based on accurate, timely, complete, and relevant information—and assurances that decisions are implemented as intended. Directors are responsible for governance and they are expected to understand fundamental aspects of the organization they oversee. They are accountable for the organizations' activities and should know about the risks that represent opportunities and those that would prevent it from meeting its objectives. Directors need information to govern, and they need assurance of that information.

Information governance addresses this need. It includes requirements for assurance. Information governance directs the oversight of risk management activities and the system of internal control intended to ensure the integrity and resiliency of mission-critical information and the supporting technologies and infrastructure.

With increasing demand for information and with the threat of fines and lawsuits and the impact on brand and reputation caused by information security breaches, identity theft, and technology failures, corporate leaders are becoming more aware of the importance of managing information risk. It appears, however, that this awareness does not necessarily translate into effective information governance.

A study sponsored by the Information Assurance Advisory Council (IAAC) in 2004 concluded that, at that time, boards generally regarded information security as a low-level technical issue and cited communication gaps as impairments to effective relations between technologists and directors.[10] KPMG reported in 2007 that audit committee members admitted they were ill-equipped to ask management and auditors the right questions about their company's IT risk.[11]

Referring to a 2008 survey by the National Association of Corporate Directors of 703 sitting directors of US public companies, Carnegie Mellon University's CyLab reported that, in general, board members were unclear on the link between IT risk and a company's overall risk posture. Directors and officers were not devoting resources or attention to the business-critical implications of faulty information security processes. CyLab reported the following statistics and concluded that boards still identify security as a technical issue.[12]

- Thirty-eight percent of the respondents said they only occasionally or rarely reviewed privacy, security, or risk-management budgets. An additional 40 percent said they never did.

- Fifty-five percent of respondents indicated they only occasionally or rarely reviewed and approved roles and responsibilities of personnel responsible for privacy and security risks. Twenty-eight percent said they never did.

- Sixty-two percent said they only occasionally or rarely received reports from senior management regarding privacy and security risks, An additional 15 percent said they never received these reports.

- Fifty-six percent said they only occasionally or rarely reviewed top-level security and privacy policies, and 23 percent said they never review these policies.

The IT Governance Institute advises board members that they can be exposed to their own set of information risks:[13]

- Being unaware of risk exposures.

- Being unaware of legal and regulatory requirements.

- Failing to understand the impact of security failures on the business.

- Being unable to monitor management's performance in managing information (and security) risks.

- Failing to set the tone at the top with regard to the importance of information management.

- Failing to judge the value of information and security investment proposals.

Healthcare systems and hospitals need an effective information governance program—one with clearly established and committed leadership, a holistic approach, a portfolio view, coordinated execution, and constant monitoring. A strong program is needed to meet the increasing demands of stakeholders and requirements for healthcare reform and corporate survival.

Directors do not require IT expertise, although it is critical that they have knowledge of the major technologies that support clinical and business operations. This knowledge should include information about significant risks. Consulting groups recommend that the board gain understanding from the CIO of the IT platform that the business operates under and the applications that support core functions.

A REPEATABLE, SCALABLE INFORMATION ASSURANCE PROCESS

In its publication *An Introduction to Computer Security: The NIST Handbook,* NIST defines computer security assurance as "the degree of confidence, based on sufficient evidence, that administrative, technical, and operational safeguards work as intended to protect the system and the information it processes." NIST warns that "Assurance is not, however, an absolute guarantee that the measures work as intended."[14]

IAAC defines information assurance as "a holistic approach towards protecting corporate information and systems (and, therefore, business continuity) by ensuring their availability, integrity, authentication, confidentiality, and nonrepudiation."[10]

The Committee on National Security Systems (CNSS) defines information assurance as "the measures that protect and defend information and information systems by ensuring their availability, integrity, authentication, confidentiality, and non-repudiation. These measures include providing for restoration and information systems by incorporating protection, detection, and reaction capabilities."[15]

The Information Systems Audit and Control Association (ISACA) views information assurance as the foundation for enterprise decision making to the extent that, without assurance, an enterprise lacks confidence that sensitive information remains secure and that reliable information is available when needed.[16]

A Wikipedia entry describes information assurance as a formal process that begins with an inventory and classification of the information assets to be protected, followed by a risk assessment and the development of a risk management plan. Frameworks including CobiT, PCI DSS, ISO 17799 or ISO/IEC 27002 are useful tools for designing a risk-management plan.[17]

Strict adherence to one of these frameworks is discouraged. A better approach to developing the risk assessment and management plans combines, from multiple sources, those elements most relevant to the organization and information assets targeted by the assurance process. Ideally, the assurance process is tailored to the organization.

This risk management plan identifies the countermeasures that would mitigate, eliminate, or transfer unacceptable risks. The plan should include cost estimates and provide a summarization of risks and rewards. Countermeasures identified in the plan can include firewalls, antivirus software, policies, procedures, regular backups, configuration hardening, training, security-awareness education and requirements for security incident and emergency response teams.[17]

The intent is to devise a plan to manage risk as efficiently and cost effectively as is possible. The entire process is cyclical. Both the risk assessment and risk management plans should be periodically reviewed and revised to address new risks and changes in business processes and information workflows.

Layered Responsibilities and Feedback Loops

Information assurances, like other assurances of internal control, can typically originate from a number of sources. One of the most important sources is the board itself. Consulting firms offer corporate governance services to assist a board in determining its effectiveness. The services include an assessment of the risks the board faces and the quality of information used by the board in making its decisions. Deliverables (feedback) include a risk-management plan. Having an external firm provide assurance of the board's own governance practices is, in a sense, the board's way of avoiding the practice of "self medicating."

Among the board's most fundamental roles is selecting a CEO, providing strategic direction, delegating responsibilities, and monitoring this individual's performance. The board's first step in satisfying its own expectation for information governance and assurance is to define and communicate the CEO's role in this governance activity. The board also establishes a monitoring capability (a feedback loop) to assess the CEO's performance in meeting the board's expectations. This monitoring capability, like others exercised by the board, is designed to avoid micromanaging and being overly dependent on information provided by the CEO.[18]

A board typically exercises its monitoring activities through one or more committees. The audit committee derives assurances from a mix of sources both within and outside the organization and with differing levels of objectivity and independence. The committee selects, on behalf of the board, an external audit firm to audit the financial statements. The extent, however, to which the firm examines information security controls is usually limited to controls affecting the financial systems.

The audit committee would expect the CEO to report on information assurance and would expect internal auditors to provide independent evaluation. The CEO, in turn, would communicate to executive management expectations for securing information and providing feedback in the form of assurances. This delegation of responsibility and corresponding requirements for feedback of assurance is communicated—from executive management to senior management and on and on through deeper layers of the organization and eventually to LOB managers. Essentially, management must assure the board's audit committee, through tangible evidence, that information security risks are clearly identified and efficiently managed.[9]

The board, through its audit committee, should be assured that management has implemented countermeasures (policy, standards, procedural and automated controls, etc.) addressing those risks that could significantly and adversely impact the health system or hospital's financial, operational, or reputational position. The audit committee should be prepared to question the controls, the checks and balances, and the tests implemented by the management team.

Management is responsible for the entire organization's internal control system, including the information assurance and security programs. Management should verify that programs are comprehensive, robust, and meet stakeholders' (including the board's) demands. Management is responsible for assuring that the programs target the most valuable information—including personally identifiable information, proprietary information, and research data. Management should identify those responsible for implementing information assurance processes and make clear their expectations for providing feedback.

LOB managers should be able to certify the validity, reliability, and integrity of the sensitive and business-critical information under their stewardship. Managers should routinely report their information governance activities to senior management and identify significant problems within the IT environment and the corrective measures being implemented. Through layered feedback loops, the CEO and, by extension, the board should be made aware of the reliance placed on the information assets (those owned and entrusted to) the organization.[26]

Feedback loops should ensure that plans are executed as designed and they should enforce quality. Performing a process without providing feedback creates an "open loop" and these processes are more likely to degrade over time. Effective feedback loops provide the assurance required to maintain quality data, processes, and patient care. Futurist Joe Flower foresees the value of feedback loops in a health provider environment. "Malpractice suits are a huge problem in healthcare largely because there is no other feedback loop enforcing quality. In a context in which providers work in teams, using evidence-based guidelines, standardized practices, except where an individual case calls for variation, and digital records that communicate clearly between different providers and document each decision, malpractice would simply not be the problem it is today."[19]

All feed-back mechanisms that provide assurances (from external and internal auditors, the CEO, other members of executive management, and line management) contribute to the overall picture on how well an organization is managing the delivery of its objectives and the risks (including information risks) that might jeopardize those objectives.

SUMMARY

For those organizations lacking strong information governance and assurance programs, cultural changes are required. Board members can affect significant changes in the organizations' security posture using one of their most powerful tools—"tone at the top." Executive and line management must take a more active role. Merely endorsing policy and standards and with the expectation that a workforce will adhere has proven ineffective. Standards become standards when they are adopted, not because they are published. Management should set clear, measurable expectations for information risk management and verify through meaningful feedback loops that their expectations are met.

IT and security professionals can affect change by continuing their risk assessment and control monitoring activities, by implementing modifications based on these processes, and providing assurances to executive management (and possibly the board).

Discussion Questions

1. American hospitals and healthcare systems are bracing for changes resulting from congressional efforts to reduce costs and improve patient care. In what ways can information security help to achieve these objectives within your organization?
2. In what ways can you broaden your perspective of information governance?
3. What steps can you take to convince your organization's financial leadership team that information assets represent a growing percentage of the organization's overall asset portfolio?
4. You and your immediate management understand the importance of layered responsibilities and feedback loops. Although executive management and the board approved your position neither group has requested information or shown interest in the security program. What efforts can you and your immediate management make to establish routine reporting requirements? (Hint: Consider Legal, Compliance, and Internal Audit teams as allies.)

References

1. Information Security and Control Association. ISACA glossary of terms. Accessed July 14, 2009. Available at: www.isaca.org/glossary.pdf.
2. Carver J, Carver M. Carver's policy governance® model in nonprofit organizations. PolicyGovernance.com. March 2009. Accessed July 14, 2009. Available at: www.carvergovernance.com/pg-np.htm.

3. KPMG Healthcare & Pharmaceutical Institute. Briefing for audit committee members of not-for-profit healthcare systems and hospitals: industry insights. November 2008. Accessed July 14, 2009. Available at: www.kpmghealthcarepharmainstitute.com/documents/HPI/8132009143010HC_AC%20Briefing_WEB_v07.pdf.

4. KPMG Healthcare & Pharmaceutical Institute. The path to value: enhancing the relevance, reliability, and transparency of reporting in the healthcare industry. *KPMG Health Care Insider.* October 10, 2008. Accessed July 14, 2009. Available at: www.kpmginsiders.com/display_analysis.asp?cs_id=229396.

5. Bigalke J, Rudish R, Hisey T, Keckley P. 2009 industry outlook: health sciences, challenging times, emerging opportunities. Deloitte LLC. January 2009. Accessed July 14, 2009. Available at: www.deloitte.com/assets/Dcom-UnitedStates/Local%20Assets/Documents/us_industryoutlook_2009OutlookHealthSciences_January2009.pdf.

6. Laney D. Information accounting and asset management. *Data Strat J* [online]. Accessed July 14, 2009. Available at:
www.datastrategyjournal.com/index.php?option=com_content&task=view&id=49&Itemid=76.

7. FlowerJ. What must be done: cheaper medicine means better medicine; make your organization efficient. Hospitals & Health Networks [online]. March 11, 2008. Accessed July 14, 2009. Available at: www.hhnmag.com/hhnmag_app/jsp/articledisplay.jsp?dcrpath=HHNMAG/Article/data/03MAR2008/080311HHN_Online_Flower&domain=HHNMAG.

8. Flower J. Does cheaper future healthcare mean lost jobs? ImagineWhatIf.com. September 12, 2008. Accessed July 14, 2009. Available at: www.imaginewhatif.com.

9. The Institute of Internal Auditors. Information security management and assurance: a call to action for corporate governance. April 2000. Accessed July 14, 2009. Available at: www.theiia.org/download.cfm?file=22398.

10. Anhal A, Daman S, O'Brien K, Rathmell A. *Engaging the Board: Corporate Governance and Information Assurance.* Rand. Santa Monica, CA: 2003.

11. Larkin G. Audit committees in search of good IT governance. *KPMG Audit Committee Insights.* April 4, 2007. Accessed July 14, 2009. Available at: www.kpmginsiders.com/display_search.asp?content_id=915262&segment_id=1&cs_id=.

12. Westby JR, Power R. Governance of enterprise security survey: CyLab 2008 report. Carnegie Mellon CyLab. Pittsburgh, PA: December 2008.

13. IT Governance Institute. *CobiT Security Baseline: An Information Security Survival Kit.* ITGI. Rolling Meadows, IL: 2007.

14. National Institute of Standards and Technology. An introduction to computer security: the NIST handbook. NIST. Special Publication 800-12; February 1996. Accessed July 14, 2009. Available at: http://csrc.nist.gov/publications/nistpubs/800-12/handbook.pdf.

15. National Information Assurance (IA) Glossary, Committee on National Security Systems. June 2006, http://www.cnss.gov/Assets/pdf/cnssi_4009.pdf.

16. ISACA. Glossary of terms [online]. ISACA. June 2008. Accessed July 14, 2009. Available at: www.isaca.org/Template.cfm?Section=Glossary&Template=/CustomSource/glossary.cfm.

17. Wikipedia. Information assurance. [online]. Accessed July 14, 2009. Available at: http://en.wikipedia.org/wiki/Information_assurance.

18. Amundson W. Enhancing the board's monitoring role…without micro-managing. The Canadian Association. March 2004. Accessed July 14, 2009. Available at: www.axi.ca/TCA/Mar2004/featurearticle.shtml.

19. Flower J. Reforming health care for cost, quality and value. Hospitals & Health Networks [online]. January 2009. Accessed July 14, 2009. Available at: www.hhnmag.com/hhnmag_app/jsp/articledisplay.jsp?dcrpath=HHNMAG/Article/data/01JAN2009/090127HHN_Online_Flower&domain=HHNMAG.

CHAPTER 18

Personal Health Records

Lory Wood

PERSONAL HEALTH RECORDS

Personal health records (PHR) are tools that empower the healthcare consumer/patient to participate in managing their family's health. As a comprehensive instrument, it assists the primary caretaker in improving the quality of living for family and friends. With the significant diversity found in the current PHR industry, it is important that the consumer is aware of the types of PHRs that are available and which best meets their needs, while also preserving their privacy and confidentiality. Some models offer the consumer more control than others.

In December 2008, HHS's Office of the National Coordinator for Health Information Technology (ONC) released the HIPAA Privacy Rule and Electronic Health Information Exchange in a Networked Environment and the Nationwide Privacy and Security Framework for Electronic Exchange of Individually Identifiable Health Information (also referred to as the Privacy and Security Framework). The latter provided a scope for guiding the actions of all healthcare-related persons and entities that participate in a network for the purpose of electronic exchange of individually identifiable health information. This model includes PHRs. On this, the document states, "The PHR market continues to evolve at a rapid pace, with new types of PHRs continually emerging…the universe of PHRs can be broken down into two categories: those subject to the (HIPAA) Privacy Rule and those that fall outside of its scope. PHRs that are subject to the Privacy Rule are those that a covered healthcare provider or health plan offers. Examples of PHRs that fall outside the scope of the Privacy Rule are those offered by an employer (separate from the employer's group health plan) or those made available directly to an individual by a PHR vendor that is not a HIPAA-covered entity."[1]

The core principles of this Security and Privacy Framework are individual access; correction, openness and transparency; individual choice; collection, use and disclosure limitations, data quality and integrity; safeguards; and accountability.

Year 2009 will be the first that the CCHIT will accept PHR systems for testing and potential certification. CCHIT is the recognized certification body for electronic health records and their networks, and a private, nonprofit initiative. Their mission is to accelerate the adoption of robust, interoperable health information technology (HIT) by creating a credible, efficient certification process.[2]

In an effort to provide broader consumer and industry strategic guidance for its new PHR certification development, the CCHIT assembled a special PHR Advisory Task Force (ATF). The ATF made its recommendations[3] of PHR attributes to certify for security, privacy, interoperability, and general functionality. This may seem like a small number of criteria, but it is exponentially complex when the various PHR models are factored into the formula. PHR information and news for consumers from CCHIT is available online with a "Q&A" section and special articles that address the key issues with privacy, security and interoperability.[4]

The ATF gave clear guidance to "accommodate diverse PHR models in certification," as seen in Figure 18-1.

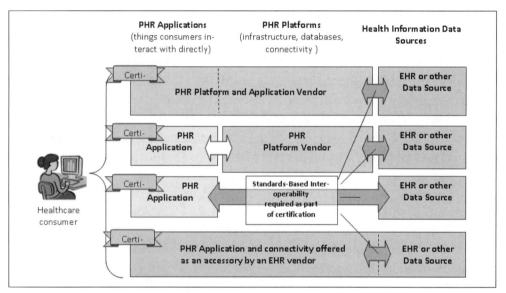

Figure 18-1: CCHIT ATF PHR Models for Certification. (Reprinted with permission from the Certification Commission for Healthcare Information Technology. Copyright 2008.)

There are two models for each of the two categories that HHS identified in their PHRs and the HIPAA Privacy Rule documentation; the categories delineate those subject to the Privacy Rule and those that are not. The four models include a PHR application provided by: 1.) independent vendors; 2.) employers or employer coalitions—which are not covered entities under the Security Rule; 3.) payors; and 4.) providers. There are benefits and innate functionality unique to each model. The independent vendor model is usually referred to as "untethered" or "unlinked." These systems are usually fully controlled and owned by the consumer/patient. By the very nature of being independent, this model uses an opt-in consent and authorization process. Consents and authorizations are the permissions that consumers give the vendor on how they may use their data.

The three other models are usually referred to as "tethered" or "linked." They are typically dependent on the parent entity, which may or may not be a covered entity under the HIPAA regulations, for their data. Some of the models transfer a subset of their data to the consumer application, while others only allow the consumer to "view" portions of their data from the central data repository. Most of the dependent models also require the users to opt-out of participation, as opposed to choosing to opt-in.

Because there are very different PHR models available in the industry and these are ever changing, there are no uniform or consistent definitions within the government or industry. This lack of standing definitions is also a result of not having any standards available, specifically for PHRs. However, HL7 balloted and vetted standards for the PHR-S Functionality Model in 2008.[5] And CCHIT, on the average, allows 12 to 18 months from the publishing of a standard before it is included as certification criteria. Therefore, general and robust functionality will begin to be tested in 2010.

The HIMSS definition for ePHR is a:

> universally accessible, layperson comprehensible, lifelong tool for managing relevant health information, promoting health maintenance and assisting with chronic disease management via an interactive, common data set of electronic health information and e-health tools. The ePHR is owned, managed, and shared by the individual or his or her legal proxy(s) and must be secure to protect the privacy and confidentiality of the health information it contains. It is not a legal record unless so defined and is subject to various legal limitations.[6]

The HHS defines PHRs as "electronic application[s] through which individuals can maintain and manage their health information (and that of others for whom they are authorized) in a private, secure, and confidential environment."[7] A confidential and easy-to-use tool for managing information about your health. A PHR is usually an electronic file or record of your health information and recent services, such as allergies, medications, personal medical facts, and doctor or hospital visits that can be stored in one place, and then shared with others, as you see fit.[8]

HHS/CMS continues by describing the advantages in using a PHR.

Key points to remember about Personal Health Records[8]:

- You control the health information in your PHR.

- If your PHR is Internet-based, you can access it from any place at any time, and easily share it with others.

- You can update your health information to make sure it stays current.

- You will be able to use tools to get information about your health conditions and learn what to expect from medications you are taking.

- You may even be able to request prescription refills, schedule appointments, or send an e-mail to your doctor with certain kinds of PHRs.

- You can keep information on your PHR that could help in an emergency situation, and give others limited access to the PHR for just this purpose.

The National Health Information Infrastructure Workgroup of the National Committee on Vital and Health Statistics (NCVHS) held six hearings on PHRs and PHR systems between 2002 and 2005. In September 2005, the NCVHS workgroup submitted a letter report on PHR systems to HHS Secretary, Michael Leavitt.[9] The report covered key potential benefits and identified the need for privacy, security and interoperability.

Interoperability

Figure 18-2, which was generated from a 2001 NCVHS report and included in the 2008 letter report, illustrates how the information needs of each area may be either unique or shared and identify potential opportunities for interoperability.

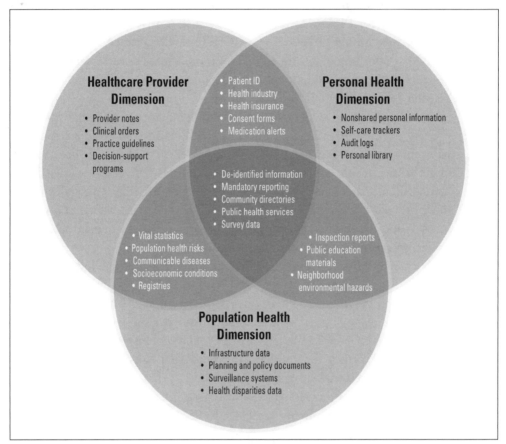

Figure 18-2: Examples of Content for the Three Dimensions and Their Overlap. (From National Committee on Vital and Health Statistics, *Information for Health: a Strategy for Building the National Health Information Infrastructure*, Washington, DC, 2001. Used by permission.)

The privacy considerations of PHR systems are complex, yet addressing them adequately is vital for PHR systems to succeed. Consumers want to be able to control access to their personal health information... While HIPAA compels covered entities to provide notice of their privacy practices to consumers, not all PHR vendors are HIPAA covered entities. The Committee is unaware of any requirement that compels the PHR vendor not covered by HIPAA to provide to consumers the terms and conditions governing the privacy of the consumers' data. While the Committee does not suggest that HIPAA or a HIPAA-like framework is necessarily the most appropriate for safeguarding privacy in PHR systems, the Committee does believe that privacy measures at least equal to those in HIPAA should apply to all PHR systems, whether or not they are managed by covered entities. The Committee also believes that it is vital for PHR systems vendors to provide clearly stated, easily understood, up-front privacy notices to consumers of their privacy policies and practices, and that these notices should be translated into other languages. [10]

Interoperability functionality is a critical component to PHRs being a viable tool for the consumer to participate on the National Health Information Network (NHIN). [11] The HHS Office of the National Coordinator states, "the NHIN is being developed to provide a secure, nationwide, interoperable health information infrastructure that will connect providers, consumers, and others involved in supporting health and healthcare. This critical part of the national health IT agenda will enable health information to follow the consumer, be available for clinical decision making, and support appropriate use of healthcare information beyond direct patient care so as to improve health….The ONC is advancing the NHIN as a 'network of networks,' which will connect diverse entities that need to exchange health information, such as state and regional HIEs, integrated delivery systems, health plans that provide care, personally controlled health records, federal agencies, and other networks as well as the systems they, in turn, connect.

Security

The NHIN is a formable and necessary goal for health information to be shared among all healthcare providers, patients, government, and industry partners. Interoperability among systems is crucial for the network to succeed. Security and privacy are critical to the success factors of network interoperability. For the information to be shared in a secure manner on the network, the network members have to be known to each other and have to be deemed authorized users with appropriate privileges to access the appropriate information.

There are multiple methods that can be used to authorize or verify a potential member or user. This process is usually called *identity proofing*. We perform this function many times in our ordinary schedules of day-to-day life. When people apply for a driver's license, as one example, they are required to bring in an original birth certificate and proof of residential address.

The Immigration Reform and Control Act of 1986 (IRCA) requires employers to certify employees by maintaining a DHS-issued Employment Eligibility Verification Form (Form I-9) for each employee. [12] When starting work at a new employer, as our second example, the new employee is required to bring in his or her social security card and a government-issued photo identification card (i.e., driver's license or passport) as part of the I-9 process. A third example is when you are seen at a physician's office for the first time. During registration the receptionist usually asks for your driver's license and insurance card, which he or she photocopies or scans into their system. All of these examples are face-to-face identity proofing or credentialing.

Face-to-face credentialing gives the organization a high level of assurance (LoA) that the person who is presenting is truly who they say they are. Budget is a major consideration when selecting the LoA that is appropriate for your organization. There is a direct correlation with a higher level of assurance and a higher level of cost. These costs include the maintenance of the user credentials, audit trails, and security infrastructure; policies; and procedures. Applications that have low levels of assurance usually only require a username and password and no verification of identity during registration. Figure 18-3 shows the correlation of LoA and cost.

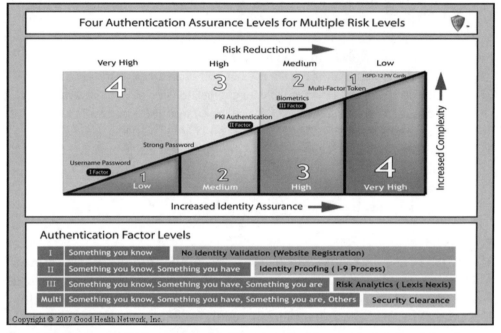

Figure 18-3: Security Risk Assessment. (Reprinted with permission from Good Health Network Inc. Copyright 2007.)

Both the financial and the banking industry are currently working to solve a similar problem. With online banking and bill-paying, individuals need to be able to prove they are who they say they are when presenting their electronic credentials over the Internet. Financial institutions need to be able to get as close to two-factor authentication as they can. Public key infrastructures (PKI) are very expensive to deploy and not realistic alternatives unless the debit and credit cards issued become smart cards with digital certificates. PKI does have the advantages of allowing roles-based access control and typically open and transparent audit trails. Roles-based access control limits the user to the application functionality and data that are actually necessary to perform his or her job function or role (i.e., proxy). Figure 18-4 is an example of one PHR application that allows consumers or account owners to grant access privilege to those they allow to access their PHR.

PKI also allows for open and transparent audit trails, which allow an account owner to monitor who has had access and to what data. This is seen in the PHR application in Figure 18-5. This journal color-codes entries based on roles.

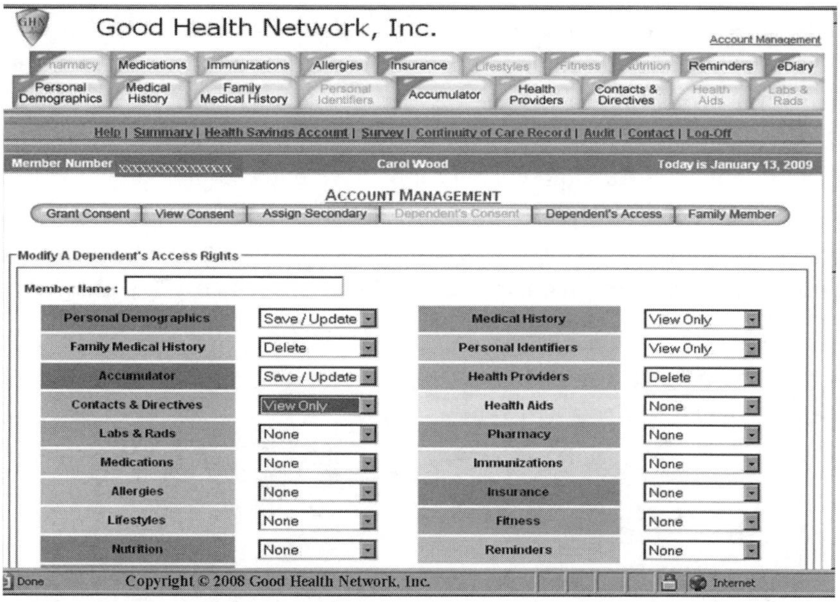

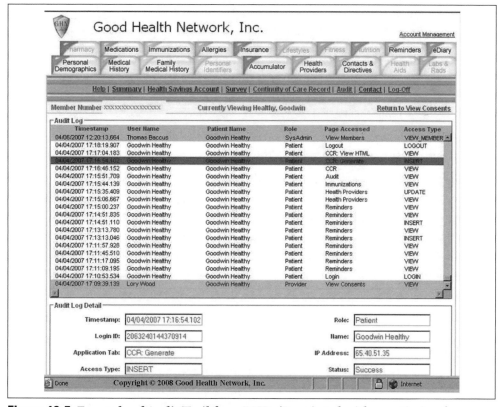

Figure 18-4: Example of a PHR–Good Health Network. (Reprinted with permission from Good Health Network Inc. Copyright 2008.)

Figure 18-5: Example of Audit Trail for a PHR. (Reprinted with permission from Good Health Network Inc. Copyright 2008.)

An alternative to the expensive PKI implementation, used by Bank of America, is the "SiteKey," which is a secure cookie. This allows the user to be confident they are at the valid online banking site and not a spoof. The SiteKey also ensures that the user is identified as the owner of the account.

Other HIT initiatives have various security methods for authenticating users into their systems. Some entities and corporations have budgets that allow them to have specialized security equipment and methods that allow for sometimes highly complex security systems with very high levels of assurance, as depicted in Figure 18-6. Most of those systems have two- or three-factor authentication protocols.

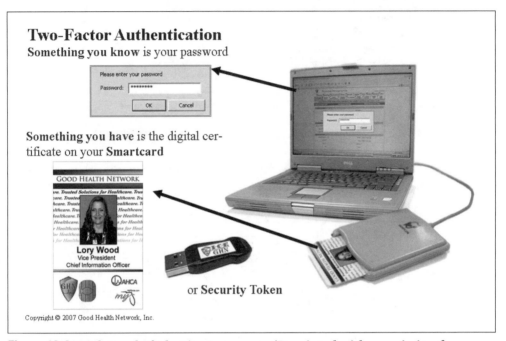

Figure 18-6: High Level of Identity Assurance. (Reprinted with permission from Good Health Network Inc. Copyright 2007.)

Healthcare consumers, especially elderly persons or those on fixed incomes, may not have card readers or computers with USB ports and high-speed Internet connection. Alternative methods will be necessary to accommodate the greatest number of users for the NHIN. Some of the methods being used in the banking industry may be very useful for these low technology users. Rather than using a full two-factor authentication method, it may be more appropriate to have a 1½ or a 1¾ factor authentication, such as the SiteKey.

HIPAA

The tethered or linked PHR models are usually associated with a covered entity. HIPAA regulations are very specific about the privacy and security requirements of a covered entity or any of their Business Associates. The independent, or untethered PHR model usually is not a covered entity under the HIPAA definition. That does not necessarily mean that these organizations do not fully comply with or exceed the HIPAA requirements, but it does mean that no federal regulations require them to be compliant and currently, no penalties or fines exist for non-compliance. Figure 18-7 is a high-level summary of the HIPAA Security and Privacy regulations.

Privacy	Security

•Consumer Amendments(§164.526)
•Right to Restrict & Access (§164.522,
    §164.524)
•BAA (§164.308, §164.314)
•Consumer Mitigation (§164.530)
•Disclosure and Auditing (§164.528)
•HIPAA Training (§164.530)
•Limiting Data & Research (§164.514)
•Opt-in Marketing (§164.508)
•Privacy Policies (§164.316)
•Privacy Statement (§164.520)
•Consents and Authorizations (§164.506,
    §164.508, §164.510)
•User/Entity Directories (§164.510)
	•Security Management Process (§164.308)
	•Assigned Security Responsibility (§164.308)
	•Workforce Security (§164.308)
	•Information Access Management (§164.308)
	•Security Awareness and Training (§164.308)
	•BAA (§164.308, §164.314)
	•Facility Access Control (§164.310)
	•Access and Audit Controls (§164.312)
	•Transmission Security (§164.312)
	•Documentation, Policies and Procedures
	    (§164.316)

Figure 18-7: HIPAA Rules Summarized.

HIPAA compliance does not seem like a big issue on the surface, but on further review, it can actually be a show-stopper to the interoperability of the NHIN and all of the PHR models. Those that are covered entities do not want to put their organizations and their infrastructure at risk by connecting with a non-covered entity. That means that a community hospital or a physician's office may refuse to allow a patient to send data to their HIS or EMR from a PHR. The covered entity's concerns may be valid. Some physicians fear even having e-mail or secure messages exchanged with a patient because there is not a high LoA that the patient or his or her valid proxy is the one receiving or reading the message. This could potentially lead to a confidentiality problem or complaint.

One potential solution to this concern would be to increase the level of identity-proofing that is being done for the patients. Physician's offices already perform a face-to-face verification at the initial visit, with the patient's credentials issued or validated by the physician's front office staff during registration, as previously discussed. Identity-proofing has become important and could potentially be required for PHRs to be allowed to participate in the NHIN. Laboratories, hospitals, and PBMs, to name a few, would be willing to exchange information with a patient who has an independent, untethered PHR if there was a credible face-to-face credentialing process like the physician office registration.

Medical Identity Theft

In May 2008, the Office of the National Coordinator for Health Information Technology (ONC) awarded a contract to Booz Allen Hamilton, a strategist and technology consultant, available at http://www.boozallen.com, to assess and evaluate the scope of the medical identity theft problem in the United States.[14] The initial phase was a comprehensive environmental scan. A one-day Medical Identity Theft Town Hall Meeting was held at the FTC. The panels discussed the identified issues of medical identity theft, quantified the impact on the healthcare industry, and identified gaps for which no reliable measures were in place. The panel also began discussing recommendations for prevention, detection, remediation and potential legislation similar to that available for the financial industry. To report medical identity theft, consumers should check the FTC site available at http://www.ftc.gov/bcp/edu/microsites/idtheft/

The PHR can be a highly effective tool to reduce the level of medical identity theft in the United States. Most victims report that the way they found out about the theft was from insurance company benefits reports or from a facility not receiving payment for services given in good faith to the wrong patient. Making the data available to patients and their families would allow for earlier detection and potential remediation. This would equate to a cost saving industrywide by reducing fraud, and with early intervention, hopefully increasing convictions.

NHIN, HIEs, AND RHIOs

Connecting nodes to the NHIN will be HIE and RHIOs in the local communities. PHRs become the connection point for patients. A precursor to the patient's full implementation and participation with the HIE/RHIO may be the emergency dataset. The full emergency dataset would include demographics (name, address, DOB), medication list, problem list, allergies, current providers, insurance information, blood type, and whether females are pregnant. These are all the same categories of data referred to in the ONC AHIC Consumer Empowerment Use Case also referred to as the "doctor's clipboard." This is all of the data a doctor's office typically requests the patient provide on the initial registration forms. This is a valid use case for emergency information because it will give a provider adequate information to treat the patient even if this is the first time the provider has seen this patient.

There is an even smaller amount of emergency contact information that could be used in an emergency situation. This dataset is used in the ONC AHIC Emergency Responder–Electronic Health Record (ER-EHR) Use Case, the IHE ID/ECON white paper (Template for Law Enforcement to Hand Over Crash Victim Identity (ID) and Emergency Contact Information (ECON) to EMS Providers Following a Motor Vehicle Crash), and the HITSP IS-04–HITSP Emergency Responder Electronic Record Interoperability Specification. Florida is hosting a pilot implementation of this use case and has generated a white paper with an HIE using PHRs. Figure 18-8 is the HITSP EMS Operational System Diagram.

Privacy
Ensuring privacy is a critical enabler to the NHIN, especially in PHR interoperability and information sharing with other health information technologies. Patient privacy is of paramount concern and a potential deterrent if it is not properly addressed. All PHR systems have a Privacy Statement and a Terms of Use agreement for which the subscriber is required to accept the terms to be granted the privileges to login. The main concern of the consumer is having Privacy Statements and Terms of Use agreements that are easily understandable, instead of those marbled in legalese, the type typically used by most software application license agreements. Most users do not take the time to read these agreements because they are so lengthy and confusing.

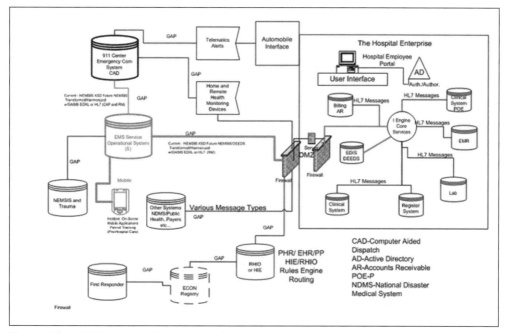

Figure 18-8: HITSP EMS Operational System Diagram.

The Markle Foundation has developed guidelines for "Connecting for Health Common Framework for Networked Personal Health Information."[13] The guidelines are based on "a flexible, 21st-century privacy approach, articulating clear national expectations for health IT: 1.) Core privacy principles, 2.) Sound network design, and 3.) Oversight and accountability. Both public and private entities will have a role in implementing and using such a framework." The guidelines include both technology and policy briefs that detail of the consumer's needs and expectations. Within the privacy domain, there are nine core principles. They are presented in Figure 18-9.

In June 2008, HHS began a multiphase and iterative research project to develop a model for presenting easy-to-understand information about PHRs to consumers (see Figure 18-10).

> The project purpose is to develop a 'plain language' model PHR fact sheet that will enable consumers to clearly understand and compare privacy policies across PHRs. The final product is envisioned to be a template for a web-based PHR fact sheet for vendors to use to deliver complex PHR privacy and security information simply and clearly so that consumers can make informed decisions. This would be similar to the nutrition label that provides a format for consumers to quickly learn nutritional information about a food or the financial services industry model privacy notice that dictates how the financial institutions inform consumers about financial privacy information practices.

PHRs IN 2009 AND BEYOND

The HITECH Act' is contained in the Stimulus Bill now being called ARRA, the American Recovery and Reinvestment Act which was passed and signed into legislation in February 2009. The HITECH portion contains several references and requirements for PHRs and PHR vendors. The following is a summary of the impact of this legislation on the PHR industry.

CORE PRIVACY PRINCIPLES
– Every information-sharing effort must provide:
Openness and Transparency

  – Communicate policies to participants and individuals

  – Provide privacy notices to consumers

  – Involve stakeholders in developing information sharing policies

Purpose Specification

  – Specify the purpose of the data collection effort clearly and make it narrowly suited to the need

Collection Limitation and Minimization

  – Assure that only data needed for specified purposes are being collected and shared

Use Limitation

  – Establish processes to ensure that data are only used for the agreed upon and stated purposes

  – Establish what data access is permitted for each user

Individual Participation and Control

  – Allow individuals to find out what data have been collected and who has access, and exercise meaningful control over data sharing

  – Give individuals access to information about them, and the ability to request corrections and see audit logs

Data Integrity and Quality

  – Provide that data are relevant, accurate, complete and up-to-date

Security Safeguards and Controls

  – Establish tools and mechanisms to provide that data are secured against breaches, loss or unauthorized access

  – Establish tools and approaches for user authentication and access

Accountability and Oversight

  – Establish who monitors compliance with policies and procedures for handling breach

  – Produce and make available audit logs

Remedies

  – Establish mechanisms for complaints

  – Establish remedies for affected parties to compensate for harm caused by breach

Figure 18-9: Connecting for Health Common Framework.

Under the definitions section of the legislation, the term *PHR* means "an electronic record of PHR identifiable health information on an individual that can be drawn from multiple sources and that is managed, shared, and controlled by or primarily for the individual." The term *vendor of PHRs* means "an entity, other than a covered entity, that offers or maintains a personal health record." The term *breach* means "unauthorized acquisition, access, use, or disclosure of" PHI.

New Business Associates Agreements
When HIPAA legislation was written, entities such as HIEs, RHIOs, and vendors of PHRs were not in existence. This new legislation ensures that they will now be under the HIPAA umbrella. The biggest change that impacts the PHR industry is that PHRs that are not offered by a covered entity may now be subject to HIPAA security and

privacy regulations through a new BAA. The BAA will now be subject to the HIPAA Security Rule, ensuring they are in compliance with administrative, technical and physical safeguards, and other applicable security procedures will be required to be incorporated into the BAA between the partner and the covered entity.

Facts about your personal information

Why do we provide you with this information?

We provide this information because we want you to clearly understand [Vendor]'s policies, practices, and procedures for using, securing, and protecting the personal information in your PHR. The table below provides you a snapshot. You can link to more detailed information by clicking on any of the areas below.

PHR Facts At-A-Glance		Our Practices
PHR Type	Provided by	
	Fee	
Who can view your personal information?	You	
	Family and friends	
	Healthcare providers	
	Insurers	
	Employers	
	Pharmacies	
	Additional health programs and services	
	[Vendor]	
	Others	
How may we use your personal information?	For [Vendor]'s business practices	
	For marketing	
	For medical research	
	For selling to others	
	For legal reasons	
What are our policies about closing your PHR?	Ability to close PHR	
	Data retention by [Vendor]	
	Ability to transfer to another PHR	
When will you be notified?	If [Vendor] is sold/merged/out of business	
	If there is a change in these policies	
	If there is a security breach	
How do we store and protect your personal information?	Geographic location of data storage	
	Logs of all PHR views for customer review	
Full printable version		
Contact information		

Disclaimer: This is a blank template. This document is a preliminary draft that is under development and provided solely for informational purposes. The information in this draft document may not be complete, comprehensive, or represent all of the legal obligations with which an entity needs to comply. Any reliance on the presentation or content provided in this document, in its current form, may pose legal risk.

| Home | Terminology | Contact Us |

Figure 18-10: Facts About Your Personal Information.

Breach Notification Requirement

ARRA includes a requirement for breach notification[2] and states, "Each vendor of personal health records, following the discovery of a breach of security of unsecured PHR identifiable health information that is in a personal health record maintained or offered by such vendor, shall first notify each individual who is a citizen or resident of the United States whose unsecured PHR identifiable health information was acquired by an unauthorized person as a result of such a breach of security;" and states also **that vendors must** "notify the Federal Trade Commission."

In addition, this requirement of notification also applies to "a third-party service provider that provides services to a vendor of personal health records or to an entity described as: (1) entities that offer products or services through the Web site of a vendor of personal health records; (2) entities that are not covered entities and that offer products or services through the websites of covered entities that offer individuals personal health records; or (3) entities that are not covered entities and that access information in a personal health record or send information to a personal health record."

This legislation additionally requires that "in connection with the offering or maintenance of a personal health record or a related product or service and that accesses, maintains, retains, modifies, records, stores, destroys, or otherwise holds, uses, or discloses unsecured PHR identifiable health information in such a record as a result of such services shall, following the discovery of a breach of security of such information, notify such vendor or entity, respectively, of such breach. Such notice shall include the identification of each individual whose unsecured PHR identifiable health information has been, or is reasonably believed to have been, accessed, acquired, or disclosed during such breach."

Application of Requirements for Timeliness, Method, and Content of Notifications

The notice of breach to the individual must be made without unreasonable delay and within 60 days of the discovery of the breach. The breach notification must include the date of the breach, the date of the discovery of the breach, the recommended steps the individuals should take to protect themselves from further harm, and the steps that the organization is taking to remediate.

Accounting of Disclosures

Consumers have the right to request an audit log of disclosures of the health information in their electronic records. The interest of the individuals vs. the administrative cost of accounting for the disclosures is taken into account. Useful as reasonable checks and balances, Accounting of Disclosures can be reviewed by consumers to reduce their fear that their PHI is being misused or used for discrimination.

Sale or Marketing of PHI

The ARRA legislation provides new restrictions on how the PHI that resides in electronic records can be used. ARRA determines the new restrictions on marketing directly to the consumer that was determined using information that resides in their electronic record. There is a limitation on the information that is allowed to be purchased for public health and research based on actual incurred cost.

Access and Portability

Lastly, individuals have the right to request and obtain an electronic copy of their EHR. The applicable charges are limited to the entity's labor costs. Individuals also have the right to designate or request that a third party, such as a PHR, be the recipient of the electronic copy from the EHR. It is required to be delivered in a standardized format.

The HITECH Act (ARRA) is an opportunity to formalize the foundation of the NHIN. It increases and standardizes the requirements to connect to the network and gives funding to jumpstart the initiative. The rights and concerns of individuals have been addressed, a definite encouragement to get the patients involved in the management of their family's healthcare.

SUMMARY

The PHR industry has had a very steady but slow adoption rate over the last five years. Because the industry has allowed for very innovative systems to be developed, patients have a myriad of choices and freedom to move between various models. Portability of data is now possible by using the ASTM Continuity of Care Record[14] or the HL7 Continuity of Care Document.[16] Both standards create an XML file that systems can use to import the data. America's Health Insurance Plans[15] has also vetted standards within HL7 that will allow for portability between and out of payor systems. The ASTM CCR standards' technical committee is working on the ability to digitally sign the record for full nonrepudiation. The following PHR application (Figure 18-11) was used for beta testing with digital healthcare certificates.

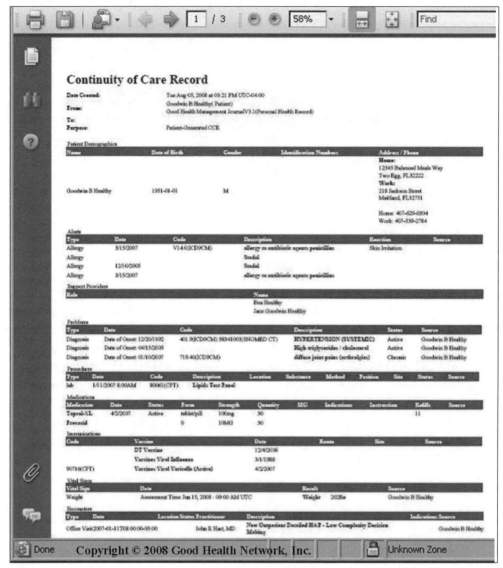

Figure 18-11: PHR Application Used for Beta Testing with Digital Healthcare Certificates. (Reprinted with permission from Good Health Network Inc. Copyright 2008.)

Discussion Questions

1. Discuss how Personal Health Records may impower healthcare consumers.
2. Discuss some of the national efforts to standardize PHRs. Describe some of the existing standards and what role they play in the PHR.
3. What role will HIPAA play in the implementation and adoption of PHRs?
4. Discuss the barriers involved with the transfer of information contained with PHRs.
5. Discuss the role of the PHR and Medical Identity Theft.

References

1. Accessed January 19, 2009. Page 7.
   http://www.hhs.gov/ocr/privacy/hipaa/understanding/special/healthit/phrs.pdf

2. Certification Commission for Health Information Technology. Work groups [online]. Accessed January 19, 2009. Available at: www.cchit.org/phr/.

3. http://www.cchit.org/node/951. Certification Commission for Health Information Technology PHR Advisory Task Force Minutes. Date accessed – January 19, 2009.

4. Certification Commission for Health Information Technology. Personal health records (PHR) information and news for consumers from CCHIT. [Web site]. Accessed January 19, 2009. Available at: http://phrdecisions.com/.

5. Health Level 7. [Web site]. Accessed January 19, 2009. Available at: www.hl7.org/.

6. Healthcare Information and Management Systems Society. HIMSS' PHR, ePHR, definition. [online] Accessed January 19, 2009. Available at: www.himss.org/ASP/topics_FocusDynamic.asp?faid=228.

7. http://healthit.hhs.gov/portal/server.pt?open=512&objID=1256&parentname=CommunityPage&parentid=2&mode=2&in_hi_userid=10741&cached=true Date accessed - January 19, 2009.

8. U.S. Department of Health & Human Services. Medicare. Personal health records. Accessed January 19, 2009. Available at: www.medicare.gov/PHR/overview.asp.

9. National Committee on Health and Vital Statistics. Date accessed – January 19, 2009.
   http://ncvhs.hhs.gov/050909lt.htm

10. Ibid.

11. U.S. Department of Health & Human Services. Nationwide Health Information Network (NHIN): Background & Scope. Accessed July 24, 2009. Available at: http://healthit.hhs.gov/portal/server.pt?open=512&objID=1142&parentname=CommunityPage&parentid=3&mode=2&in_hi_userid=10741&cached=true.

12. U.S. Department of Homeland Security. U.S. Citizenship and Immigration Services. Employment Eligibility Verification. [Web site]. Accessed January 19, 2009. Available at:
    www.dhs.gov/ximgtn/gc_1179350066521.shtm.

13. Markle Foundation. Common framework for networked personal health information. Accessed July 24, 2009. Available at: www.connectingforhealth.org/phti/.

14. ASTM International. Standard Specification for the Continuity of Care. Accessed July 24, 2009. Available at: www.astm.org/Standards/E2369.htm.

15. Date accessed - January 19, 2009. http://www.hl7.org/Library/General/HL7_CCD_final.zip.

16. Standard for Electronic Data Interchange – Personal Health Record Data Transfer Between Health Plans. Accessed January 19, 2009. Available at: www.ahip.org/content/default.aspx?bc=39|341|18427|20076.

Appendix A

Resources for Information Privacy and Security in Healthcare

The intent of this appendix is to provide links to sites containing regulation, guidance or information regarding privacy and security "best practices" for healthcare.

AMERICAN HEALTH INFORMATION MANAGEMENT ASSOCIATION (AHIMA)

The American Health Information Management Association (AHIMA) is the premier association of health information management (HIM) professionals. AHIMA's more than 53,000 members are dedicated to the effective management of personal health information required to deliver quality healthcare to the public. Founded in 1928 to improve the quality of medical records, AHIMA is committed to advancing the HIM profession in an increasingly electronic and global environment through leadership in advocacy, education, certification, and lifelong learning.

- **Primary Web site**
  www.ahima.org
- **Industry Activities and Emerging Issues**
  www.ahima.org/emerging_issues/
- **Privacy and Security**
  www.ahima.org/emerging_issues/PrivacyandSecurity.asp
- **Practice Briefs and Tools**
  www.ahima.org/infocenter/practice_tools.asp
- **Toolkits**
  www.ahima.org/infocenter/practice_tools.asp#Kits

AGENCY FOR HEALTHCARE RESEARCH AND QUALITY (AHRQ)

The Agency for Healthcare Research and Quality's (AHRQ) mission is to improve the quality, safety, efficiency, and effectiveness of healthcare for all Americans. Information from AHRQ's research helps people make more informed decisions and improves the quality of healthcare services. AHRQ was formerly known as the Agency for Health Care Policy and Research.

- **Primary Web site**
  www.ahrq.gov

AMERICAN RECOVERY AND REINVESTMENT ACT OF 2009 (ARRA)

The American Recovery and Reinvestment Act (ARRA) of 2009 (Pub.L. 111-5) is an economic stimulus package enacted by the 111th US Congress and signed into law by President Barack Obama on February 17, 2009. The Act of Congress was based largely on proposals made by President Obama and is intended to provide a stimulus to the US economy in the wake of the economic downturn. The measures are nominally worth $787 billion. The act includes federal tax relief, expansion of unemployment benefits, and other social welfare provisions, and domestic spending in education, healthcare, and infrastructure, including the energy sector.

- **Primary Web site**
  http://frwebgate.access.gpo.gov/cgi-bin/getdoc.cgi?dbname=111_cong_public_laws&docid=f:publ005.111

Relevant Privacy and Security Sections:
TITLE XIII—HEALTH INFORMATION TECHNOLOGY-HITECH

- Sec. 13101. ONCHIT; standards development and adoption

- Sec. 13201. NATIONAL INSTITUTE FOR STANDARDS AND TECHNOLOGY TESTING.

- Sec. 13400. Definition of the term "Breach"

- SEC. 13401. APPLICATION OF SECURITY PROVISIONS AND PENALTIES TO Business AssociateS OF COVERED ENTITIES; ANNUAL GUIDANCE ON SECURITY PROVISIONS

- SEC. 13402. NOTIFICATION IN THE CASE OF BREACH

- SEC. 13403. EDUCATION ON HEALTH INFORMATION PRIVACY

- SEC. 13404. APPLICATION OF PRIVACY PROVISIONS AND PENALTIES TO Business AssociateS OF COVERED ENTITIES

- SEC. 13405. RESTRICTIONS ON CERTAIN DISCLOSURES AND SALES OF HEALTH INFORMATION; ACCOUNTING OF CERTAIN PROTECTED HEALTH INFORMATION DISCLOSURES; ACCESS TO CERTAIN INFORMATION IN ELECTRONIC FORMAT

- SEC. 13406. CONDITIONS ON CERTAIN CONTACTS AS PART OF HEALTH CARE OPERATIONS
- SEC. 13407. TEMPORARY BREACH NOTIFICATION REQUIREMENT FOR VENDORS OF PERSONAL HEALTH RECORDS AND OTHER NON-HIPAA COVERED ENTITIES
- SEC. 13408. Business Associate CONTRACTS REQUIRED FOR CERTAIN ENTITIES
- SEC. 13409. CLARIFICATION OF APPLICATION OF WRONGFUL DISCLOSURES CRIMINAL PENALTIES
- SEC. 13410. IMPROVED ENFORCEMENT
- SEC. 13411. AUDITS
- SEC. 13412. RELATIONSHIP TO OTHER LAWS

CERTIFICATION COMMISSION FOR HEALTH INFORMATION TECHNOLOGY (CCHIT)

The Certification Commission for Healthcare Information Technology (CCHIT) is a recognized certification body for electronic health records and their networks, and a private, nonprofit initiative.

The commission operates with a nine-member volunteer board of Trustees, 21 volunteer Commissioners who represent all sectors of health IT and provide strategic guidance and oversight for the certification process and criteria, and 170 volunteers who serve on 15 work groups and bring their expertise to the process of creating the certification criteria.

- **Primary Web site**
  www.cchit.org/index.asp

CENTERS FOR MEDICARE & MEDICAID SERVICES (CMS)

Security Standard

The Administrative Simplification provisions of the Health Insurance Portability and Accountability Act of 1996 (HIPAA, Title II) required the Department of Health and Human Services (HHS) to establish national standards for the security of electronic healthcare information. The final rule adopting HIPAA standards for security was published in the Federal Register on February 20, 2003. This final rule specifies a series of administrative, technical, and physical security procedures for covered entities to use to assure the confidentiality of electronic protected health information. The standards are delineated into either required or addressable implementation specifications.

- **Web site**
  www.cms.hhs.gov/SecurityStandard/

HIPAA SECURITY GUIDANCE FOR THE REMOTE USE OF AND ACCESS TO ELECTRONIC PROTECTED HEALTH INFORMATION

This guidance document has been prepared with the main objective of reinforcing some of the ways a covered entity may protect EPHI when it is accessed or used outside of the organization's physical purview. In so doing, this document sets forth strategies that may be reasonable and appropriate for organizations that conduct any of their business activities through 1.) the use of portable media/devices (such as USB flash drives) that store EPHI; and 2.) offsite access or transport of EPHI via laptops, personal digital assistants (PDAs), home computers, or other non corporate equipment.

- **Web site**
  www.cms.hhs.gov/SecurityStandard/Downloads/
  SecurityGuidanceforRemoteUseFinal122806.pdf

HIPAA Security Materials

This area of the CMS site offers guidance and educational materials aimed at implementing HIPAA Security.

- **Web site**
  www.cms.hhs.gov/EducationMaterials

- **Security 101 for Covered Entities**
  www.cms.hhs.gov/EducationMaterials/Downloads/
  Security101forCoveredEntities.pdf

- **Security Standards: Administrative Safeguards**
  www.cms.hhs.gov/EducationMaterials/Downloads/
  SecurityStandardsAdministrativeSafeguards.pdf

- **Security Standards: Physical Safeguards**
  www.cms.hhs.gov/EducationMaterials/Downloads/
  SecurityStandardsPhysicalSafeguards.pdf

- **Security Standards: Technical Safeguards**
  www.cms.hhs.gov/EducationMaterials/Downloads/
  SecurityStandardsTechnicalSafeguards.pdf

- **Security Standards: Organizational, Policies and Procedures and Documentation Requirements**
  www.cms.hhs.gov/EducationMaterials/Downloads/
  SecurityStandardsOrganizationalPolicies.pdf

- **Security Standards: Basics of Security Risk Analysis and Risk Management**
  www.cms.hhs.gov/EducationMaterials/Downloads/
  BasicsofRiskAnalysisandRiskManagement.pdf

- **Security Standards: Implementation for the Small Provider**
  www.cms.hhs.gov/EducationMaterials/Downloads/SmallProvider4final.pdf

HIPAA Security Final Rule

45 CFR Parts 160, 162, and 164 Health Insurance Reform: Security Standards; Final Rule. 68 *Federal Register* 34 (20 February 2003); 8334-8381.

- **Web site**
  www.cms.hhs.gov/SecurityStandard/Downloads/securityfinalrule.pdf

Office of Civil Rights

Privacy Standards

The Office of Civil Rights (OCR), within the Department of Health & Human Services (DHHS), has the responsibility for enforcing the HIPAA Privacy Standards.

- **Web site**
  www.hhs.gov/ocr/privacy/index.html

The Privacy Rule

The HIPAA Privacy Rule establishes national standards to protect individuals' medical records and other personal health information and applies to health plans, healthcare clearinghouses, and those healthcare providers that conduct certain healthcare transactions electronically. The rule requires appropriate safeguards to protect the privacy of personal health information and sets limits and conditions on the uses and disclosures that may be made of such information without patient authorization. The rule also gives patients rights over their health information, including rights to examine and obtain a copy of their health records, and to request corrections.

- **Web site**
  www.hhs.gov/ocr/privacy/hipaa/administrative/privacyrule/index.html
    The Privacy Rule-Final

- **Web site**
  www.hhs.gov/ocr/privacy/hipaa/administrative/privacyrule/adminsimpregtext.pdf

The HIPAA Enforcement Rule

The HIPAA Enforcement Rule contains provisions related to compliance and investigations, the imposition of civil money penalties for violations of the HIPAA Administrative Simplification Rules, and procedures for hearings. The HIPAA Enforcement Rule is codified at: 45 CFR Part 160, Subparts C, D, and E.

71 *Federal Register* 32 (16 February 2006); 8390-8433.

- **Web site**
  www.hhs.gov/ocr/privacy/hipaa/administrative/privacyrule/
  finalenforcementrule06.pdf

HIPAA - Frequently Asked Questions

A searchable Web page for questions regarding the Privacy Rule.

- **Web site**
  www.hhs.gov/ocr/privacy/hipaa/faq/index.html

OFFICE OF THE NATIONAL COORDINATOR (ONC)

On April 27, 2004, President Bush issued Executive Order (EO) 13335 "to provide leadership for the development and nationwide implementation of an interoperable health information technology infrastructure to improve the quality and efficiency of health care." EO 13335 established the position of a National Coordinator for Health Information Technology (IT) within the Office of the Secretary of Health and Human Services.

EO 13335 also charged the National Coordinator with developing, maintaining, and directing

> "...the implementation of a strategic plan to guide the nationwide implementation of interoperable health information technology in both the public and private health care sectors that will reduce medical errors, improve quality, and produce greater value for health care expenditures."

Accordingly, the Office of the National Coordinator for Health Information Technology (ONC) has worked across the federal government to develop this ONC-coordinated Federal Health IT Strategic Plan (the Plan), which identifies the federal activities necessary to achieve the nationwide implementation of this technology infrastructure throughout both the public and private sectors. The timeframe of the Plan is 2008-2012.

- **Web site**
  http://healthit.hhs.gov/portal/server.pt?open=512&objID=1211&parentname=Com munityPage&parentid=2&mode=2&in_hi_userid=10741&cached=true

Privacy and Security Toolkit

The materials listed next are the HIPAA privacy components of the *Privacy and Security Toolkit* developed in conjunction with the Office of the National Coordinator. The *Privacy and Security Toolkit* implements the principles in *The Nationwide Privacy and Security Framework for Electronic Exchange of Individually Identifiable Health Information* (Privacy and Security Framework). These new guidance documents discuss how the Privacy Rule can facilitate the electronic exchange of health information.

- **Web site**
  www.hhs.gov/ocr/privacy/hipaa/understanding/special/healthit/index.html

Privacy Components

- **Privacy and Security Framework: Introduction**
  www.hhs.gov/ocr/privacy/hipaa/understanding/special/healthit/introduction.pdf

- **Privacy and Security Framework: Corrections**
  www.hhs.gov/ocr/privacy/hipaa/understanding/special/healthit/correction.pdf

- **Privacy and Security Framework: Transparency**
  www.hhs.gov/ocr/privacy/hipaa/understanding/special/healthit/
  opennesstransparency.pdf

- **Privacy and Security Framework: Individual Choice**

www.hhs.gov/ocr/privacy/hipaa/understanding/special/healthit/individualchoice.
pdf

- **Privacy and Security Framework: Collection**
www.hhs.gov/ocr/privacy/hipaa/understanding/special/healthit/
collectionusedisclosure.pdf

- **Privacy and Security Framework: Safeguards**
www.hhs.gov/ocr/privacy/hipaa/understanding/special/healthit/safeguards.pdf

- **Privacy and Security Framework: Accountability**
www.hhs.gov/ocr/privacy/hipaa/understanding/special/healthit/accountability.pdf

- **Privacy and Security Framework: Right of Access**
www.hhs.gov/ocr/privacy/hipaa/understanding/special/healthit/eaccess.pdf

- **Personal Health Records**
www.hhs.gov/ocr/privacy/hipaa/understanding/special/healthit/phrs.pdf

Nationwide Privacy and Security Framework for the Exchange of PHI

- **Web site**
http://healthit.hhs.gov/portal/server.pt/gateway/
PTARGS_0_10731_848088_0_0_18/NationwidePS_Framework-5.pdf

HEALTHCARE INFORMATION AND MANAGEMENT SYSTEMS SOCIETY

The Healthcare Information and Management Systems Society (HIMSS) is the healthcare industry's membership organization exclusively focused on providing global leadership for the optimal use of healthcare information technology (IT) and management systems for the betterment of healthcare. Founded in 1961 with offices in Chicago, Washington D.C., Brussels, Singapore, and other locations across the United States, HIMSS represents more than 23,000 individual members and over 380 corporate members that collectively represent organizations employing millions of people. HIMSS frames and leads healthcare public policy and industry practices through its advocacy, educational and professional development initiatives designed to promote information and management systems' contributions to ensuring quality patient care.

- **Web site**
www.himss.org

PORTALS AND TOOLS

Electronic Health Record

The Electronic Health Record (EHR) is a longitudinal electronic record of patient health information generated by one or more encounters in any care delivery setting. Included in this information are patient demographics, progress notes, problems, medications, vital signs, past medical history, immunizations, laboratory data, and radiology reports.

- **Web site**
  www.himss.org/ASP/topics_ehr.asp

Healthcare Information Technology Standards Panel (HITSP)

The Office of the National Coordinator for Health Information Technology (ONC) has as its mission the implementation of President Bush's vision for widespread adoption of interoperable electronic health records (EHRs) by 2014. In 2005, ONC awarded multiple contracts to advance this goal. Among these were contracts for creating processes to harmonize standards, certify EHR applications, develop nationwide health information network (HIN) prototypes, and recommend necessary changes to standardize diverse security and privacy policies. ANSI—in cooperation with strategic partners HIMSS, Booz Allen Hamilton, and Advanced Technology Institute—was awarded this contract. This standards harmonization collaborative established the Healthcare Information Technology Standards Panel (HITSP).

- **Web site**
  www.hitsp.org

Privacy and Security

The HIMSS Privacy & Security Toolkit (formerly known as the HIMSS CPRI Toolkit) offers new insights and up-to-date information in many areas, including a timely discussion of some national-level initiatives from DHHS' Office of the National Coordinator for Health Information Technology (ONC), such as CCHIT and HITSP.

- **Web site**
  www.himss.org/ASP/privacySecurityTree.asp?faid=78&tid=4

Privacy and Security for RHIOs/HIEs

Information and data exchange is critical to the delivery of quality patient care services and the effectiveness of healthcare organizations. The benefits of appropriate sharing of health information among patients, physicians, and other authorized participants in the healthcare delivery value chain are nearly universally understood and desired. A RHIO, or regional health information organization, is a group of organizations with a business stake in improving the quality, safety, and efficiency of healthcare delivery that comes together to exchange information for these purposes. The terms RHIO and Health Information Exchange (HIE) are often used interchangeably.

- **Web site**
  www.himss.org/ASP/topics_FocusDynamic.asp?faid=226

Privacy and Security for Personal Health Records

A personal health record (PHR) is an electronic repository in which a patient can store his or her health data privately and securely and can share these data with healthcare providers and others at the patient's discretion. This section features reports, white papers, and other documents and tools that discuss P&S issues relating to PHRs. Refer also to HIMSS PHR content page for HIMSS ePHR definition and other general information on PHRs.

- **Web site**

www.himss.org/ASP/topics_FocusDynamic.asp?faid=225

Privacy and Security Workgroups, Committees, and Task Forces

The Privacy and Security Steering Committee provides oversight and strategic directions for HIMSS projects, policies, and other matters related to privacy and security issues associated with the exchange and storage of electronic health information.

- **Web site**

  www.himss.org/ASP/topics_privacy_committees.asp?faid=83&tid=4

Legal and Regulatory

Privacy and security are key policy topics in the healthcare industry and therefore at the top of the agenda for discussion and action by the administration, congress, the federal government, and the healthcare industry.

- **Web site**

  www.himss.org/ASP/topics_FocusDynamic.asp?faid=62

Medical Identity Theft

Medical identity theft is a specific type of identity theft which occurs when a person uses someone else's personal health identifiable information, such as insurance information, Social Security number, healthcare file, or medical records; without the individual's knowledge or consent to obtain medical goods or services, or to submit false claims for medical services. There is limited information available about the scope, depth, and breadth of medical identity theft.

- **Web site**

  www.himss.org/ASP/topics_FocusDynamic.asp?faid=281

Medical Device Security

Medical devices and systems represent a growing risk with respect to the security of the medical data they contain. Hospitals and similar healthcare organizations typically have 300 percent to 400 percent more medical equipment than IT devices and two trends are contributing to the increasing significance of this security risk:

1. Medical devices and systems are being designed and operated as special purpose computers … more features are being automated, increasing amounts of medical data are being collected, analyzed and stored in these devices.
2. There has been a rapidly growing integration and interconnection of disparate medical (and information) technology devices and systems where medical data is being increasingly exchanged.

- **Web site**

  www.himss.org/ASP/topics_medicalDevice.asp

HIMSS RHIO/HIE

The terms "RHIO" and "Health Information Exchange" or "HIE" are often used interchangeably. RHIO (regional health information organization) is a group of organizations with a business stake in improving the quality, safety, and efficiency of healthcare delivery. RHIOs are the building blocks of the proposed National Health Information Network (NHIN) initiative proposed by David Brailer, MD, and his team at the Office of the National Coordinator for Health Information Technology (ONCHIT).

- **Web site**
  www.himss.org/ASP/topics_rhio.asp

THE HEALTH INFORMATION SECURITY AND PRIVACY COLLABORATION (HISPC)

Established in June 2006 by RTI International, through a contract with the DHHS, the Health Information Security and Privacy Collaboration (HISPC) originally comprised 34 states and territories. HISPC phase 3 began in April 2008, and HISPC now comprises 42 states and territories and aims to address the privacy and security challenges presented by electronic health information exchange through multistate collaboration. Each HISPC participant continues to have the support of its state or territorial governor and maintains a steering committee and contact with a range of local stakeholders to ensure that developed solutions accurately reflect local preferences. The third phase, comprises seven multistate collaborative privacy and security projects focused on analyzing consent data elements in state law; studying intrastate and interstate consent policies; developing tools to help harmonize state privacy laws; developing tools and strategies to educate and engage consumers; developing a toolkit to educate providers; recommending basic security policy requirements; and developing inter-organizational agreements. Each project is designed to develop common, replicable multistate solutions that have the potential to reduce variation in and harmonize privacy and security practices; policies; and laws. For more information about HISPC's background or what each multistate collaborative is working on, click on the following links.

- **Web site**
  http://healthit.hhs.gov/portal/server.pt?open=512&objID=1175&parentname=Com
  munityPage&parentid=22&mode=2&in_hi_userid=10741&cached=true

- **HISPC Executive Summary**
  http://healthit.hhs.gov/portal/server.pt/gateway/
  PTARGS_0_10731_848334_0_0_18/HISPC_Flyer_ExecSumm_508.pdf

- **HISPC-Adoption of Standard Policies for Authentication and Audit Collaborative**
  http://healthit.hhs.gov/portal/server.pt/gateway/
  PTARGS_0_10731_848246_0_0_18/HISPCStandardPolicies-1.pdf

- **HISPC-Interstate Disclosure and Patient Consent Requirements**
  http://healthit.hhs.gov/portal/server.pt/gateway/
  PTARGS_0_10731_848243_0_0_18/HISPCInterStateDisclosure-1.pdf

- **HISPC-Interstate and Intrastate Consent Policy Options**
  http://healthit.hhs.gov/portal/server.pt/gateway/
  PTARGS_0_10731_848357_0_0_18/HISPCConsent2v6.pdf

- **HISPC-Consumer Education and Engagement Collaborative**
  http://healthit.hhs.gov/portal/server.pt/gateway/
  PTARGS_0_10731_848240_0_0_18/HISPCConsumerEd-1.pdf

- **HISPC-Harmonizing State Privacy Law Collaborative**
  http://healthit.hhs.gov/portal/server.pt/gateway/
  PTARGS_0_10731_848241_0_0_18/HISPCHarmonizing-1.pdf

- **HISPC-Interorganizational Agreements Collaborative**
  http://healthit.hhs.gov/portal/server.pt/gateway/
  PTARGS_0_10731_848242_0_0_18/HISPCInterOrg-1.pdf

- **HISPC-Provider Education Collaborative**
  http://healthit.hhs.gov/portal/server.pt/gateway/
  PTARGS_0_10731_848245_0_0_18/HISPCProviderEd-1.pdf

HEALTH INFORMATION TECHNOLOGY STANDARDS PANEL (HITSP)

Data & Technical Standards: Health Information Technology Standards Panel
The Office of the National Coordinator established the Health Information Technology Standards Panel (HITSP), a public-private partnership with broad participation across more than 300 health related organizations, to identify and harmonize data and technical standards for healthcare. HITSP operates with an inclusive governance model established through the American National Standards Institute (ANSI).

- **Web site**
  www.hitsp.org/

HITSP works to:

- Harmonize standards to use for specific priorities advanced by the American Health Information Community (AHIC).

- Work with standard development organizations (SDO) to ensure that standards exist to meet health needs.

- Ensure specific guidance exists to unambiguously implement harmonized standards.

- Foster the availability and use of health information technology standards nationally.

ISO/IEC 17799:2005 Code of Practice for Information Security Management
ISO/IEC 17799:2005 Code of Practice for Information Security Management is an internationally recognized set of controls that focus on the best practices for information security. BS 7799-2:2002 provides instructions on how to apply ISO/IEC 17799 and to construct, run, sustain, and advance an information security management program.

- **Web site**

www.iso.org/iso/support/faqs/faqs_widely_used_standards/widely_used_
standards_other/information_security.htm

NATIONAL COMMITTEE ON VITAL AND HEALTH STATISTICS (NCVHS)

The National Committee on Vital and Health Statistics was established by Congress to serve as an advisory body to the Department of Health and Human Services on health data, statistics, and national health information policy. It fulfills important review and advisory functions relative to health data and statistical problems of national and international interest, stimulates or conducts studies of such problems, and makes proposals for improvement of the nation's health statistics and information systems. In 1996, the committee was restructured to meet expanded responsibilities under the Health Insurance Portability and Accountability Act of 1996 (HIPAA).

- **Web site**
  www.ncvhs.hhs.gov/intro.htm

Relevant Works:

- **Enhancing Protections for Uses of Health Data: A Stewardship Framework**
  www.ncvhs.hhs.gov/080424rpt.pdf

- **Enhanced Protections for Uses of Health Data: A Stewardship Framework for "Secondary Uses" of Electronically Collected and Transmitted Health Data**
  www.ncvhs.hhs.gov/071221lt.pdf

NATIONAL INSTITUTE OF STANDARDS AND TECHNOLOGY (NIST)

Founded in 1901, NIST is a non-regulatory federal agency within the US Department of Commerce. NIST's mission is to promote US innovation and industrial competitiveness by advancing measurement science, standards, and technology in ways that enhance economic security and improve our quality of life.

- **Web site**
  www.nist.gov

The Computer Security Division (CSD)-(893)

The Computer Security Division Responds to the Federal Information Security Management Act of 2002

The E-Government Act [Public Law 107-347] passed by the 107th US Congress and signed into law by President George W. Bush in December 2002 recognized the importance of information security to the economic and national security interests of the United States. Title III of the E-Government Act, entitled the Federal Information Security Management Act of 2002 (FISMA), included duties and responsibilities for the Computer Security Division in Section 303 "National Institute of Standards and Technology." Work to date includes:

- **Provide assistance in using NIST guides to comply with FISMA.** Information Technology Laboratory (ITL) Computer Security Bulletin *Understanding the New NIST Standards and Guidelines Required by FISMA: How Three Mandated Documents Are Changing the Dynamic of Information Security for the Federal Government* (**issued November 2004**).

- **Provide a specification for minimum security requirements for federal information and information systems using a standardized, risk-based approach.** Developed FIPS 200, *Minimum Security Requirements for Federal Information and Information Systems* (**issued March 2006**).

- **Define minimum information security requirements (management, operational, and technical security controls) for information and information systems in each such category.** Developed SP 800-53, *Recommended Security Controls for Federal Information Systems* (**revision 1 issued December 2006**).

- **Identify methods for assessing effectiveness of security requirements.** SP 800-53A, *Guide for Assessing the Security Controls in Federal Information Systems* (**second public draft issued April 2006**).

- **Bring the security planning process up-to-date with key standards and guidelines developed by NIST.** SP 800-18 Revision 1, *Guide for Developing Security Plans for Federal Information Systems* (**issued February 2006**).

- **Provide assistance to agencies and private sector.** Conduct ongoing, substantial reimbursable and nonreimbursable assistance support, including many outreach efforts such as the Federal Information Systems Security Educators' Association (FISSEA), the Federal Computer Security Program Managers' Forum (FCSM Forum), the Small Business Corner, and the Program Review for Information Security Management Assistance (PRISMA).

- **Evaluate security policies and technologies from the private sector and national security systems for potential federal agency use.** Host a growing repository of federal agency security practices, public/private security practices, and security configuration checklists for IT products. In conjunction with the government of Canada's Communications Security Establishment, CSD leads the Cryptographic Module Validation Program (CMVP). The Common Criteria Evaluation and Validation Scheme (CCEVS) and CMVP facilitate security testing of IT products usable by the Federal government.

- **Solicit recommendations of the Information Security and Privacy Advisory Board on draft standards and guidelines.** Solicit recommendations of the board regularly at quarterly meetings.

- **Provide outreach, workshops, and briefings.** Conduct ongoing awareness briefings and outreach to our customer community and beyond to ensure comprehension of guidance and awareness of planned and future activities. We also hold workshops to identify areas our customer community wishes addressed and to scope guidance in a collaborative and open format.

- **Satisfy annual NIST reporting requirement.** Produce an annual report as a NIST Interagency Report (IR). The 2003-2006 Annual Reports are available via the Web or upon request.

  Web site
  http://csrc.nist.gov/about/index.html

A large amount of HIPAA relies on the practices developed as part of the FISMA requirements. Work continues to help identify technologies, standards, and processes to enable the secure use of sensitive information. The recent passage of the American Recovery and Reinvestment Act (ARRA) specifically looks to the efforts of NIST in determining appropriate technology for encryption.

This section of Appendix A will include links to NIST documentation that may be of particular interest to privacy and security needs related to healthcare.

Where to start

Readers unfamiliar with the NIST Security site will probably wish to review the following two documents:

- **Guide to NIST Information Security Documents**
  http://csrc.nist.gov/publications/CSD_DocsGuide.pdf

- **NIST Information Security Document Roadmap**
  http://csrc.nist.gov/publications/CSD_DocsGuide_Trifold.pdf

Special publications

Good starting points to implement HIPAA:

- **An Introductory Resource Guide for Implementing the Health Insurance Portability and Accountability Act (HIPAA) Security Rule.**
  http://csrc.nist.gov/publications/nistpubs/800-66-Rev1/SP-800-66-Revision1.pdf

- **SP 800-53 Rev. 3 DRAFT Recommended Security Controls for Federal Information Systems and Organizations.**
  http://csrc.nist.gov/publications/drafts/800-53/800-53-rev3-IPD.pdf

- **SP 800-122 DRAFT Guide to Protecting the Confidentiality of Personally Identifiable Information (PII).**
  http://csrc.nist.gov/publications/drafts/800-122/Draft-SP800-122.pdf

- **NIST IR-7497 DRAFT Security Architecture Design Process for Health Information Exchanges (HIE).**
  http://csrc.nist.gov/publications/drafts/nistir-7497/Draft-NISTIR-7497.pdf

Health Information Privacy & Security

SP 800-111	Nov 2007	Guide to Storage Encryption Technologies for End User Devices. http://csrc.nist.gov/publications/nistpubs/800-111/SP800-111.pdf
SP 800-98	Apr 2007	Guidelines for Securing Radio Frequency Identification (RFID) Systems. http://csrc.nist.gov/publications/nistpubs/800-98/SP800-98_RFID-2007.pdf
NIST IR 7497	Jan 2009	DRAFT Security Architecture Design Process for Health Information Exchanges (HIE). http://csrc.nist.gov/publications/drafts/nistir-7497/Draft-NISTIR-7497.pdf
ITL October 2006	Oct 2006	Log Management: Using Computer And Network Records To Improve Information Security - ITL Security Bulletin. http://csrc.nist.gov/publications/nistbul/b-10-06.pdf
SP 800-34	Jun 2002	Contingency Planning Guide for Information Technology Systems.
SP 800-30	Jul 2002	Risk Management Guide for Information Technology Systems.
SP 800-48 Rev. 1	Jul 2008	Guide to Securing Legacy IEEE 802.11 Wireless Networks.
SP 800-46 Rev. 1	Feb. 24, 2009	DRAFT Guide to Enterprise Telework and Remote Access Security. http://csrc.nist.gov/publications/drafts/800-46Rev1/Draft-SP800-46r1.pdf

The reader should note that the NIST site has an enormous repository of guidance documents available to the public. Many of these documents contain information that may assist in implementing privacy and security programs. Due to the vast number of available documents, it is not feasible to print them in this appendix. NIST takes great efforts to group their documentation in an effort to make the resources easy to find. You may wish to consult the following links:

- **NIST Publications grouped by document family:**
  http://csrc.nist.gov/publications/PubsFL.html#Access%20Control

- **NIST Publications grouped by topic clusters:**
  http://csrc.nist.gov/publications/PubsTC.html

Appendix B

Sample Security Plan

An effective information security management program must have a documented plan. Content and organization for security plans vary, as each organization develops a plan to help guide their program. The security plan should be a living document and contain more than just control documentation. It should never sit on a shelf collecting dust. In fact, it may never exist in print form as a complete document. Over the past several years, I have observed many security plans develop from spreadsheets, databases, and word documents. If you choose the electronic route, don't forget the best practices of backups and contingency planning.

The framework provided next is just that: a framework. It should be tailored to the organization's mission, strategic plan, and operational practices.

SAMPLE SECURITY PLAN
REVISION INFORMATION
DATE
WHOM TO CONTACT FOR QUESTIONS/CONCERNS

1. **Purpose and Scope**

    This section should define the purpose of the document and the applicable scope. Examples of content for this section include who prepared the document, who authorized it, and the scope of its applicability (department-, hospital-, or health systemwide?) This section should also provide the contact information for the individuals or group responsible for the maintenance of the plan.

    As this plan will contain highly sensitive information, document the restrictions on distribution.

    Some plans will document applicable state and federal laws and regulatory issues within this section.

2. Risk Assessment Information and Asset Inventory

Risk assessment. Document thoroughly your risk assessment practices. Include any surveys and their results. The results should be documented with mitigation strategies and priority, as they will become action items.

Key concept. Information security management is risk management. Identifying the risk and level of threat is key to prioritizing your mitigation and management program.

Asset inventory. Include a listing of assets (a separate document or an appendix). This list should include assets such as software, hardware, databases, information data flows, connectivity dependencies, printers, portable devices, network equipment, desktop workstations, server farms, remote terminals, VLAN architectures, and personnel. Asset inventories often result from a thorough business impact assessment. A business impact assessment can be a critical source of documentation for business continuity programs.

3. Security Planning

After performing the risk assessment, devise a plan that takes into account the acceptable level of risks for systems and processes. This plan should be consistent with organizational goals and efforts to mitigate the risks.

Policies, standards, guidances, and procedures: Document all applicable policies, standards, guidances, and procedure documents. It is not unusual for these documents to be maintained in a central location. It is helpful to include links to the sites at which the complete documents can be found.

Define sensitive and restricted data. This section should include guidance on the appropriate handling and destruction of sensitive information.

Document appropriate safeguards and mechanisms relative to the security objectives determined by the risk assessment. Controls selected to mitigate risks should include administrative, operational, physical, and technical measures.

3.1. Administrative Controls

Workforce controls include the appropriate assignment of responsibilities within the organization and the need for access for the workforce member to complete his or her job responsibilities.

This section should consider controls for the following items:

3.1.1. Hiring and termination practices
3.1.1.1. Background checks
3.1.1.2. Hostile and non-hostile terminations
3.1.2. Acceptable use of IT resources
3.1.3. Violations and sanctions

3.2. Operational and Technical Controls

This section should document the controls in place for safeguarding access to sensitive resources through operational or technical measures (passwords, two-factor authentication, certificates, software and network controls, software development, and change management practices, malicious software, etc.)

3.2.1. Identity and access management

This section would include information regarding assigning accounts, authorization procedures, and authentication practices. Remember the importance remote access and vendor accounts when developing this section.

3.2.2 Access controls

This section should contain documentation related to the technical controls that restrict access to individuals with an authorized access.

3.2.2.1 Passwords

Address password controls such as requirements (length, use of special characters, etc.) If additional authentication mechanisms are required, information related to those mechanisms go in this section.

3.2.2.2 Session protection mechanisms

Include information about screen locks, automatic logouts, etc.

3.2.2.3 Administrator-level access

This section should address controls for system administrators and the need for "root" level or administrator access. Who can perform privileged operations and under what conditions? How will password accounts be managed?

3.2.3 Systems and application security

3.2.3.1 Backup and retention

This section should contain information related to the backup and restoration of applications and the data associated with them. This area could also include media rotation plans, offsite storage plans and documentation, and the cycling of media.

If the organization has a formal archive and retention plan, this would be the appropriate section in which to include that documentation.

3.2.3.2 System protection

Measures that should be employed to protect systems with sensitive information are the focus of this section. Include measures used to protect against "malware."

3.2.3.3 Patch and vulnerability management

Identify the controls and mechanisms to patch systems and mitigate software vulnerabilities.

3.2.3.4 Software development

Software development should follow an approved engineering life cycle. This section should include the life-cycle standards approved for use of, and the related controls for, software development. Be sure to include controls related to software development by a third party or software changes made on the part of a vendor.

3.2.4 Network security

This part of the security plan should thoroughly document all network infrastructure controls. These include firewalls, network access controls, content filters, virtual LANs, dedicated leased circuits, intrusion detection, and other network controls.

3.2.5 Change management

To maintain system integrity, all system changes should be conducted according to a planned and supervised process. This section should document the change management program and related controls, such as change logs, detection of unauthorized changes, testing and the movement of code from test to production environments, movement of hardware and infrastructure components, back out plans, and so on.

3.2.6 Log management

Most systems and software components produce logs of activity. Logs that provide details related to the performance of the host or application or security activities related to logins and authentication can be indispensable tools in the event of a problem or security incident.

3.2.7 Encryption

Encryption technologies should be employed to make sensitive information unreadable in the event of a compromise. This section should contain documentation detailing encryption controls for data at rest and in transit and how the keys to such encryption technologies are to be managed.

3.3 Physical Security

Physical security should be employed to protect sensitive systems and data from theft and environmental threats.

3.3.2 Physical access controls

Controls documented in this section include items such as locks, badge readers, sign in/out logs, CCTV monitoring, power conditioning, flood and fire controls, and other physical controls.

3.3.3 Inventory controls

It is difficult to secure systems and equipment if you are not aware of what the organization owns and uses daily. Equipment is often moved and/or reused and eventually discarded. This section should define the controls used to track the movement of devices.

3.3.4 Portable devices

Portable devices such as laptops, PDAs, cell phones, and other similar equipment pose significant risks for the loss of data and the potential for a breach. This section should document controls for the authorization and use of portable devices, the minimal security configurations required, and encryption technologies to be employed.

3.3.5 Media

Controls related to the use of media such as CDs, DVDs, flash cards, and other smart media are contained in this part of the security plan.

3.3.6 Destruction of equipment and media

This section should have procedures and controls related to the disposal of media and computing equipment. Be sure to include procedures for the destruction of hard drives, non-volatile memory, such as found in printers and multifunction devices, the premature failure of components in need of return for repair or replacement, and equipment that may have been used for demonstration purposes.

3.4 Incident Response

This section should contain detailed plans and procedures for the investigation and response to security incidents.

3.4.2 Notification involving breaches

In the event of a breach, detailed plans should be in place to document who will require notification, the methods of notification, working with external agencies and media, and so on.

3.4.3 Investigation and response plans

The security plan must detail the procedures related to whom has investigative authority, investigative procedures, chain of custody and evidence, notification and interaction with law enforcement, and the organization's legal team for these occurrences.

3.5 Security Awareness and Training

This portion should contain procedures for the training and education of all workforce members. The training program should include reviews of policy, standards, guidances, and procedures. The training program should also include frequent updates to make workforce members aware of new threats and safeguards, appropriate use of technology, and sensitive information.

3.5.2 Workforce members

3.5.3 Temporary staffing

3.5.4 Vendors and Business Associates

3.6 Contracts and Business Associates

When contracts are established with contractors, consultants, or external vendors, the agreements should contain satisfactory assurances that the third party will appropriately safeguard the information entrusted to them.

3.7 Continuity Planning

This section should include all procedures, controls, and contact information related to continuity of operations.

3.7.2 Disaster recovery

3.7.3 Emergency operations

4. Minimum Acceptable Configurations for Operations

All systems and devices should meet a minimum set of standards before the system or device is placed into a production environment. At a minimum, standards should exist for the areas listed next.

4.2 Host-based firewall configurations

4.3 Malware configurations

4.4 Auto-updates or patch management configurations

4.5 Authentication

4.6 Removal of unnecessary services

4.7 Encryption

5. Appendices

Index